an introduction to Physical Education

9th edition

John E. Nixon, Ed. D.
Professor of Education
and Physical Education
Stanford University
Stanford, California

Ann E. Jewett, Ed. D.
Professor of Health and
Physical Education
University of Georgia
Athens, Georgia

1980
SAUNDERS COLLEGE
Philadelphia

Saunders College
West Washington Square
Philadelphia, PA   19105

Cover photo by Laurie Usher.

An Introduction to Physical Education   ISBN   0-03-056778-5

0123   038   9 8 7 6 5 4 3 2 1

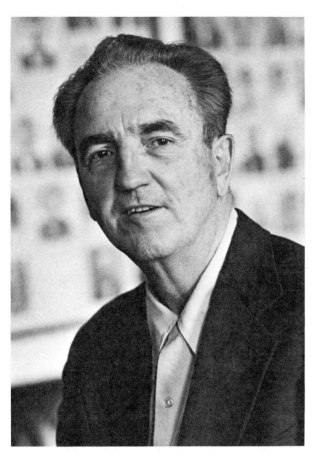

Dr. John E. Nixon is Professor of Education and Physical Education at Stanford University, where he is Director of Graduate Programs in Physical Education. Among Dr. Nixon's contributions to his field are three books and many academic and professional articles.

Dr. Nixon brings to this book a wide range of experience. He has coached and officiated in several sports at the college and secondary school levels and, through invitations from several foreign countries, has taught and coached around the world. Dr. Nixon has held national offices in professional organizations and has received state, district, and national honors, including the R. Tait McKenzie Award, given to the most outstanding physical educator in America. He also has been the recipient of two Fulbright Lectureships. These experiences and activities qualify Dr. Nixon to observe, analyze, and evaluate the complex areas of physical education, sport, and dance in broad perspective.

As senior author of this textbook for the past four editions, Dr. Nixon again joins with Dr. Ann Jewett to explore, illuminate, and interpret the meaning and significance of physical education, sport, and dance in their fullest sense. Now in its 9th edition, An Introduction to Physical Education is the longest continuously published physical education text in the United States, having originated with Dr. Nixon's father, Professor Eugene W. Nixon, and Professor Frederick Cozens in 1934.

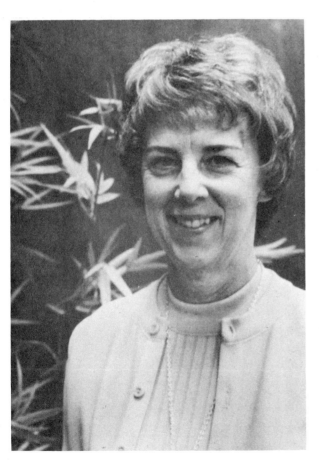

Dr. Ann E. Jewett is Professor and Head of the Division of Health, Physical Education, and Recreation at the University of Georgia. Among her previous professional titles are Director of Women's Physical Education at Springfield College, Chairperson of the Physical Education Graduate Faculty at the University of Wisconsin—Madison, and visiting professorships at several universities. Dr. Jewett served two years of active duty with the United States Navy and currently holds the rank of Captain in the U.S. Naval Reserve.

Recognition for Dr. Jewett's achievements in her area of study includes election to numerous offices in various physical education associations and membership in distinguished sororities. She was awarded a Fulbright Lectureship in The Netherlands and has been selected Piedmont University Visiting Scholar, Laura J. Huelster Lecturer, and 1980 Amy Morris Homans Lecturer. She is a recipient of the Honor Award of the American Alliance for Health, Physical Education, Recreation, and Dance and of the Woman of the Year Golden Award in Athens, Georgia.

Dr. Jewett's publications are primarily in the areas of physical education curriculum, professional preparation, and education theory. Her most recent major contribution is *Curriculum Design: Purposes and Processes in Physical Education Teaching—Learning*, a report of the AAHPERD Physical Education Research Project co-authored with Marie R. Mullan. Earlier publications include a physical education curriculum textbook co-authored with Dr. Nixon.

PREFACE

Physical education as an academic discipline and as a profession continues to develop and expand at a rapid rate in most countries of the world. In America, in some states, a larger number of children are enrolled in physical education classes than in any other subject in junior and senior high schools. There is a participant "boom" in sport, dance, and exercise throughout our country. Research results are proliferating in exercise physiology, in the biomechanics of human movement, and in motor learning. Inquiry into effective teaching, development of curriculum theory, careful curriculum planning, and valid curriculum evaluation are becoming more sophisticated. Large numbers of college students continue to enroll in physical education major programs in hundreds of colleges and universities across America. Many of them receive their start in the professional and academic study of physical education in that unique, and most effective, American two-year educational institution known as the community college.

The ninth edition of *An Introduction to Physical Education* has been completely revised and enlarged to meet the needs resulting from the continued expansion of physical education throughout America. Physical education is becoming a pluralistic and more diverse profession, including several rapidly expanding specializations. Young scholars and practitioners are concentrating their efforts in one or two components of physical education. The shift in professional preparation toward emphasizing more narrowly defined specializations has created a serious scarcity of generalists who are competent to study and interpret the ever-evolving new specializations and their interrelationships within the total context of physical education as an academic discipline and as a field of professional study and practice. At the same time, the dramatically increasing awareness of the significant societal roles of the movement arts and sports sciences in health and fitness, social service, communications, leisure and recreation, and business and economics has opened up many career options beyond teaching and outside traditional school and college environments. Both of these trends underscore the need for a broader, more general foundation for young professionals beginning their undergraduate specialized professional education.

We, the authors of this book, are generalists in the sense that the roles and responsibilities we have held over the years were and are diversified; these roles include teacher, coach, sport official, teacher educator, program administrator, scholar, researcher, and professional leader. Our purpose in writing the ninth edition is to bring to the physical education field an integrated description and analysis of the exciting, complex, ever-changing field of physical education—a purpose that has prevailed throughout the previous editions of this book, first written in 1934 by Professors Eugene W. Nixon and Frederick W. Cozens. This ninth edition qualifies as the oldest continuing textbook in physical education in the United States.

The rapid proliferation of (1) programs and activities, which may be labeled the "professional" aspects, and (2) knowledge, theory, and concepts, which constitute the "academic" subject matter, requires a complete and careful revision. Consequently, the decision was made to provide greater depth and breadth in content and topical coverage than in previous editions. Basic concepts have been selected that are relevant and crucial to the understanding of the major topics in each chapter. Suggestions, usually in the form of principles, are offered for the application of selected concepts to effective curriculum planning, instruction, professional practice, and evaluation. Thus, the theoretical and practical aspects of physical education are integrated throughout the text, as indeed they are in the real world of teaching, coaching, research, and administration in a wide variety of societal institutions, roles, and settings.

The first two chapters introduce the reader to a general understanding of what physical education is all about, centered on analyses of its nature and scope and of its purposes when put to use formally or informally by individuals or groups.

Chapters Three through Six are designed to identify major concepts, generalizations, facts, theories, and practical examples of principles of physical education taken from selected recent literature in basic academic disciplines that provide normative, socio-cultural, biological, and psychological concepts upon which "foundations" of physical education are built. Pertinent literature has been identified from the broad field of education. Key concepts have been selected from recent high quality physical education literature. Concepts from the academic disciplines have been integrated into the educational and physical educational contexts within which professionals in the movement arts and sport sciences must function. We attempt to present perceptions, understandings, and interpretations of physical education as an academic discipline, and what its roles, functions, responsibilities, and opportunities are as a fundamental segment of the total school curriculum.

Then follow chapters on the physical education curriculum per se and on teaching physical education. The evidence from the preceding chapters is related to curriculum development, improvement, and evaluation and to improvement of teaching effectiveness in physical education. Chapter Seven has been expanded to accomodate developments that have taken place in physical education curriculum theory and practice since the eighth edition. Chapter Eight adds a significant additional dimension to the ninth edition, presenting for the first time an entire chapter devoted to improvement of teaching effectiveness.

Chapter Nine introduces new content that reflects the significantly broader scope of the human movement professions. Six societal roles filled by the movement arts and sports sciences are identified. Each broad role is viewed from the perspectives of its cultural significance, its relationships to the foundations fields, its relationships to school physical education programs, and its organizational leadership and professional specializations. The next chapter is devoted to a discussion of professional preparation, so that qualified leaders may conduct programs in various specializations, both in education and in the other five aspects of societal life previously identified.

The final chapter explains the vital roles of several types of evaluation for assessing the effectiveness of achieving physical education objectives. Also, the fundamental purposes of a variety of theoretical and applied research methods in physical education are described and discussed.

Thus, the ninth edition offers considerably more than the previous editions. One of the strengths of the ninth edition is the increased emphasis on depth of description of the major academic concepts upon which physical education is based. Likewise, the professional applications of these foundational concepts to more relevant curricula, more effective teaching and coaching, higher quality and longer retention of pupil learnings, and more exact evaluations of pupil behavioral changes, teacher effectiveness, and curriculum validity will result in a decidedly improved total program of physical education. In addition, more emphasis is given to professional concerns beyond formal educational contexts. Because substantially more content is included than in previous editions, the book is appropriate for use as an introductory exposure to the formal study of physical education and also can serve as a text in courses having to do with the "foundations" or "principles" of physical education.

This edition continues to provide a current, relevant list of references from a variety of sources at the end of each chapter. The footnote citations, combined with the Selected References, provide additional evidence, varied interpretations, and differing views about topics of major concern. Teachers and students alike will find their library work facilitated by use of these lists. To help make reading the text more enjoyable, a new stylistic dimension has been added to this edition, including a larger format, more headings to highlight the text, and many new photos and drawings. A teacher's guide is also available with this edition.

As authors, we worked together on the seventh and eighth editions of this text as well as on other previous publications. We have collaborated in various professional and academic projects over the years. We have our debates, our agreements, our divergent viewpoints. We maintain our faith and confidence in each other. We have the same general philosophical view of the total field of physical education and we agree on our conceptualizations about its parts and their functions. We have our differences of opinions and judgments, as well, on specific aspects of physical education. The reader may detect some slight differences in beliefs concerning particular topics. We hope our individual contributions will at least be recognizable to the reader, even if not persuasive at all times. At least they may provide "food for thought." In the final analysis, we assume equal responsibility for the content of each chapter and the views expressed therein.

Emphasis is accorded to recent research evidence that tends to support the contentions we offer. The rapid development of specializations within physical education is manifested in the extension of the content in the various chapters and is verified by the variety of recent, high quality references included in the chapter footnotes and the end-of-chapter Selected Reference lists. Perhaps the reader will be impressed by the rapid accretion of literature in all forms—magazines, books, pamphlets, research reports, audio-visual media, and so on—available in these times, not only in the United States but also in many foreign countries.

The general tenor of this book is carried over from previous editions. The book is intended to impress the reader with the rapid development, expansion, and increasing understanding and acceptance of physical education as a basic subject in the academic curriculum of schools, from nursery schools through colleges and universities. We are pleased with the progress we observe in this country and abroad concerning improved and expanded programs of physical education suited to the needs, interests, and abilities of people of all ages and varying degrees of health. We realize there are still major problems to be identified and studied intensively. We hope we are making modest contributions to these studies in our own ways. We are optimistic about the future of physical education. We believe it will continue to expand and be accepted in the family of educational disciplines. It is clearly being recognized for its contributions to the medical sciences, to individual therapies, and to general health preservation.

Finally, we hope this book will add impetus to the decision-making process that will lead outstanding young students in colleges and universities to decide on an interesting and rewarding career in physical education.

PHOTO CREDITS —————

The authors wish to express their appreciation to the following sources for permission to use the illustrations on the pages noted.

American Alliance for Health, Physical Education, Recreation, and Dance: 8, 10, 12, 15, 21, 37, 45, 50, 54, 92, 130, 138, 146, 151, 156, 182, 185, 209, 211, 240, 247, 285, 288, 299, 306, 314, 324, 335, 352, 370, 373, 407; Journal of Physical Education and Recreation: 30, 48, 282, 339; Terry Boyd: 272, 312; Chris Capolongo: 378, 384; Brian Sharkey: 30, 48

American Medical Association: 321, 387

American Museum of Natural History, New York, N.Y.: 114, 115

Bellevue Elementary School District, Washington, D.C.: 205, 252

Barton, Paul: 328

Burk Uzzle/Magnum Photos, Inc.: 160

Coakley, J.: *Sport in Society.* St. Louis: C. V. Mosby Co., 1978, p. 210: 330, 338

Diem, Liselott: 18, 62, 97, 153, 244

Fait, H. F.: *Special Physical Education: Adaptive, Corrective, Developmental.* (4th ed.). Philadelphia: W. B. Saunders Co., 1978, p. 327: 333

Florida State News Bureau: 326

Hubbard Scientific Company, Northbrook, Ill.: 152

Jewett, A. E., and Mullan, M. R.: *Curriculum Design: Purposes and Processes in Physical Education Teaching-Learning.* Washington: American Alliance for Health, Physical Education, Recreation, and Dance, 1977: 247

McCleneghan, B. A., and Gallahue, D. L.: *Fundamental Movement: A Developmental and Remedial Approach.* Philadelphia: W. B. Saunders Co., 1978, p. 130: 41

Maslow, A.: *Motivation and Personality* (2nd ed.). New York: Harper and Row, 1970: 36

Nixon, J. E., and Locke, L. F.: "Research on Teaching Physical Education." *In* Travers, R. M. W.: *Second Handbook of Research on Teaching* (2nd ed.). Chicago: Rand McNally and Company, 1973, p. 1213: 216

Paffenbarger, R. S.: "Physical Activity as an Index on Heart Attack Risk in College Alumni." *American Journal of Epidemiology*, Vol. 108 (1978), p. 171: 164

Pennsylvania State University Still Photography Services: 71, 296

Silverton Public Schools, Silverton, Colo.: 275, 324

Smith, D. W., Bierman, E. L., and Robinson, N. M.: *The Biologic Ages of Man* (2nd ed.). Philadelphia: W. B. Saunders Co., 1973, p. 188: 245

Southern Illinois University, Carbondale, Ill.: 162, 184, 316, 366

Stuber, Lynda: 199, 234, 302, 409

U.S. Army Photos: 166

Ulrich, C., and Nixon, J. E.: *Tones of Theory—A Theoretical Structure for Physical Education—A Tentative Perspective.* Washington: American Association for Health, Physical Education, and Recreation, 1972: 12

University of California, Santa Cruz, Calif.: 292, 318, 347, 381

University of Georgia, Athens, Ga., Division of Health, Physical Education, and Recreation: 6

University of Illinois, Urbana, Ill.: 226, 269, 398, 412, 413

University of Oregon, Eugene, Oreg.: 2, 4, 33, 39, 66, 112, 123, 177, 223, 240, 285, 322, 332

Usher, Laurie E.: 127, 356, Cover

Warren Central High School, Indianapolis, Ind.: 56, 78, 190, 207, 258

World Wide Photos: 163

CONTENTS

CONTENTS

Chapter 8 ─────────────────────────────────────

TEACHING PHYSICAL EDUCATION 283

Chapter 9 ─────────────────────────────────────

SOCIETAL ROLES OF THE MOVEMENT ARTS AND SPORT SCIENCES 313

an introduction to
Physical Education

9th edition

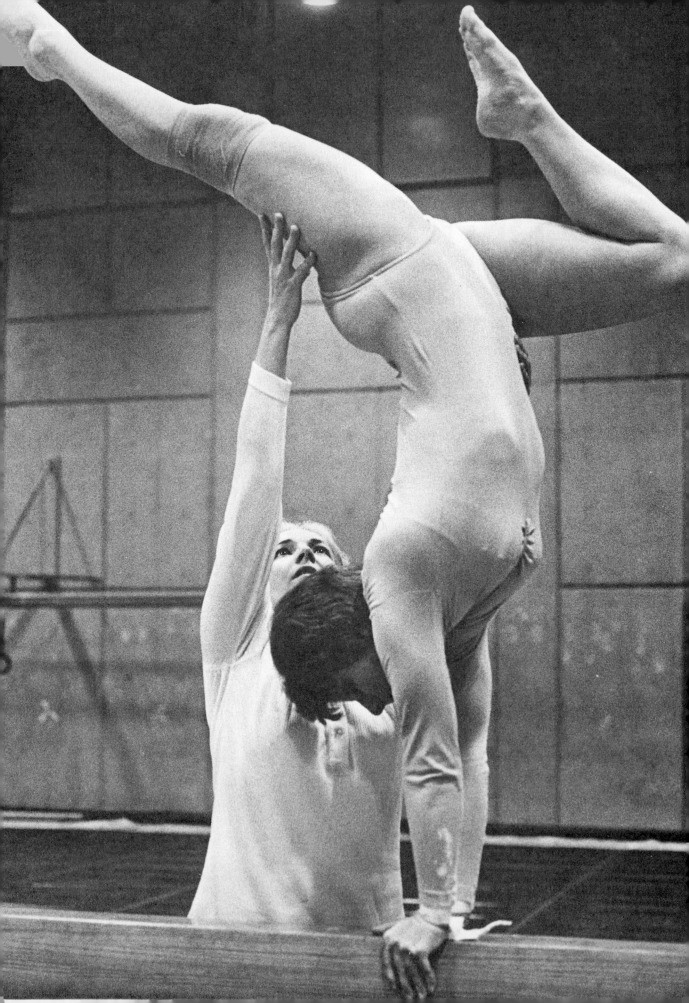

THE NATURE AND SCOPE ———— ———— OF PHYSICAL EDUCATION

Sport, dance, and physical recreation have been fundamental elements of all cultures throughout the history of the world, according to anthropological and historical research. Likewise, physical education is one of the most ancient arts of the humanities. The first physical educator was the father who taught his sons how to hunt, provide food, build protective shelters, and engage in other physical tasks required to protect the family unit from the ravages of nature and the ferocity of wild animals. From humankind's* early history to the present time, physical education in one form or another has been present in all civilizations of the world, receiving varying degrees of cultural and governmental emphasis.

In its broadest interpretation, physical education is defined as the art and science of voluntary, purposeful human movement. It focuses on selective aspects of the realm of experiences in voluntary, purposeful human movement. The physical educator basically is interested in all human movements, but because this is so encompassing, formal studies and programs of physical education today are generally concentrated in movement designated by such terms as sport, dance, gymnastics, aquatics, and exercise.

It is clear that physical education is concerned with a fundamental mode of human expression. Likewise, it is an essential form of nonverbal communication in company with art, drama, and music. The human being can, and does, express a wide range of emotions while participating in the activities of physical education.

The mores and the cultural imperatives of human societies throughout history have utilized components of physical education to inculcate basic values almost from birth in the informal and formal

*The authors use the term "man" throughout the text as a convenient and acceptable short word that connotes all human beings, male or female, or both. No discrimination between sexes is implied or intended.

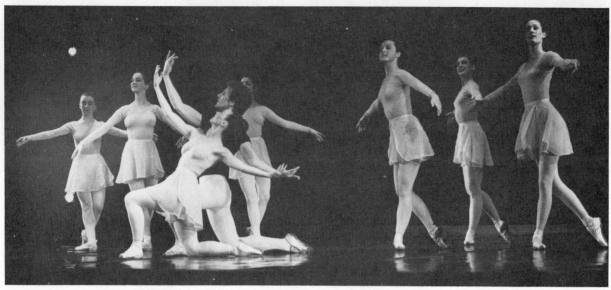

Instructional programs in dance have increased substantially in the U.S.

education of youth. Artists have depicted people and animals in scenes emphasizing movements essential to survival, artistic and emotional expression, and historical record.

The physical educator does not have unique claim to primary concern for human movements. Teachers and scholars in a variety of fields of study and research, such as human ecology, human engineering, physical medicine, physical therapy, and recreation, likewise have a primary interest in selected human movement phenomena. Rather than overlap into these areas, physical educators have generally concentrated their interests and efforts primarily in the areas of sport, dance, and exercise.

Many physical educators have chosen to join forces with scholars and practitioners in other areas of human movement of mutual interest or overlapping concerns. In the United States there is a movement at the college and university level to transfer instructional programs in dance from departments and schools of physical education to other academic units, such as the Department of the Performing Arts, the Department of Speech and Drama, the Department of Humanities, or even into a newly created Department of Dance.

The term "physical education" has been in use in America since the turn of the century. It evolved from the more restrictive phrase "physical training," used by the pioneers who developed these programs in schools and colleges in the late 1800s. The term "physical education" denoted that this subject was a bona fide field to be included in the formal studies of young people in the public schools and in the colleges and universities of the nation. The "education of the physical" became "education through the physical." Although "physical education" implies a mind-body dichotomy in human beings, a concept no longer tenable in the light of modern scientific knowledge concerning the organismic unity of the individual, the term has persisted in the educational lexicon. In recent years efforts to substitute other names for the subject of physical education have been made in the United States and other countries.

CHAPTER ONE

Thus, since its inception, physical education has been a recognized subject in the basic curriculum of American public schools and universities. Physical education also has gradually been accepted in other public, semi-private, and private agencies and organizations throughout the country. It has evolved from a school-centered program to one that serves people of all ages, in all degrees of health, in public and private educational institutions, in a large variety of social agencies, and including individuals, informal groups, and families. Perhaps none of us have fully recognized how pervasive physical education is in American life.

Many authorities have guidelines with which to define a field of study as a profession. Criteria commonly considered are:

1. The field involves a specified area of human interest and concern;
2. Individuals who render service in this field for the benefit of others must be specially qualified by training and experience relative to their unique responsibilities;
3. The motivation of the practitioners of the profession is largely intrinsic; that is, they desire to serve others and their satisfactions come primarily from the opportunity to serve rather than from external incentives such as high salary or public recognition;
4. The members of a profession regulate the conduct of each other and insist on high ethical and moral values to guide the behaviors of all concerned;
5. The practices engaged in by the leaders of the profession are based, insofar as possible, upon validated concepts developed by qualified scholars and researchers in one or more related areas of the supporting academic disciplines and supplemented by the cumulative experience and evaluations of leaders and practitioners in the profession.

This list of professional attributes clearly delineates the majority of the teachers, coaches, and administrators who have elected to devote their lives to rendering professional services in physical education, sport, dance, exercises, and other activities commonly organized in physical education programs.

Physical education also involves many professional organizations ranging from individual schools and recreational groups to school districts, counties, states, and to the national and international levels. These professional organizations constantly strive to elevate the quality of the services and programs being offered to young people and adults, whether participation is mandated by law or policy, or is voluntary because of the interest, enjoyment, and satisfaction gained.

From the time of its origin in America to the 1960s, physical education was regarded primarily as a profession, not an academic discipline. Gradually, physical education scholars, and sometimes interested specialists and researchers from other academic disciplines, began to study various conceptual aspects of physical education, such as its history, exercise physiology, kinesiology, and motor learning. Young scholars in particular became interested in emerging specializations called the sociology of sport and sport psychology. There has always been a strong interest in the philosophy of physical education

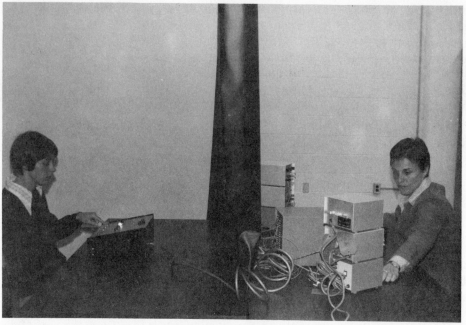

Historically regarded as primarily a profession, physical education is now established as an academic discipline, as demonstrated in this motor learning laboratory.

that combined with its history to form the so-called normative foundations of physical education.

In the 1960s, professional associations such as the American Association for Health, Physical Education, Recreation (AAHPER),* and others developed projects to define and describe the nature and scope of physical education. Concerned lay people, university physical education faculty members, and leaders of professional organizations worked to establish physical education as an academic discipline with a unique body of knowledge. In a landmark article, Franklin Henry[1] asserted that physical education is indeed an academic discipline, and he presented a persuasive argument for this viewpoint. Subsequently, many books, articles,** and speeches have interpreted physical education as an academic discipline, which it is now regarded in the scholarly community in most colleges and universities.

Nixon[2] summarized the major criteria of a discipline that are most frequently advocated by specialists on this subject:

1. A discipline has an identifiable domain; it asks vital and important questions; it deals with immensely significant questions, significant themes, a specifiable scope of inquiry, a central core of interest; it has a definite beginning point; and it has stated goals.
2. A discipline is characterized by a substantial history and a publicly recognized tradition, exemplified by time-tested works.
3. A discipline is rooted in a unique conceptual structure and employs syntactical structure; the structure organizes a body of basic

---

*As of March, 1979, the American Alliance for Health, Physical Education, Recreation, and Dance (AAHPERD).
**An entire issue of *Quest*[3] magazine discussed the nature of a discipline.

concepts; and it consists of conceptual relationships as well as appropriate relations between facts.

4. A discipline possesses an integrity and an arbitrary quality unlike any other discipline; its scope is defined by common consent of its specialists.
5. A discipline is recognized by the procedures and methods it employs; it utilizes intellectual and conceptual tools as well as technical and mechanical tools and follows a relevant set of rules leading to learning and knowing in the domain of the discipline.
6. A discipline is recognized as a process as well as being noted for its products (knowledge, generalizations, principles).
7. Finally, a discipline relies on an accurate language system to provide channels of precise, careful communication, both within and outside of the discipline.

Nixon[4] also notes that "in the final analysis of the collective behavior, the quality of the endeavors of the scholars of a field must command a sufficient respect by observers for the label 'discipline' to be truly deserved and thus bestowed on the field in academic circles."

In physical education as an academic discipline, Metheny[5] explains, study and research are directed toward understanding people, with particular reference to their ability to move, the ways in which they utilize this ability, and the ways in which their use of this ability is related to other aspects of their functioning as whole persons. Thus, Metheny says that "movement as a dynamic function of man is the area of central concern that gives physical education its unique identity as an academic discipline."

Body of Knowledge

The body of knowledge that comprises the academic discipline of physical education has six categories: (1) the history and philosophy of physical education, or the normative foundations; (2) the sociology and anthropology of sports, dance, and physical activities as an essential element in all cultures from primitive times to the present day; (3) biomechanics and kinesiology; (4) exercise physiology and sports medicine involving the adaptation of the human organism to exercise stress under a variety of environmental conditions; (5) motor development, motor learning, and related phenomena; and (6) sport and physical education pedagogy.

Dance as a Discipline

Hayes takes the view that dance should not be regarded as a "mere subdivision of physical education," but as "an independent discipline [that] offers virgin territory for research and discovery."[6]

Hayes[7] says, "The fact is that much knowledge in dance, as in any of the arts, is not factual knowledge based on scientific research; it is intuitive knowledge. But intuitive knowledge is also real knowledge based upon human sensitivity and human experience. Dance creation, appreciation, and criticism are all largely the reflection and the outcome of human intuition."

Hayes goes on to make an eloquent argument describing dance as a separate discipline, discussing knowledge of dance technique, dance as a revelation of an individual and a reflection of culture, the role of dance history in reproducing the past, dance as a form of cultural exchange, and dance as education in creativity. Hayes[8] then says:

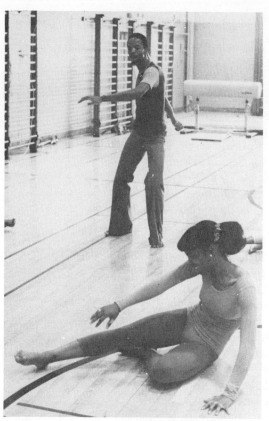

Dance — an education in creativity.

In conclusion, it must be agreed that dance as a discipline is still in its infancy in comparison to many subjects of academia, yet in recent years giant steps forward have been taken in areas in movement perception and analysis, in dance notation, in dance therapy, and in anthropological, ethnic, and historical research. Some progress is being made in developing sound programs in dance for children. Although dance philosophy has been an integral part of many college dance curricula, there is a need for increased specialization in areas of philosophy and criticism which enable dance oriented people to replace the often inept music and drama critics who attempt to pass judgment upon dance in the theatre. In all areas of knowledge we have only made beginnings. While answers are few, questions are many. The challenges of the future are bright with promise!

A major project in dance was sponsored by the United States Office of Education in 1970, when it awarded a one million dollar grant for a national experiment to involve five school systems located in various parts of the country to "find ways to infuse the arts (music, visual arts, drama, and dance) into all aspects of the school curriculum, as a means of enhancing and improving the quality and quantity of aesthetic education in the school and as a principal means for expanding the base for affective learning experience in the school program."[9] This project was called IMPACT, which stands for Interdisciplinary Model Programs in the Arts for Children and Teachers.

The area of dance is gradually separating organizationally and philosophically from physical education and is becoming recognized as an academic discipline in its own right.

CHAPTER ONE

Although there is now considerable agreement that physical education is an academic discipline, there is disagreement in the United States, and around the world, as to the focus of and the limits to its unique subject matter. Likewise, there is discontent with the term "physical education" and many leaders advocate adoption of a new name.

Bouchard[10] discusses the history of the dispute about the adequacy of the name "physical education," the need to change it, the alternative titles that have been suggested and their rationale, and finally he arrives at reasons for his own recommendation. This comprehensive discussion is recommended to all interested physical educators. Bouchard proposes the adoption of the title "physical activity sciences" to refer to study and research in the field presently known as "physical education." He says:

> We personally think that the object, physical activity, in the physical activity sciences is the sector of human activity consisting of body movements, as well as perceptual and voluntary motions as exemplified in sport, games, dance, graded exercises of development, training or education, work and some forms of housework, locomotion, physical recreation, performance and preparation for performance, physical conditioning, physical rehabilitation, physical and motor re-education. Therefore, the scope of the physical activity sciences is this portion of the reality of man in motion.[11]

Bouchard[12] also lists alternative titles that have frequently been suggested to replace the term "physical education": sport science, the science of man in motion, activity sciences, anthropokinetics, physical education sciences, kinanthropology, kinesiology, exercise sciences, homokinetics, and gymnology.

It will be noted that Bouchard's definition is broader than the one in this book, including realms of human physical activity that have been omitted from our definition. We believe that physical education as an academic discipline and field of professional activity is comprehensive and requires no elaboration or extension beyond the parameters identified in this text. When any one attempts to describe the nature, scope, and the purposes of physical education, a decision must be made on arbitrary delimitations and a rationale described. The fact that individuals do encompass different domains of human physical activity in their definitions of physical education stimulates all of us to even more intensive scrutiny and evaluation of the basic conceptions we hold about this area of study and human activity.

Sport Science. In recent years there has been a new conceptualization of the fundamental components of physical education as well as a change in its title, particularly in European countries. The term "physical education" has been virtually discarded and replaced by the term "sport science." Sport science is composed of seven theory fields: (1) sport medicine and exercise physiology, (2) sport biomechanics, (3) sport psychology, (4) sport sociology, (5) sport history, (6) sport philosophy, and (7) sport pedagogy.

"Sport pedagogy," a term not frequently used in the United States, is now becoming recognized as a legitimate subdiscipline of sport science.

Sport Pedagogy. Sport pedagogy includes formal study and research in the areas of curriculum, teaching, teacher education, evaluation, and organization and administration. The traditionalists in physical education and "academic" fields of study probably will not

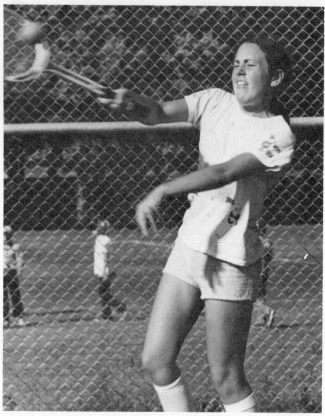

We regard "sport pedagogy" as an academic discipline.

regard the area of study currently called "sport pedagogy" as an academic discipline. We contend that sport pedagogy has advanced to the point at which it incorporates the criteria of a discipline as previously listed.

Siedentop[13] eloquently justifies the inclusion of sport pedagogy as an academic discipline:

> In our rush to embrace the growing discipline of physical education we have neglected to explore the possibility that there may be a discipline that is more immediately referential to teacher education in physical education. The primary reason why we may have neglected this is that many people do not believe this other field to be a discipline or a science: I am speaking about pedagogy. There was a time when pedagogy was considered to be a legitimate discipline. I think that at the present moment it has every bit as much right to that title as does the discipline of physical education. The level of scientific inquiry in areas such as instructional systems and teacher behaviors is just as sophisticated and meets the criteria for a discipline just as fully as do any sub-fields of the discipline of physical education. But I do not want my argument to degenerate into discussions of labels and criteria.
>
> Let our undergraduate and graduate programs reflect the central concern of the vast majority of those who choose our field for their life's work: the teaching of physical education to students in schools. But, let those programs reflect that emphasis in a competent, scholarly manner with a primary emphasis on the discipline of pedagogy so that we do not have to feel ashamed about the quality of our program or the productivity of those who are educated in our programs.
>
> There is a discipline of pedagogy waiting for us to embrace it. It

is a discipline with a rich history of scholarship, research, and theory. Its central concerns have always been those that we confront on a day to day basis, but for which we find so little help in our field. It's time to change models. It's time for teachers to demand a change in models. It's time for teacher educators to effect that model change in our universities and colleges. The need is great. Let us be about that task.

In summary, it is clear that the subject matter, or academic content, of physical education is centered on selected types of movement experiences and behavioral patterns suggested by such terms as exercise, sport, dance, gymnastics, and athletics; and in movements commonly required for daily living that portray the individual's search for purpose and identity through meaningful activity.[14]

Physical education is one of several fields of human endeavor **INTERRELATIONSHIPS** that have a primary interest in human movement phenomena. The AAHPERD publication *Tones of Theory*[15] explains the interrelationships of physical education with other aspects of human movement such as physical therapy, recreation, physical medicine, human engineering, and human ecology as illustrated in the figure on p. 12.

Physical education is concerned with two types of knowledge, process knowledge and product knowledge. These provide the bases for melding the academic discipline and the profession of physical education into one cohesive field of human endeavor.

According to Ulrich and Nixon,[16] the *process knowledge* of physical education involves the following content areas:

1. Acquisition of skill patterns through ordinative movement
2. Self-actualization through generic, ordinative, and creative movement
3. Creative patterns for physical activity emphasizing individual style
4. Conditioning and training regimens
5. Decision-making and its movement patterns
6. Experience in behavioral situations that foster interaction, social stratification, social control, self-realization, motivational understandings, social processing, interpretations of ethics and morality, making value judgments
7. Behavioral opportunities for non-verbal communication
8. Utilization of cognitive learning commensurate with motoric development

The *product knowledge* areas of physical education are:

1. Worthy use of leisure time
2. Ability to participate adequately in sports and games
3. Understanding of rules, strategies, and tactics
4. Organic integrity — usually called optimum physical fitness
5. Desirable behavioral attitudes
6. Emotional satisfaction gained through involvement
7. Maximum work results with minimum mechanical effort

Physical educators should continually seek the integration of conceptual theory and knowledge in order to promote clear understanding of physical education as an academic discipline and as a profession.

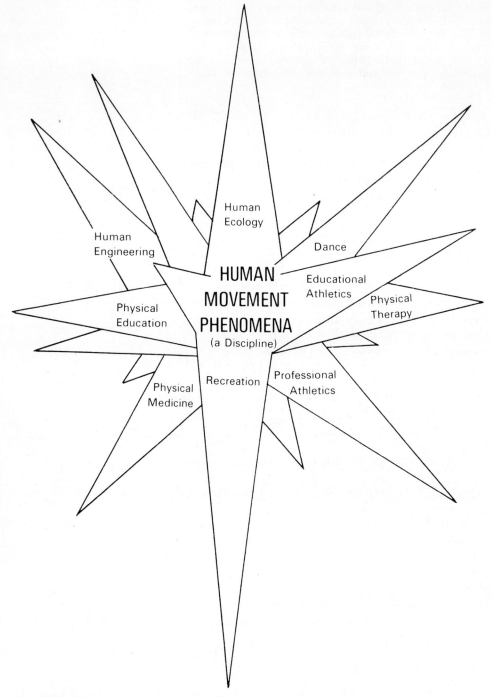

The study of human movement: A dynamic process.

The interrelationship of theory and practice is summarized by Ulrich and Nixon:[17]

> The conceptual theory of physical education should clarify for the practitioner the place of school-sponsored physical education. It should make clear the relationships of movement, fitness, play, discipline, body of knowledge, process, media, and results. It should provide an orderly scheme which can facilitate the "goodness of fit" of the varied components of physical education into a functional, viable, pattern of operation.

The relationship of the conceptual theory and knowledge defines the perimeters of physical education. It helps individuals make judgments regarding what physical education is. If the activity of surfing fits into the design, it might be considered as an addition to the program. If the activity of driving a car does not fit the structure, it is not to be considered as physical education. If the factual understandings concerning neurological integration fit the knowledge design, they should be included in the study of physical education; if the understandings of first aid for injury do not fit, they should be discarded as components of the physical education experience.

Thus, theory and knowledge are combined with the experience and judgments of teachers and administrators in determining administrative policy and developing appropriate physical education curricula for the students in the schools. Theory, knowledge, and practice are inseparable. The selecting and teaching of activities, and practicing and contesting in sports, will be aimless if not guided by enlightened physical education theory and up-to-date knowledge of the basic concepts in the physical education disciplinary subfields.

Thus, in considering the nature and scope of physical education, we may now describe it as (1) an educationally based "profession," and (2) a discrete "academic discipline" with a unique body of knowledge. These basic components are continually developed and refined with the guidance of an ever expanding and clarifying set of theories of physical education and its major elements.

SUMMARY

INTERPRETATION OF PHYSICAL EDUCATION

The term "physical education" has always been involved with confusion and misunderstandings; unfortunately, these difficulties continue to exist today. In recent years there have been intensive efforts by various members of organizations in physical education to seek an official change of name and many departments and schools of physical education have already changed their titles.

We believe that more effective interpretation of the purposes of physical education is being carried out today than in the past. However, continuous efforts still are required to convey this interpretation clearly and persuasively, not only to the members of the physical education profession, but also to their professional colleagues and administrators, to the public they serve, and most of all, to the children and adults in their programs. Some examples of the confusion that apparently exists concerning basic understanding of the nature and the purposes of physical education follow.

The individual whose concept of physical education is limited to the development of the purely physical aspects of the human organism, "body building" and "physical fitness," will scarcely understand the language of another who thinks of physical education as a process concerned primarily with the development of creative and patterned movement skills. And neither of them will be in full accord, in word or deed, with other persons who speak of physical education as an agency for the promotion of "health" or "good citizenship." The advocates of "movement education" create additional uncertainty and misconceptions in the minds of persons who have long held to the traditional view of physical education as "sports, games, and rhythms."

Also, many school administrators and curriculum coordinators are unable to distinguish between the unique purposes of physical education and health education, preferring to regard these two areas as components of one broad field of educational experience. In fact, however, health education has developed to such an extent that it is now a separate academic discipline.

One approach to the clarification of "physical education" is to state a clear and compelling rationale concerning the fundamental nature of all education as a framework within which physical education is an essential component. Of course, it must be remembered that physical education is not restricted only to the formal school program. It permeates many aspects of American life, both informally and formally, and is available in one form or another to people of all ages and degrees of health.

Before presenting our rationale for physical education as an essential component of formal education, we stress that, in our view, physical education is a broad concept encompassing more than just the formal subject called "physical education" or "physical education and athletics" in a school or college curriculum. We will elaborate on the broad perspectives we hold for physical education following the exposition of the fundamental nature of education.

EDUCATION AND PHYSICAL EDUCATION

Perceptive educators and laymen no longer regard education merely as "schooling." Obviously, formal organizations called schools, colleges, and universities are not the only sources from which individuals may learn. There are a large number of private and public agencies and organizations available to those who desire to pursue specific types of learnings, either for tuition or free. As society's agencies, schools expose young people to a series of fundamental educational experiences that are deemed necessary for the proper understanding of values of the American culture; schools train the students in the fundamental skills necessary to basic survival and successful participation in society.

"Schooling," the education received in the schools, is provided by local, county, state, and federal government agencies, both on a mandatory and an elective basis, from day-care centers to adult education programs open to anyone with the interest and physical capacity to attend.

Recently there has been widespread dissatisfaction with the curricula offered in many schools and colleges around the country. The mandatory attendance age is gradually being reduced in most states. Schools, teachers, and administrators are accused of becoming overly permissive and a decline in discipline has been noted. Students are not engaging in as much homework as in previous years, largely owing to the competing attraction of television in the evenings. Grading systems have been changed from the traditional letter grades to other less discriminating indicators. Many other complaints about the public schools are being registered.

Alternative Forms of Education. As a result, many alternative forms of education have sprung up around the country. School district personnel have been innovators in organizing alternative schools, open schools, schools without walls, parkway schools, and other provisions for stimulating educational experiences. Individual entrepre-

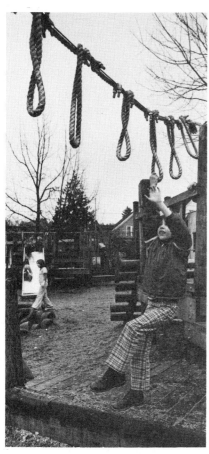

Creating a stimulating environment is an important concept in today's innovative schools.

neurs likewise have increased the number of private schools and other forms of educational opportunities as alternatives to attendance in public schools, prompting many parents to withdraw their children from the public schools and send them to these other organizations.

New schools tend to offer children more personal freedom, emphasizing self-responsibility with respect to school attendance, election of courses, and pupil goal-setting and self-evaluation; such schools attempt to adapt to relevant environmental conditions within or outside the school to promote direct personal experiences and multisensory learning opportunities. Students of professional education should become acquainted with examples of these schools in the extensive literature concerning them and visit them when possible.

"Back to Basics." Most public schools around the country have been undergoing intensive scrutiny in recent years by concerned citizens and are engaged in both internal and external examination of their objectives, programs, and instructional modes. Widespread educational changes are evident in many schools and colleges, occurring at a faster pace than ever before. Physical education is caught up in these changes, too. (In a later chapter, we will discuss selected developments that seem to hold promise for improving the quality of the physical education curriculum and instructional competence.)

This movement has been called "back to the basics." There is a clamor for the return to so-called "basic education." Debate rages as to exactly what elements constitute basic education, but generally this approach starts with requiring specific subjects of all students, as was typical 20 and 30 years ago; such subjects might include reading, spelling, arithmetic, English composition, history, geography, and civics. So-called "frills" are eliminated; national patriotism is stressed; classroom discipline is tightened. Students are assigned daily homework and must attend study halls during periods when they are not in class.

One dangerous paradox in this movement is that other valuable educational experiences such as physical education, art, music, and drama may be eliminated or relegated to the status of elective subjects, thus depriving the majority of the children of a well-rounded, "basic" education.

Competency-Based Instruction. Accompanying the "back to the basics" movement are new state laws specifying requirements that all high school seniors must meet in order to receive their diplomas. In order to ensure that students have indeed met stated requirements in specified subject fields, many state and local districts have been given mandates that state explicit graduation requirements and standards; this type of curriculum is referred to as competency-based instruction. Each student must perform at the minimum specified level in each subject in order to be eligible for graduation.

Sometimes physical education is included on the mandatory graduation subject competencies list. Examples of competency behaviors and standards in physical education could include (1) perform on the state physical fitness test at the 70th percentile or higher; (2) swim with the overhand crawl stroke 100 yards in two minutes without stopping; (3) pass a written examination on physical health questions at the 80th percentile; and (4) show evidence of having satisfactorily completed an instructional course in a lifetime sport, in a dance or rhythms course, and in a physical fitness course. Special instructional assistance should be provided to all pupils who are unable to meet the various competence standards.

One strong reservation many critics have about the competency policy is that it emphasizes only those educational experiences that are amenable to objective measurement and neglects many other equally valuable educational activities, such as aesthetic experiences in art, music, dance, and drama. There is no objective way to measure a student's performance in these humanistic fields, which contribute significantly to the aesthetic and contemplative life of the participant. As a compromise, the policy might require successful course participation in these areas for graduation, without specific competency measurement.

"Concept Learning." Traditionally, education has been thought of by the layman, and even by some educators, as a process of acquiring knowledge through the school. In recent years, in such subjects as mathematics, biology, physics, chemistry, and more recently in the social studies, health education, and physical education, a strong emphasis has been developed on "concept" learning, which suggests that the body of knowledge in each discipline should be organized around a unique conceptual structure. Thus we hear the phrase "structure of knowledge" as the central element in teaching the new math, the new science, and so forth. Children learn selected "key concepts" and the most important lower level concepts in the hierarchy of a given subject.

Today's schools place great stress on acquiring knowledge of "concepts" as the most effective means for the human central nervous system to receive, classify, store, retrieve, and utilize essential elements from the vast reservoir of rapidly increasing and ever changing human knowledge. Also, pupils are given practice in using some of the basic modes of inquiry germane to a field of knowledge at a rudimentary level. The idea is that students will learn to think like researchers or scholars in the disciplines.

A few forward-looking curriculum experts believe this trend fragments the educational experience and places too much emphasis on subject matter areas per se, at the expense of equal concern for the nature of the individual child and the child's cultural milieu. These leaders predict that the school curriculum will evolve in the direction of a more "humanistic" approach, which will seek a balance between the subject matter, the pupil, and the environment, and that the focus will be on the optimum development of the potential of the student, mentally, physically, socially, emotionally, and spiritually, in the humanistic tradition. It is pertinent to note that this book, since its initial publication in 1934, has maintained steadfastly a commitment to this humanistic philosophy of education and to the unusual opportunities physical education can contribute to this over-all aim of education in the lives of young people everywhere. This view also permeates this edition, for we believe most sincerely that the physical educator can assist many students in highly significant ways through personal example and commitment as a humanistic educator.

LEARNING

DEFINITION

Learning is generally defined as the process by which one's behavior is changed. In formal learning the change is relatively stable as the pupil acquires a totally new response or a change in the frequency or type of previous responses.

It should be recognized that not all of our behaviors are learned. We are born with response tendencies, some of which are evident in prenatal life. For example, the pupil of the eye innately contracts as more light is suddenly cast upon it. Babies can swallow, they can "make a face" when they taste something bitter, and they can clutch objects placed in their hands.

Learning, a process, should be differentiated from performance, which is a single act. Learning is inferred from a series of individual performances over a period of time during which the individual appears to change the performance significantly from what it was on the original attempt. Learning has taken place when the newly acquired behavior persists over time. Learned performances in sport and dance can be observed and in many cases can be objectively measured.

There are three elements in the definition of learning:

1. Learning indicates relatively permanent changes in the ability, tendency, or capacity to respond.
2. Relatively permanent change in a specific behavior occurs over time.
3. Modifications of neurophysiological structures cause changes in the capacity to respond or behave differently.

In summary, the three criteria of learning refer to change in ca-

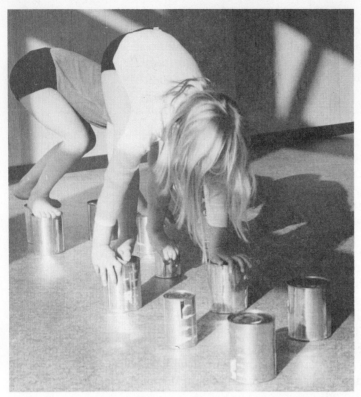

Learning can occur without directly imposed formal instruction.

pacity to respond, change in specific behavior, and change in neural structure.

The obvious purpose of schools is to provide direct, formal instruction in order to promote what society deems to be desirable educational objectives. However, sometimes learning does not occur as a result of experience or exposure to certain phenomena; likewise, learning can occur without directly imposed formal instruction. Recognizing this, teachers arrange learning conditions in school classrooms and laboratories in order to enable each child to achieve the specified learning objectives.

Klausmeier and Ripple[18] describe six steps that are essential to purposeful learning. The learner:

1. Becomes motivated; sets a goal.
2. Appraises situation; evaluates the means and goal relationship.
3. Tries to attain goal; engages in productive thinking and physical activity.
4. Confirms or rejects initial responses.
5. Reaches goal or does not reach goal.
6. Experiences satisfaction; remembers and applies learning. Or modifies goal, modifies responses, or withdraws.

Four learning theories are prominent in the psychological literature today. These are (1) conditioning, (2) modeling and imitation, (3) cognitive restructuring, and (4) information processing. A brief summary of each follows. As space does not permit a detailed explanation of the theories, references concerning each have been placed at the end of this chapter. The physical education major will be exposed to more intensive study of learning theories later in the professional preparation program.

Conditioning. Conditioning theory usually is divided into two components, classical and operant. In classical conditioning, learning is acquired through the building of an association between an external stimulus and a response when no such connection existed prior to learning. The response can be a physiological reaction such as a change in the heart rate, or it can be an external movement such as withdrawing the hand from a hot stove. The main point is that the reaction is a natural reflex to a particular stimulus. A new stimulus, called the "conditioned" stimulus, is inserted closely preceding the original stimulus. After repeated exposures of the new and original stimuli in close association, resulting in a consistent response, the new response becomes predominant and occurs even when the original stimulus is removed. The new response is provoked by the conditioned stimulus. This response is called the *conditioned response*.

Operant conditioning, made famous by the work of B. F. Skinner,[19] differs from classical conditioning in that the operant response is not a reflex but is freely given. Whenever appropriate responses occur, the subject is rewarded in some way. The person's individual response is instrumental (operant) in receiving a reward, hence the term instrumental or operant conditioning. Note that the reinforcing stimulus (reinforcer) is deliberately introduced soon *after* a subject has made a desirable response — behavior that indicates student progress toward the attainment of a desirable learning goal.

Klausmeier and Ripple[20] summarize main generalizations about operant conditioning as follows:

> When a positive reinforcer closely follows a certain response, the probability that the response will occur again is increased. When a negative reinforcer is removed soon after a certain response that led to the removal, the probability that the response will occur again is also increased. Higher-order conditioning occurs in operant conditioning. When a neutral stimulus is paired with a positive reinforcing stimulus, the neutral stimulus, after repeated pairing, itself acquires reinforcing power.

In summary, operant conditioning theorists contend that prompt, positive reinforcement of desirable behaviors influences the learner to attempt to display the desired behavior again and again. It is believed that conditioning is most applicable to affective learning that deals with emotional feelings, values, interests, attitudes, and similar concepts relative to human learning and motivation. Conditioning also has its place in cognitive learning and in motor learning and is well known in connection with programmed learning.

Modeling and Imitation. This learning theory is based on the learner's observation of accurate teaching models. The learner attempts to make responses learned from observing the performance of the model being emulated. Models can be actual persons, such as the teacher, a pupil who is an expert performer, parents, siblings, and others, or symbolic representations presented through pictures, drawings, book illustrations, TV tapes, motion pictures, loop films, and oral and written instructions. Bandura[21] states that "virtually all learning phenomena resulting from direct experiences can occur on a vicarious basis through observation of other persons' behaviors and the consequences of them. Modeling procedures are therefore ideally suited for effective, diverse outcomes including elimination of behavioral deficits, reduction of excessive fears and inhibitions, transmission of self-regulating systems, and social facilitation of behavioral patterns on a group-wide scale." Although Bandura does not mention complex motor skills learning per se, it is obvious from his strong conclusion that modeling and imitation have a central role to play in this type of learning.

Because very few studies have been done on this topic in motor learning, data on the use of imitation and modeling in the acquisition and performance of various types of motor skills are scarce. Therefore, we must be tentative about the use of conclusions drawn by Bandura and Walters.[22] Martens, Burwitz, and Zuckerman[23] indicate that physical education teachers and athletic coaches frequently use models of skilled individuals performing complex motor acts.

Theory indicates that a model facilitates improved performance information concerning the appropriate and inappropriate responses, and also improves the motivational state of the student. In four experiments Martens and colleagues[24] reported, "Evidence indicates that modeling a correct performance facilitated performance on early practice trials for a relatively simple motor skill." Also, data indicated that information about the correct performance was indeed communicated to the learner who was observing the model. More of this type of research is urgently needed in physical education.

It is important that the real-life model be prestigious, or highly regarded by the learners; it is also desirable that the model have the authority to bestow rewards on learners who improve through this process of imitation. Although rewards can take many intrinsic and extrinsic forms, two of the most effective are positive reinforcement and self-satisfaction. It is obvious that the teacher must provide a model of desired behavior so students can understand the performance. They can then reproduce the series of behaviors that moves them in the direction of the learning goal. Finally, students from differing cultural and educational backgrounds must be provided with appropriate models with whom they empathize and associate; one model may not suffice for all members of a large, culturally diverse class of students.

Cognitive Restructuring. In complex learning situations the roles of perception and knowledge are crucial. Cognitive learning is the term applied to the phase of over-all learning theory that concentrates on explaining and describing relationships and means. It suggests that learners develop a cognitive structure within their memory that organizes information and retains it for future retention and use.

One aspect of cognitive learning is insight. The learner must perceive fundamental relationships that underlie the solution to a problem. A certain degree of insight is present in all human learning. We all know of an individual who, through "sudden insight," evolves a solution to a major problem. Apparently, once a solution has been developed through insight, it can be repeated promptly and also transferred to similar situations. Teachers should emphasize insightful learning rather than pure memorization or mechanical skills, and thus encourage problem-solving behaviors.

Another aspect of cognitive learning is known as sign learning. It is defined by Hilgard et al.[25] as "an acquired expectation that one stimulus will be followed by another in a particular context." It is an expectation that is acquired; it is not a chained sequence of responses. What is learned is a set of expectations or a cognitive map of the situation rather than precise responses. Therefore, sign learning is based on understanding rather than on conditioning.

In cognitive structuring the teacher assists pupils to associate new knowledge with existing knowledge stored in their neural systems. Each new segment of information is seen in the light of previously learned concepts. This melding of new knowledge with the existing conceptual system is described as *cognitive restructuring*. Concepts, principles, generalizations, theories, facts, laws, and other forms of cognitive input are arranged in meaningful relationships that promote desirable learning results. The teacher assists the learner to recognize the relationship or choose other concepts or principles having the potential to solve a problem.

Experienced teachers present a variety of learning materials to the students, such as books, motion pictures, TV film, teacher-prepared notes and memoranda, movement experiences, and other teaching aids. This theory of learning applies only to learning materials that can be presented to the learner in final form, such as the correct answer to a multiplication problem in arithmetic. It does not replace or substitute for the conditioning theory or modeling and imitation theory. Research needs to be undertaken to distinguish concepts that are best learned through movement experiences from those best assimilated from books or pictures; and to determine how such concepts are restructured into the existing cognitive system of the learner.

Hilgard[26] provides an excellent summary of the three learning theories we have discussed so far.

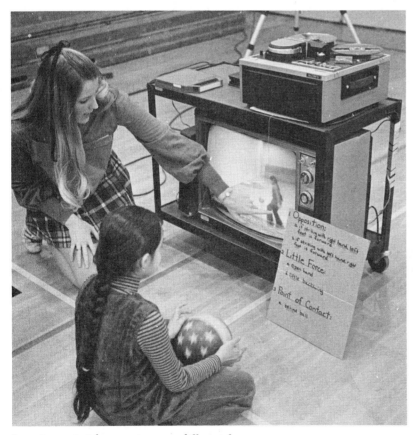

Learning materials come in many different forms.

It is possible to grade examples of learning on a crude scale, with the most automatic kind of learning (explained best as S-R [Stimulus–Response] associations) at one end and the most insightful and rational kind at the other (explained best according to cognitive principles). Those habits learned by classical conditioning, and without awareness, would be at one extreme of the scale. Perhaps learning to salivate when we see a delicious meal or becoming anxious when we encounter a situation that has proved dangerous in the past would be examples of such conditioning. Toward the middle of the scale would be tasks learned with full awareness but still somewhat automatically, as when we learn a foreign language vocabulary or skill like swimming. At the other end of the scale fall tasks that require reasoning about many facts in complex relationships. Most learning would probably fall somewhere in the middle range of the scale, a kind of mixture between simple association and understanding. . . .

For most practical applications it may be best to adopt a conservative position that pays attention to associative aspects of the learning process as well as to problems of cognitive organization.

Information Processing.   In recent years psychologists have developed models of human thinking based on the concepts and procedures that underlie modern-day computer systems and programs, hence the term *information-processing.* Gagné[27] describes this new theory.

Recent research demonstrates that incoming stimuli are processed in the central nervous system (CNS) in a variety of complex ways. Stimuli received through the various sensory organs are labeled as information. It is now believed that when the sensory systems initially register incoming information it is stored for approximately 30 seconds in its original form in the brain. This information is not immediately altered, as was formerly believed. It is held in *short-term store.* Because our sensory systems constantly bombard the CNS with new incoming information, the old information is forced out of the short-term storage area. While in the short-term storage area, a "rehearsal buffer" acts upon the new information to organize and rehearse it. From the short-term store the rehearsed information is transferred into *long-term store* by a process called *coding,* which prepares it for economical long-term storing and later retrieval.

Apparently information processing occurs in a serial manner. Only a few abstract symbols can be processed at a time and held temporarily in the short-term memory storage. At this time, the content can be rapidly reorganized and changed. The short-term memory has a very small storage capacity, so there is a severe limitation on the ability of the individual to employ efficient strategies to retrieve and utilize the knowledge that is in the short-term store. Also, a relatively long period of time is required to transfer information from short-term to long-term memory. The information processing model is much more complicated than indicated above, but brief mention of these major components serves to introduce this recent theory, which is gaining wide acceptance.

Gagné believes that the key element in learning is "the prior learning of prerequisite capabilities." Spaced reviews are vital to long-term retention, whether a mental task or a motor learning task. Reviews must be made with the deliberate intention to remember them over a period of time. The individual must learn coding and retrieval strategies. The use of "advance organizers" and "anchoring ideas" as a basis for connecting and retaining new information is extremely important. At the same time, this theory tends to weaken previously held beliefs that practice and repetition result in improved retention.

Gagné[28] relates the above theory to instruction by teachers as follows:

> Instruction becomes not primarily a matter of communicating something that is to be stored. Instead, it is the matter of stimulating the use of capabilities the learner already has at his disposal, and making sure he has the requisite capabilities for the present learning task, as well as for more to come.

Summary. The physical education teacher, the athletic coach, and the dance instructor should be knowledgeable about the major elements of the preceding learning theories. These theories provide an acceptable basis not only for selecting desirable learning opportunities for pupils, but also for deriving principles of teaching that most effectively facilitate pupils' achievement of educational goals.

TRANSFER OF LEARNING

One of the major purposes of instruction in schools is to enable the individual to apply what has been learned to the complex variety of situations and problems in life in general. Therefore, the transfer of learning is a fundamental topic for teachers. It refers to the ability of the individual to make use of previous educational experiences to learn something new and different and thereby optimize the learning experience. When the learning of one task has a positive effect on the learning of a subsequent task, this phenomenon is called *positive transfer*. However, if there is an interference between the original learning and the attempt to apply it to another learning situation, then it is called *negative transfer*. For example, in learning to hit a tennis forehand drive the player is taught to maintain a firm wrist as the ball strikes the racket. In hitting a badminton bird the student is taught to "snap the wrist" at the moment of impact with the shuttle cock. A student should not receive instruction in tennis and badminton on alternating days because negative transfer will impede the correct learning of either stroke.

Even though tasks previously learned may not be identical to a new task, the pupil may develop an approach to the learning of the new task that facilitates its performance. In effect, the student is learning to learn. Obviously, this capability should be encouraged and reinforced by teachers.

Transfer of learning also helps the student understand and apply principles from an original learning experience to a similar situation in a new circumstance. An advantage is that the learner can more easily master and remember a set of principles than recall all the details of many discrete specifics involved in original learning situations. Likewise, the more thoroughly the students have mastered the original knowledges and principles, the more likely they are to be transferred to the new learning situation.[29]

FUNDAMENTAL GENERALIZATIONS

Education. The brief explanations about schools, schooling, education, and learning theories provide a background for a definition of the term "education." In our view, education is a continuous, lifelong process of change, modification, or adjustment of the individual — in school or out of it — resulting from responses to the stimuli and conditions of the external and internal* environments. These persistent changes in behav-

---

*The internal environment consists of the conditions, influences, and forces within the organism itself, particularly within the blood and lymph. For example, the hormones are powerful influences.

ior, resulting from the learner's own activities, affect the mental, physical, emotional, moral, and ethical aspects of life in significant ways. Societal values and cultural and subcultural norms determine the extent to which these behavioral changes are desirable or are "valued."

Generalizations. Substantial evidence from biology, psychology, physiology, and neurology provides a basis for the above concept of education and is summarized by the following generalizations.

1. *All Educational Changes and Modifications in Behavior Come About Through the Individual's Own Activities.* Some changes occur through the influence of normal growth and development based on hereditary predispositions and maturational processes. These changes are not regarded as educational modifications. Many educational changes are deliberately selected and sought by the teacher, and are stated as educational objectives. The pupil is engaged in a series of planned educational experiences having as their purpose "learning": stable changes in behavior that approximate the behavioral changes described in the objectives.

The student must be engaged, directly and actively, in this learning process. The learner must define clear, realistic, attainable goals. Conditions that facilitate viable learning experiences and motivate the learner are essential ingredients in this process of significant stable behavior change. The learner must participate in frequent repetition of learning experiences that provide multisensory stimulation and that result in the neural integration of a variety of stimuli for long-term retention and retrieval.

Not all specific changes in pupil behaviors are planned in advance and encouraged by instructors. Artistic teachers in any field will provide learning opportunities that encourage divergent, creative behaviors. Problem-solving situations are formulated that encourage students to find novel and creative responses or solutions through their own intellectual efforts. Self-discovery and heuristic learning experiences are fundamental to curriculum and instruction at all levels of formal education. In this type of open-ended learning there is no one predictable or required solution; rather, a range of possible responses of equal "correctness" is encouraged. Boys and girls should be urged to engage in expressive behaviors that reflect their feelings and emotions. Non-verbal behaviors that communicate and express ideas, moods, preferences, and idiosyncratic personality traits are to be encouraged. None of the above behavioral changes are preplanned to the extent of specifying performance objectives in advance, but all are valuable, potential educational outcomes in pupil behaviors nurtured and developed under the guidance of a sensitive, receptive teacher.

2. *Planned Educational Opportunities Provide Experiences for Developing Guided Behavioral Responses to Stimuli Presented in the Internal and External Environments.* Stimuli, in the sense employed in the above generalization, refers to total learning situations, not to isolated, unplanned stimulus–response reflexes or reactions.

Basketball players spend hours of practice time learning cues for instantaneously recognizing various defensive maneuvers such as "switches," "presses," "over-playing," and other stratagems. Thus, the player learns to respond automatically with a countermove that takes advantage of a weakness in the opponent's move. Long distance runners learn from their coaches the causes and effects of physical fatigue upon performance in their events. In planned practices the runners learn to cope with, and to react favorably to, both external and internal influences during an official race. Golfers estimate the width of the fairway, the distance of the fairway trap in front of the tee, the direction of the prevailing wind, and the best position on the fairway for the second shot toward the green before making their drive, by developing a mental plan that they hope to execute accurately.

Individual responses to total learning situations are based upon prior opportunities for practice and participation in varied contexts, thus enhancing the likelihood of discriminating responses in later environments. The term discrimination means that the fundamental movement response the athlete has learned can be adapted and utilized effectively under specific conditions that vary throughout the course of a contest.

There is a risk that reference to "stimulus" and "response" as used in the above generalization will imply a type of rote, automatic learning of only one correct response. This is incorrect. Teachers should organize learning opportunities so that comprehension and understanding of the total situation confronting the learner are integral aspects of the experience. Likewise, students should be encouraged and rewarded (reinforced) for attempts to think and act divergently or creatively, as well as convergently or logically, as the specific instance requires. The full human potential for learning will not be realized if it is restricted to logical, expected, predicted responses.

3. *All Responses to Learning Opportunities Change, Modify, or "Educate" the Individual.* The basketball players, the long distance runners, and the golfers have reacted in various total learning experiences to different types of stimuli, and thus their behaviors are changed or modified in several ways. As these athletes undergo significant behavioral changes or modifications, it may be generally assumed that they therefore become increasingly more effective in attaining their specific objectives. If they are "learning" they are more nearly approximating the ideal behaviors described in the objectives formulated by their coaches and themselves. Athletes should be consulted by the coaches, and their views should be considered as these objectives are developed and evaluated. Likewise, students who engage in creative, problem-solving, expressive, and non-verbal communicative behaviors are changing during these educational episodes, and their behaviors are modified as a result of these experiences. Obviously, competent instruction contributes significantly to these educational achievements.

4. *All Responses Involve the Integrated Human Organism.* All the behaviors an individual exhibits at any given time are organized into a complex, unique system called personality. Each person attempts to organize and structure patterns of behavior that promote successful adaptation to society. All responses of the individual are subject to a continual process of neural integration. Education is concerned with the individual as a whole. We may observe that an experimental subject's pulse rate rises to 200 beats per minute on the bicycle ergometer, and we may thoughtlessly believe that this performance represents an isolated physiological response. A quarterback may be heard issuing an audible change in signal at the line of scrimmage, which superficially seems only to be a rapid mental adjustment and response. The girl who wins the 100 yard freestyle race in the conference swimming meet shows her happiness by waving her arms and her swimming cap at the audience and smiling broadly, surely an emotional response. Yet , in each case, modern knowledge about the totally integrated functioning of all the organic systems of the human being assures us that each of the above experiences

modifies these athletes in some way. It is the cumulative state of these integrated responses that determines the individual's personality at any given time.

Application. The four generalizations discussed can be summarized by the statement that all education fundamentally is concerned with (1) the *individual,* in terms of purposes, needs, abilities, aptitudes, interests, attitudes, and personality; (2) the *situation* (or stimulus) as perceived by the individual and the *setting* (learning environment) in which the educational experience occurs; (3) the *response* (reaction) of the individual, and the interaction between the individual and the situation (or stimulus); (4) the *changes,* modifications, stable adaptations, and behaviors that are brought about as a result of responses to the situation (or stimulus); and (5) the total *integration* of these responses and subsequent *altered behaviors* that mold the human personality.

These generalizations and conclusions apply to physical education as well as to any other form or phase of education. Fundamentally, physical education is concerned with individuals, situations, responses, and modifications of behavior. In the final analysis the only distinction between physical education and other forms of education is that physical education is concerned largely with learning situations and pupil responses that are characterized by overt movement activities, such as sports, aquatics, and exercises. It is recognized that all responses of the individual involve the integrated human organism; and that certain responses are characterized mainly by intellectual activity, others by emotional activity, and still others by vigorous physical movement. Physical education learning activities are characterized by vigorous, skilled movements through which students learn to make intellectual, social, emotional, and physical changes and adaptations in their behaviors and personalities.

It must be emphasized that physical education is not concerned exclusively with muscular reactions and the resultant physiological and anatomical changes in the individual. It is true that rational muscular exercise, among other effects, promotes growth and development, strengthens and enlarges muscles, improves muscle tone, and increases the power and vigor of the organic system. But it would be a rare program of physical education indeed that could be conducted without involving the individual in situations calling for mental and emotional responses, with resultant modifications in habits, attitudes, appreciations, and skills. The nearest approach to such a barren and limited program is to be found in "systems" in which the individual gains physical education, or, more accurately, physical training, through drills, dumbbells, wands, gripping devices, mechanical horses, or vibrating belts driven by electric motors.

Studies in neurophysiology and kinesiology are producing evidence that leads us to believe that the contribution of kinesthesis to intellectual development is more crucial than previously realized. Steinhaus[30] says:

> Every movement, every body position, every tension in muscle, tendon, and joint structure contributes to the formation of concepts or ideas that form the building stones with which we construct our thought life.

In a more recent review of current research in neurology and physiological psychology, Steinhaus also expresses the startling notion that "your muscles see more than your eyes"![31] A person who is unfortunately almost completely paralyzed cannot cope with the external environment as well as a blind person. More concepts are learned through proprioception and kinesthesis than through vision.

DEFINITION OF PHYSICAL EDUCATION

We believe physical education is most appropriately defined as *that phase of the total process of education that is concerned with the development and utilization of the individual's voluntary, purposeful, movement capabilities, and with directly related mental, emotional and social responses*. Stable behavior modifications in the individual result from these movement-centered responses and thus the individual *learns* through physical education.

This definition asserts that the school program of physical education consists fundamentally of a specialized learning environment, characterized by many planned conditions and stimuli specifically intended to induce or provide opportunities for physical, social, emotional, intellectual, and other beneficial responses through which the student may become changed, modified, or educated in desirable ways. The dance studio, the tennis courts, the gymnastics apparatus, other appropriate equipment and supplies, and the facilities and spaces required for their use, are essential parts of the specialized physical educational environment, as are the teacher, the coach, the scheduled contest, and the standards and traditions of the school physical education and athletic programs. The quality of physical education learning outcomes in the students in any school will depend upon the responses and attitudes induced in the participants. Hence, it is of vital importance to select, periodically evaluate, and retain physical education teachers and athletic coaches of high moral standards and outstanding personal character.

If the total school physical education and sports environment is restricted to exercises performed to command, to regimented, militaristic physical fitness activities, and to highly structured competitive activities, the program will be narrow indeed and, in fact, can be labeled as a "physical training" program. On the other hand, if the total physical education environment presents learning opportunities that result in frequent and desirable responses and interactions of an intellectual, social, and moral nature, along with a physical performance emphasis, the program is of vital educational significance.

When planned and conducted according to the above philosophy, physical education is now accepted as an essential educational experience in which all pupils in the school engage regularly throughout elementary, secondary, and higher education programs. Physical education is an integral phase of the total institutional academic curriculum.

SUMMARY

The physical educator of today must be fully informed and deeply concerned about the proper roles and contributions of physical education programs in relation to the full range of human activities, for persons of all ages, and for individuals in varying degrees of health. Physical educators must broaden their horizons concerning the contributions this field can make to human health, happiness, and welfare through a more accurate and widespread understanding and public interpretation. Physical education should provide vigorous leadership to develop and expand programs based on current knowledge and understanding about the significance and the meaning of purposeful, physical movements and skilled activities in the lives of children, youths, and adults.

The term "physical education" evolved from the more restrictive phrase, "physical training." Thus, the emphasis was transferred from the "education of the physical" to "education through the physical."

In describing physical education as an academic discipline, Metheny says that "movement as a dynamic function of man is the area of central concern that gives physical education its unique identity as an academic discipline."

The discussion about physical education as an academic discipline and as physical activity science is centered on selected types of movement experiences and behavioral patterns suggested by such terms as exercise, sport, dance, gymnastics, athletics, and movements commonly required for the essential activities of daily living.

We may describe the nature and scope of physical education as (1) a discrete academic discipline with a unique body of knowledge, and (2) an educationally based profession.

One danger in the "back to the basics" movement in education is that certain valuable educational experiences, such as physical education, art, music, and drama, may be eliminated from the curriculum or relegated to the status of elective subjects. This policy would deprive the majority of children of a well-rounded education, which to be truly "basic" must include experiences in these areas of human endeavor.

Education is defined as a continuous, lifelong process of change, modification, or adjustment of the individual — in school or out of it — resulting from responses to the stimuli and conditions of the external and internal environments. These persistent changes in behaviors, which result from the learner's activities, affect the mental, physical, emotional, moral, and ethical aspects of life in many significant ways.

The only distinction between physical education and other forms of education is that physical education is concerned largely with learning situations and pupil responses characterized by overt movement activities such as sports, aquatics, dance, and exercises.

Physical education is defined as that phase of the total process of education that is concerned with the development and utilization of the individual's voluntary, purposeful movement capabilities, and with directly related mental, emotional, and social responses. Stable behavior modifications result from these movement-centered responses and thus the individual *learns* through physical education.

FOOTNOTES

[1]Franklin M. Henry, "Physical Education, An Academic Discipline," *JOHPER*, 35:32–33, 69 (September 1964).

[2]John E. Nixon, "The Criteria of a Discipline," *Quest*, IX:42–48 (December 1967).

[3]"The Nature of a Discipline," *Quest*, IX:87 (December 1967).

[4]John E. Nixon, op. cit.

[5]Eleanor Metheny, *Connotations of Movement in Sport and Dance*. Dubuque, Iowa: Wm. C. Brown and Company, 1965.

[6]Elizabeth R. Hayes, "Dance as a Discipline: Past, Present and Future," The Academy Papers No. 10, *Beyond Research – Solutions to Human Problems*. Louisville, KY: American Academy of Physical Education, November 1976, 56–66, p. 57.

[7]Ibid., p. 58.

[8]Ibid., p. 65.

[9]Joel Lydia, "The Impact of IMPACT – Dance Artists Are Catalysts for Change in Education," *Dance Scope*, VI:8 (Spring/Summer 1972).

[10]Claude Bouchard, "Physical Activity Sciences: A Basic Concept for the Organization of the Discipline and the Profession," *International Journal of Physical Education*, XII:10–15 (Winter 1976).

[11]Ibid., p. 11.

[12]Ibid.

[13]Daryl Siedentop, *Developing Teaching Skills in Physical Education*. Boston: Houghton-Mifflin Company, 1976, pp. 12–14.

[14]Eleanor Metheny, "The Unique Meaning Inherent in Human Movement," *The Physical Educator*, 18:3–7 (March 1961).

[15]Celeste Ulrich and John E. Nixon, *Tones of Theory — A Theoretical Structure for Physical Education — A Tentative Perspective*. Washington, D.C.: American Association for Health, Physical Education, and Recreation, 1972.

[16]Ibid.

[17]Ibid, p. 24.

[18]Herbert J. Klausmeier and Richard E. Ripple, *Learning and Human Abilities: Educational Psychology* (3rd ed.). New York: Harper and Row, 1971, p. 33.

[19]B. F. Skinner, *The Technology of Teaching*. New York: Appleton-Century-Crofts, Inc., 1968.

[20]Herbert J. Klausmeier and Richard E. Ripple, op. cit., p. 45.

[21]Albert Bandura, *Principles of Behavior Modification*. New York: Holt, Rinehart and Winston, 1969, p. 118.

[22]Albert Bandura and Richard H. Walters, *Social Learning and Personality Development*. New York: Holt, Rinehart and Winston, 1963.

[23]Rainer Martens, Les Burwitz, and Joshua Zuckerman, "Modeling Effects on Motor Performance," *Research Quarterly*, 47:227–291 (May 1976), pp. 289, 290.

[24]Ibid., p. 290.

[25]Ernest R. Hilgard, Richard C. Atkinson, and Rita L. Atkinson, *Introduction to Psychology* (6th ed.). New York: Harcourt, Brace, Jovanovich, Inc., 1975, p. 217.

[26]Ibid., pp. 218, 219.

[27]Robert M. Gagné, "Some New Views of Learning and Instruction," *Phi Delta Kappan*, 43:468–472 (May 1970).

[28]Ibid., p. 469.

[29]Ernest R. Hilgard, Richard C. Atkinson, and Rita L. Atkinson, op. cit., p. 75.

[30]Arthur H. Steinhaus, *Toward an Understanding of Health and Physical Education*. Dubuque, Iowa: Wm. C. Brown and Company, 1963, p. 10.

[31]Arthur H. Steinhaus, "Your Muscles See More than Your Eyes," *JOHPER*, 37:48–50 (September 1966).

SELECTED REFERENCES

American Academy of Physical Education, *Relationships in Physical Education*. The Academy Papers, No. 11, Washington, D.C. 1977.

American Academy of Physical Education, *Realms of Meaning*. The Academy Papers, No. 9, Washington, D.C., 1975.

AAHPER, *Encyclopedia of Physical Education, Fitness and Sports*. Washington, D.C.: American Association for Health, Physical Education, and Recreation, 1977.

Brown, Camille, and Cassidy, Rosalind, *Theory in Physical Education: A Guide to Program Change*. Philadelphia: Lea & Febiger, 1963.

Cheffers, John T., and Evaul, Thomas, *Introduction to Physical Education: Concepts of Human Movement*. Englewood Cliffs, N.J.: Prentice-Hall, Inc., 1978.

Freeman, William H., *Physical Education in a Changing Society*. Boston, MA: Houghton-Mifflin, 1977.

Haag, Herbert (Ed.), *Sport Pedagogy, Content and Methodology*. Baltimore: University Park Press, 1978.

Henry, Franklin M., "Physical Education, an Academic Discipline." *Journal of Health, Physical Education, and Recreation*, 35:32–33 (September 1964).

Henry, Franklin M., "The Academic Discipline of Physical Education," *Quest*, 29:13–29 (November 1978).

Hilgard, Ernest R., Atkinson, Richard C., and Atkinson, Rita L., *Introduction to Psychology* (6th Ed.). New York: Harcourt, Brace, Jovanovich, Inc., 1975.

Jewett, Ann E., and Mullan, Marie R., *Curriculum Design: Purposes and Processes in Physical Education Teaching-Learning*. Washington, D.C.: American Alliance for Health, Physical Education, Recreation, and Dance, 1977.

Johnson, Perry B., Updyke, Wynn, Schaefer, and Stolberg, Donald, *Sport, Exercise, and You*. New York: Holt, Rinehart and Winston, 1975.

Metheny, Eleanor, *Movement and Meaning*. New York: McGraw-Hill Book Company, 1968.

Quest, IX, 1967, "The Nature of a Discipline."

Quest, XXIII, 1975, "The Language of Movement."

Rivenes, Richard S., *Foundations of Physical Education: A Scientific Approach*. Boston, MA: Houghton-Mifflin, 1978.

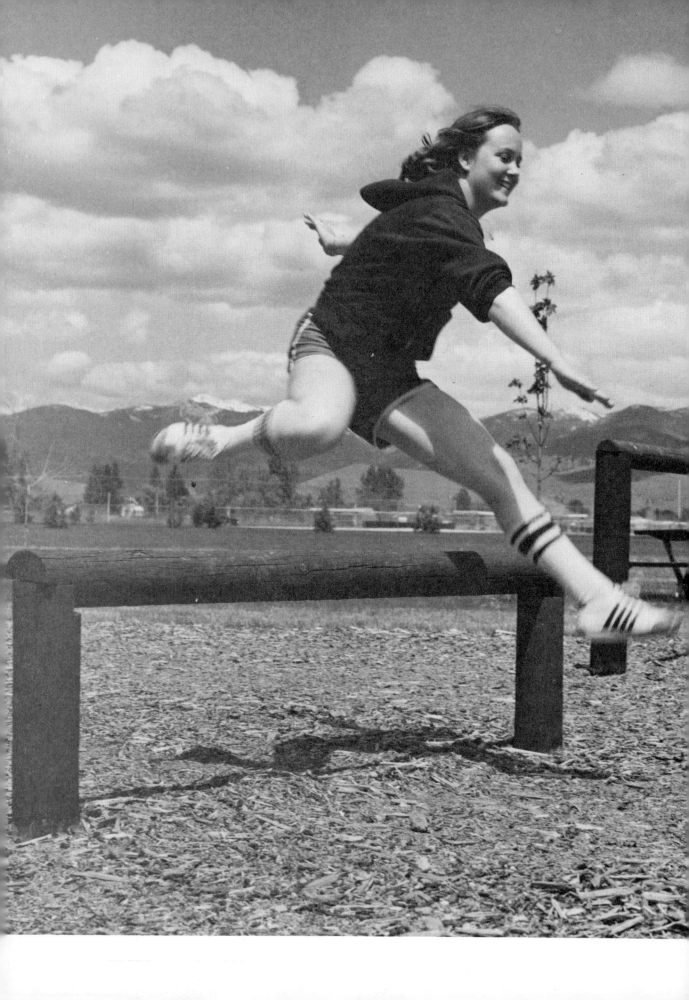

THE PURPOSES OF ———
——— PHYSICAL EDUCATION

This chapter presents an approach to the understanding and conceptual organization of the purposes of physical education as conceived by the authors. The term "purposes" is used in the inclusive sense and will be elucidated in detail through a definition and description of such terms as aim, objectives (general, instructional, performance, specific, and behavioral), and goals.

Obviously, there is more than one acceptable framework for viewing the value of physical education experiences. Therefore, frequent reference is made to the publications of other individuals and professional organizations proposing alternative conceptual structures. The professional student should be exposed to a variety of these views as a basis for developing a personal conceptual framework within which to organize thoughts and understanding about the objectives of physical education. Personal objectives and values influence virtually every pedagogical act performed by the physical educator, though this effect may not be apparent in the course of the planning, teaching, coaching, or evaluating.

There is no consistent use among authors of terms such as "aims," "purposes," "objectives," "goals," and "outcomes."; often two or more are used interchangeably or synonymously. Since there is no standard acceptance or agreement for each of these terms, it is indeed difficult to order one's thinking about the objectives of physical education, and to compare and contrast varying shades of philosophical exposition that have accumulated in recent years in the professional literature. We believe that a consistent understanding and use of these terms is desirable and possible. Our organizational structure of basic purpose concepts involves the following categories: aim, general objectives, instructional objectives, behavioral and performance objectives, formative and summative objectives, goals, and outcomes. Each of these concepts is discussed in more detail in this chapter.

BASIC AIM

American public education at various school levels still faces the dilemma of ambiguous, vague, and widely divergent aims proposed by state legislatures, school boards, educational writers, curriculum com-

31

missions, and other sources. One can readily see a diversity of aims in the following:

"to train the mind"

"to develop the intellect"

"to master prescribed bodies of knowledge"

"to learn the basic concepts of selected disciplines"

"to develop the character"

"to develop the human potentialities so the individual will become an effective, participating member of the democratic society"

"to develop the rational power"

"to develop the ability to think"

"to develop the capacity to make wise decisions, in order to become an effective citizen in the democratic processes upon which this free country depends"

"to learn to learn for a lifetime"

Perhaps the task of deriving an over-all aim of physical education can best be accomplished by analyzing two fundamental concepts about education in general that are substantiated by carefully validated scientific research. These two basic generalizations, which were described in more detail in the previous chapter, are (1) that education is a process of stable change in, or modification of, the behavior of the individual resulting from activities, reactions, and interactions with different environments; and (2) that formal education promotes modifications enabling the individual to grow and develop in all phases of life and to attain a satisfactory degree of social adjustment.

Sheppard and Willoughby[1] state a laudable aim for education in general:

> A growing commitment to the full realization of human potential will place permanent emphasis upon the development of competent, productive, responsible, inquiring, questioning, value-judging, sensitive, compassionate, loving, humane individuals and their individuality as expressed by the concept of self: self-esteem, self-direction, self-control, and self-actualization. Along with this will go the preparation to play many and varied societal roles — citizen, spouse, lover, parent, colleague, worker, player — and an emphasis on skills which are of life-long importance. Schools will actually attempt to prepare students to live a life, not merely to educate them.

Statements of purposes of physical education found in recent literature generally agree on the importance of providing opportunities in school programs for individuals to engage in selected movement activities (such as sports, dance, exercises, gymnastics, and aquatics). These statements also stress the need for adequate facilities and for exemplary leadership, thus providing favorable environments for educational activities best suited to produce desirable changes in behavior, growth, and development. Following this line of reasoning, we may define the *aim* of physical education as follows:

> *The aim of organized physical education programs is to create an environment that stimulates selected movement experiences, resulting in desirable responses that contribute to the optimal development of the individual's potentialities in all phases of life.*

The aim of physical education consists of several general objectives and their components. Innumerable books, pamphlets, curriculum guides, and magazine articles contain descriptions of general physical education objectives. It is startling and instructive to construct a list of physical education objectives from selected sources and to categorize each under various topical headings. First, one is impressed with the diverse terminology used to express each author's precise meaning. Attaching clear meanings to these many descriptions naturally leads to an attempt to classify them for inherent similarity and for distinctiveness. It soon becomes apparent that physical education objectives from various sources cover a wide range of expectations for changing human behavior. *Determining Objectives*

This diversity of claims works to the detriment of the field. One of the most frequent charges leveled against physical education is that it claims too much, that it purports to be all things to all people, and that it puts itself on a pedestal of unattainable virtue. Indeed, certain objectives appear to be self-serving. An exaggerated list of objectives weakens the position of physical education and underlines the need for interpretation and understanding.

Objectives should be tentatively held, even though some of them are strongly advocated at the moment and seem to be well substantiated. New evidence and varied experience, combined with increasing ability to examine them critically, undoubtedly will cause each physical educator to revise objectives, and even, at times, to alter the selection of them. A continual revision of objectives is a fact of professional life for the perceptive physical educator and is to be encouraged. Every educational decision concerning curriculum planning, selecting and carrying out instructional strategies, choosing and employing teaching techniques, and evaluating procedures and conclusions about pupil learning emanates from clarity of the program objectives and teachers' commitments to them.

The objectives of school physical educational programs should be developed cooperatively by the staff and the administration. Many educators advocate that pupil representatives, parents, and citizen committees recommend educational philosophy and curriculum. Some school districts appoint citizens' advisory committees for each subject in a school curriculum. These committees, if wise, will start their study with a pupil–needs assessment.

The aim of physical education is to maximize an individual's potential in all phases of life.

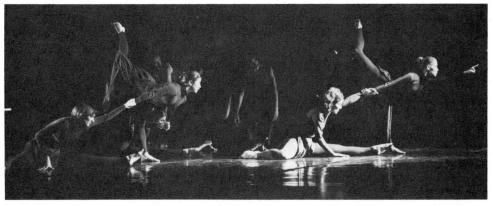

Physical education objectives grow out of the needs of the individuals served by the program, and the needs of the society of which they are a part. Therefore, these needs, as with societal values, must be determined and described as accurately as possible.

Having identified the needs and values, and having set the objectives, learning activities are then selected to facilitate the attainment of the objectives, and from these a program is organized and conducted that will best satisfy the needs and values, and attain the educational objectives.

We may restate these curriculum development procedures as a series of questions to be answered:

1. What are the needs in terms of growth, development, and adjustment of the individuals to be "educated"?
2. What are the basic personal and societal values held by the citizens in the school district?
3. What educational activities will best contribute to the satisfaction of these specific needs and the promotion of the community values?
4. What are the characteristics of the school environment in which we can best provide these desirable educational opportunities?
5. To what extent do formal and informal evaluation procedures reveal the accomplishment of the educational objectives and the acquisition of societal values?

One of the major problems facing the school physical education program is how to provide individualized programs that best meet the *needs* of each student. Far too often in the past we have lumped all students together into heterogeneous classes, directed these students in an authoritarian manner, and forced them through a standard curriculum with little regard for their individual differences, needs, and interests. By such practices we seem to assume that one prescribed program of activities is equally valuable (educative) for all pupils.

DETERMINING THE NEEDS OF PUPILS

The teacher who genuinely believes that individualized learning experiences should be based on needs and interests has an obligation to understand the nature of needs and interests, their relationships to motives and to the goals that we have previously discussed. McDonald[2] aptly weaves these three concepts together:

> Curriculum organization has profited from the conception of basing the curriculum on the needs of children. . . . Modern educators have built a curriculum derived from conceptions of what the majority of children will need in order to be useful members of society, with provisions for the needs of particular groups of children. This reorganization of the curriculum has not simplified or resolved the problem that has always confronted teachers — the problem of motivating students to work for specific goals. The teacher faces children with varying needs and learned goal expectations. The teacher's task is to broaden children's conceptions of their goals, foster the acquisition of new needs, and through this process enhance the total development of the child.

Definitions. We define personal *needs* as relatively stable and permanent dispositions or tendencies that are amenable to specific types of motivation. Unsatisfied needs, developed either from external environmental stimuli or from internal bodily changes, may arouse or direct activity toward goals that will presumably satisfy those needs.

CHAPTER TWO

The current status of research and theory on the concept of needs is too complex and extensive to summarize here. Hilgard, Atkinson, and Atkinson[3] provide a detailed basic discussion about needs and related concepts such as drives, motives, incentives, appetites, aversions, and other highly interrelated concepts. The physical educator should study these topics as a basis for understanding current knowledge and theory and their relationships to teaching and coaching principles and practices.

The following brief summary of recent evidence concerning the nature of motivation and human needs by Hilgard, Atkinson, and Atkinson[4] is useful:

> Motivation refers to the factors that *energize* and *direct* behavior. Attempts to explain motivated acts have had various emphases. (a) *Instinct theory* postulates innate predispositions to specific actions. (b) *Drive-reduction theory* bases motivation on bodily *needs* that create a state of tension or *drive* which the organism seeks to reduce by doing something to satisfy the need. Tissue needs prompt action because the body tends to maintain a constant internal environment or *homeostasis*. (c) *Incentive theory* emphasizes the importance of external conditions as a source of motivation. These may be *positive incentives* which the organism will approach or *negative incentives* which he will avoid. Incentives can arouse behavior as well as direct it.
>
> Motives with no known physiological basis are the needs to *explore* new environments and to *manipulate* objects. The organism requires a certain amount of stimulation; *sensory deprivation* can be very aversive.
>
> Central to current approaches to motivation is the notion of *arousal*. Internal or external stimulation that produces too severe a change from the optimal arousal level motivates the organism to do something to restore equilibrium.

Today many physical educators are attracted to a theory of needs that emphasizes self-actualization as pioneered by Maslow.[5] According to Alderman,[6] Maslow postulates that humankind's basic nature is "inherent goodness." The individual constantly strives to become a person who adequately functions in society according to the potential he or she possesses for developing appropriate adaptive behaviors. Persons who succeed in meeting this self-actualization need in a relatively satisfactory manner are judged to be healthy and well adjusted in our society.

SELF-ACTUALIZATION

Alderman[7] interprets Maslow as contending that life consists of (1) a strong desire to meet basic human needs for physical and psychological survival and (2) a continual attempt to fulfill one's "inherent potentialities i.e., the meta-needs of justice, goodness, beauty, order, and so on." These two need systems are hierarchical in that the meta-needs develop from the basic survival needs.

The basic structure of Maslow's hierarchy of needs can be seen on page 36. In general, the individual must find adequate need satisfaction at all lower levels before a higher need can be met completely. Satisfaction of higher needs is based on fulfillment of lower needs. Most normal individuals are both partially satisfied and partially unsatisfied at each level, but in varying degrees. It is not a matter of all-or-none. However, it is generally observed that the degree and numbers of unmet wants or needs increase in each higher category; thus, it can be said that human beings are a continually "wanting" organism.

Alderman[8] makes an interesting assessment of the application of

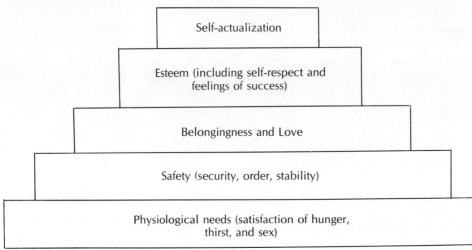

Maslow's hierarchy of needs.

Maslow's theory to self-actualization in sport. He indicates that it is improbable that humans reflect physiological needs in physical activities and sports, at least in the western world. Undoubtedly there are many people who elect to participate in sport and other physical activities at a level that will assure them of physical safety and expose them to few accidents. Jogging, bowling, dancing, and similar safe activities are examples.

There are many individuals who participate in sport and dance because of the need to be closely associated wtih other people engaging in these activities. They may care little as to the expertise they display in particular sport skills; rather, these people are attempting to meet a fundamental need for affection and group approval.

Many individuals in sport and dance are striving to meet self-esteem needs, as indicated by the way they drive themselves through intense practice and heated competition. Being a winner attracts attention of others immediately. Social approval bestowed by spectators at the contest, and indirectly through newspaper reports, helps to meet the needs of these individuals.

The ultimate goal of some people is reached through what Maslow calls "peak experiences."[9] In many areas of human endeavor, including sports, an individual becomes so involved and derives such personal satisfaction, as well as social approval, that a state of self-actualization can be achieved in which the athlete becomes one with the sport. The ultimate is the "peak experience," for as Alderman[10] says, "some people can become so involved in their play or sports participation that they completely lose touch with reality — they totally transcend themselves — and though initially their participation was in terms of a lower basic need, they are now so totally involved that they are actually performing at a metaphysical level."

It is evident that the basic needs of each individual student are of primary concern to dedicated, perceptive teachers as a basis for effective curriculum planning and assignment and to facilitate economical learning. The following examples of developmental and adjustment needs have been found common to a high percentage of American youth and can be used as guides for physical education teachers.

Physiological Needs. In early childhood and preadolescence children require several hours daily of physical activity to promote normal growth and development. Actually, regular physical activity is a basic developmental and maintenance need of all individuals throughout their lifetime. Young children play and exercise in one way or another in almost any environment; however, in many cases the amount and type of physical activities are too limited to be fully beneficial. The constraints of inner city life are particularly significant in this respect.[10] Specific physiological needs arise from:

1. Lack of regular habits of exercise, which are necessary under modern conditions of living. The marked trend toward sedentary living in America is generally regarded as a serious menace to the health status of our citizens.
2. Abnormalities in bodily growth and development are often attributable, at least in part, to lack of sufficient muscular activity on a regular basis.
3. Lack of adequate muscle tone, and accompanying defects in posture, may be largely attributable to inadequate muscular activity.

The continual trend of American families moving into large metropolitan areas and crowding into inner cities has tended to reduce, if not eliminate, the survival activities characteristic of former years. Thus, a large percentage of American youth is deprived of normal opportunities to engage in a variety of challenging and exciting vigorous physical activities under professional leadership and involving adequate and safe equipment and facilities. Regular vigorous physical activity is the only means of developing and maintaining organic power and vigor.[11]

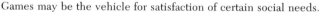
Games may be the vehicle for satisfaction of certain social needs.

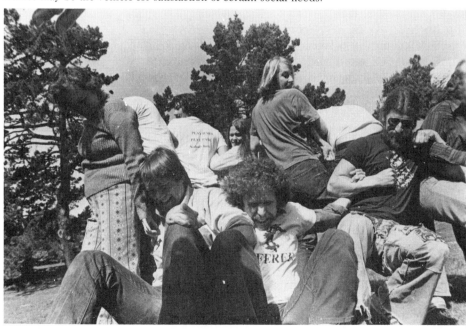

Psychological Needs. These needs are characterized by the following:

1. The human being has an innate tendency to be physically and socially active. Thus the need can be viewed as an opportunity for the wholesome expression of human tendencies through appropriate acts of individual and social actions and interactions. Many abnormalities of personality and a variety of forms of antisocial behavior are apparently related to insufficient fulfillment of this need. Teachers should urge shy children to participate in group games, sports, dances and exercises.
2. The need for the development of resourcefulness, initiative, and the capacity for quick and accurate mental reactions under conditions of stress.
3. The need for the development of satisfactory, socially acceptable emotional control.
4. The need to overcome awkward movements in the efficient performance of daily activities.
5. The need to develop interest in a variety of wholesome recreational activities contributing to the joy of living and as a means of release from the mental and emotional strains engendered by the pressures of modern life.
6. The need to engage in creative, divergent thinking and novel activities frequently throughout life. It is stultifying, restrictive, and psychologically detrimental to be conditioned and to be expected to habitually act and think in conforming, logical, and predictable ways.

Social Needs. Human beings rarely live alone. Much of our life is spent in interaction with others in familial, social, recreational, and work relationships. Thus, societal needs exist that require fulfillment by all youth. Cultural influences operate on children almost from the day of birth. Several important social needs of children and youth are:

1. The need to develop an interest in a spectrum of stimulating and interesting human activities, many of which contain a strong emotional element. Such diversity of participation is required to counteract the pervasive influence of television, radio, motion pictures, and other sedentary forms of entertainment that expose young people to vicarious emotional experiences and synthetic participation, to the detriment of their physical and mental health.
2. The need to rapidly assess, and quickly adjust, to the perceived needs, motives and intentions of other persons with whom we interact in work, play, and in social life in general.
3. The need to cultivate an attitude of fairness and display good sportsmanship when playing with or competing against others in various social activities, thereby taking into account the rights and welfare of others.
4. The need, especially in adolescent youth, to acquire a variety of physical skills in recreational activities to a level of competence that will result in continued participation as an enjoyable social activity.

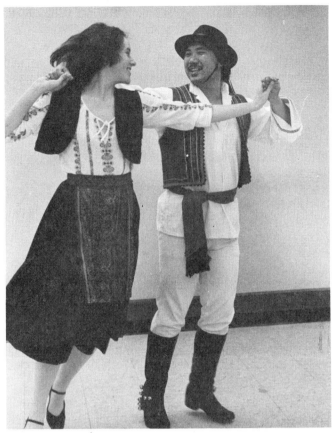

A knowledge of physical skills in recreational activities often results in enjoyable social activity.

The following procedures are suggested for determining the individual needs of students in physical education settings: *Criteria*

1. A thorough medical examination for each student should be required by the school in the year of original entry into the school system and at the fourth grade, the seventh grade, and the tenth grade. The child's educational program and individual health status and remediation should be guided by the results of these examinations.
2. Periodic evaluation of each individual's social characteristics and needs.
3. Evaluation of changing social, cultural, and economic conditions in America in terms of human needs now and as predicted for the future.
4. Tentative determination of the probable social, cultural, and occupational status of the individual in later years, with a view to determining probable future needs in forms of recreation, exercise, and desirable health habits.
5. Evaluation of the individual's interest in physical education and recreational activities in relation to other interests (on the basis of observation and an interest inventory).
6. Evaluation of the individual's cultural and occupational situations outside the physical education environment.
7. Frequent tests of the individual's skills in physical activities and the ability to properly control bodily movements.

Selectivity and Priority. Because physical education is such a vast endeavor, the public schools in general have undertaken too large a commitment, considering their limited time and financial resources. It is therefore important that physical education instructors determine the major objectives that are believed to be most beneficial to the largest number of students, both during the time they are enrolled in school and in the years following graduation.

Perhaps too often in the past it was typical for a physical education department to list a set of educational objectives and to imply, if not to state explicitly, that each objective was of equal value. Then the department would set out to teach all the pupils on the basis of this assumption. Modern thought holds that the school should demand more selectivity from the departments, and that departments should concentrate on fulfilling those responsibilities for which they are uniquely qualified.

Physical education objectives can be stated at several levels of abstraction. Inability to express objectives clearly and accurately at different levels compounds the problem of understanding the fundamental nature and purposes of this field. The following section presents one schema for stating physical education objectives at various levels of theoretical and concrete precision. If educational objectives are stated only in general and abstract terms, at least two major difficulties ensue. First, there are many problems in the selection and planning of comprehensive and efficient learning experiences to achieve such broad purposes. Second, difficulties of implementation occur because the concepts and descriptions of the behavioral goals are so vague. In order to overcome these problems, it becomes necessary to subdivide the general and specific objectives into more operational statements.

The aim we defined earlier in this chapter is the most abstract type of program purpose; however, it is a useful way of describing the role of the school and its program as an agency of society. As the term indicates, the aim acts as the guide, giving direction to the educational process.

General objectives reflect the values of the community, the state, and the nation; they separate and clarify the essential elements of the over-all aim. Though more specific than the aim, they have the same essential function as a guide.

The authors subscribe to the following *general objectives* of physical education:

1. To develop the movement potentialities of each individual to an optimal level. Formal physical education instruction concentrates on the development of selected neuromuscular skills and the refinement of fundamental movement patterns comprised of these specific skills.
2. To develop a basic understanding and appreciation of human movement. This broad objective involves (a) the development of an understanding and appreciation of significant human meanings and values acquired through idea-directed movement experiences; (b) an appreciation of human movement as an essential non-verbal mode of human expression; (c) the development of a positive self-concept and body image through appropriate movement experiences; and (d) the mastery of key concepts through voluntary movement and closely related non-verbal learning activities.

Aim

GENERAL OBJECTIVES

CHAPTER TWO

3. To develop and maintain optimal individual muscular strength, muscular endurance, and cardiovascular endurance. It is customary to refer to this general objective as "physical fitness." This concept, expanded to include such factors as flexibility, balance, agility, power, and speed, is called "motor fitness." It is essential that the student acquire knowledge of basic concepts that explain the meaning of physical fitness.

4. To develop skills, knowledge, and attitudes basic to voluntary participation in satisfying, enjoyable physical recreation experiences in the course of one's lifetime. Normal mental, physical, and emotional health is enhanced by participation in voluntary physical recreation.

5. To develop personally rewarding and socially acceptable behaviors through participation in enjoyable movement activities. Physical education instruction stresses the development of enjoyable, desirable social habits, attitudes, and personal characteristics.

The authors urge physical educators to select a limited number of general objectives that are well grounded in valid evidence. These objectives should describe desirable, stable changes in human behavior (called learning) that can be expected to result from appropriate educational experiences organized and conducted by carefully selected and highly trained teachers, coaches, and administrators. Other chapters in this book present more detailed evidence, professional judgments, and rational arguments that underlie our five objectives. Extensive literature has been written about each of these objectives and is cited throughout the book.

Physical education instruction stresses the development of enjoyable, desirable social habits, attitudes and personal characteristics.

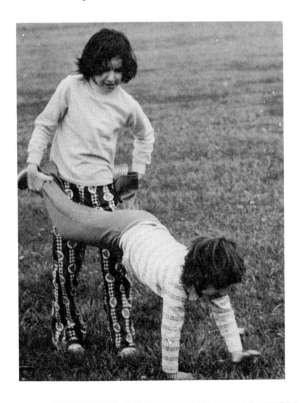

General Objectives. General objectives for physical education, such as the preceding, may be classified into three types, namely, "unique," "shared," and "primary."

Unique Objectives. Physical education has certain objectives that are unique to this area of the curriculum, such as the development and maintenance of physical fitness and the acquisition of selected movement skills in sport, dance, and healthful exercises. No other subject in the curriculum lists these particular objectives.

Shared Objectives. Other objectives to which physical education makes solid claim may be regarded as "shared" objectives, meaning that one or more of the other subjects in the curriculum also make significant contributions to the achievement of these purposes. For example, most physical educators believe that their field makes important contributions to social behaviors such as sportsmanship and cooperation, and that it exerts a favorable influence on character development. Surely teachers of other subjects feel that they, too, help develop sportsmanship, cooperation, and character. Thus, the physical educator should regard such objectives as "shared."

Primary Objectives. Primary objectives are those facets of the physical education program deemed most important. For example, most physical educators believe that muscular strength, muscular endurance, cardiovascular efficiency, flexibility, balance, and agility are essential elements, or primary objectives, of a total concept of physical fitness.

It is obvious that the above general objectives are so broad that they do not indicate types of overt behaviors. General objectives are not readily transferable into a selection of instructional activities and teaching techniques. Instructional, behavioral, and performance objectives serve this purpose of instrumentalizing objectives into teaching, learning, and evaluating processes.

INSTRUCTIONAL OBJECTIVES

Each general objective can be subdivided into numerous instructional objectives, depending upon the interests and goals of the teachers and students involved. Instructional objectives emphasize the *consequences* of instruction, the actual observable changes in pupil behaviors that result from practice under teacher direction over time. The focus is on *consequences* rather than on what the *intentions* of the teacher were prior to the start of the instructional unit.

Instructional objectives encompass behavioral and performance objectives as well as expressive objectives. Behavioral or performance objectives are stated as specific descriptions of potential, stable, behavioral changes that the student should master by the termination of the learning experience.

Popham[12] is a leading authority and advocate of the proper use of instructional, behavioral, and performance objectives. He says:

> An instructional objective stated in performance, behavioral, or measurable terms is simply an assertion of what you want to happen to learners as a consequence of instruction.

The above statement implies that a teacher must describe the learner's behaviors that are anticipated at the end of the instructional unit. These behaviors must be measurable. Popham[13] continues:

> I think there are almost no goals, however, which are not amenable to some form of operationalization in order to provide the educator with better clues as to whether the goal has been achieved.

It is commonplace to use the terms "behavioral" and "performance" objectives interchangeably. In either case, these objectives contain specific descriptions of attainable, stable *behavioral changes* that the teacher expects will be acquired by the end of the organized learning experience or instructional unit. These behaviors, described in advance with emphasis on action verbs, are amenable to direct observation. In most cases, there is some type of objective measurement, or evaluation, that indicates the degree of attainment of the objective by the student. From this planning and instructional process come the common expressions "stating objectives in behavioral terms," describing them "operationally," and formulating "performance objectives."

Behavioral and Performance Objectives

In planning instruction based on behavioral objectives the instructor must (1) determine carefully the overt and measurable behaviors of each pupil as the class progresses and (2) predict attainment by the end of the unit. Mager[14] calls this description of anticipated student performance "terminal" behaviors. The teacher's description must include not only what the pupil actually *performs* in observable ways, but must also state the *conditions* under which the behaviors are to be elicited, as well as describe an acceptable *level of performance* for each of the behaviors. It is obvious that these statements must employ action verbs that are amenable to objective measurement. Abstract verbs such as "to appreciate," "to understand," or "to know" are imprecise and not objectively measurable; they are appropriate in stating general objectives, but not behavioral objectives.

Planning Behavioral Objectives. In planning lessons based on behavioral objectives the teacher must begin with a clear description and understanding of the final, summative objectives that students are expected to demonstrate at the end of the unit. Actually, the teacher plans the instructional unit in reverse. Working back through the lesson sequence from the anticipated terminal performances, the teacher subdivides each of these performance objectives into *subordinate* or *formative* behavioral objectives that are to be accomplished in sequential order through practice and instruction over time. The teacher must be able to estimate the prior experience each pupil has had in the activities to be learned, their "entering" or original skill abilities, their understanding, and their motivation to practice and learn throughout the unit. Thus, the decisions the teacher makes about the complexity, variety, and types of smaller behavioral objectives are crucial to the success of this type of instruction. Obviously, the more the teachers know about the capabilities, interests, and motivations of each student, the more effective they will be in providing an instructional climate that will produce the desired behavioral changes.

It seems obvious that all worthwhile educational objectives are not necessarily amenable to formulation as behavioral objectives. Even Popham[15] admits that "the real worthwhile goals of education are invariably the most difficult to measure." However, he goes on to say "an outcome oriented approach to education is the only defensible stance open to the responsible educator." Rather than abandon this approach because of the difficulty in stating some highly desirable objectives in performance terms, it is preferable to plan as much instruction as possible around measurable objectives. Popham, Mager, and others explain and demonstrate how to approach the problems of stating and assessing behavioral changes related to the "more difficult to measure" objectives.

To use performance objectives to the fullest possible extent, teachers should (1) describe as objectively as possible the changes in pupil behaviors believed to be desirable by the end of the unit; (2) carefully plan and employ instructional strategies and procedures that are designed to develop most effectively the desired behaviors; and (3) locate, develop, and utilize the most valid assessment techniques available during the unit as well as at the end of the lesson or unit.

Criticism. Critics of behavioral objectives generally regard them as leading to the dehumanization of the pupil, a forced shaping of behavior and a mechanized form of learning. Eisner[16] and other critics contend that the use of behavioral objectives is not always appropriate.

Inappropriate for Evaluating Certain Types of Pupil Responses. Subjects involving suitable time and practice in motor learning behaviors (such as physical education, industrial arts, business practices, science, and language) are more appropriate for performance behavior statements than are subjects that encourage creative and unique experiences, behaviors, and responses (art, music, and dance). Likewise, certain subjects emphasize the objective of seeking out and describing unique relationships not previously apparent to the learner.

In all of the above cases, unpredictable pupil behavior is encouraged and rewarded; specific behavioral objectives cannot, and should not, be assigned or anticipated. There is no objective way to assess the impact of a poem or musical piece, or the emotional response of a person viewing a beautiful painting. So-called creative outcomes can only be judged subjectively. In terms of curiosity, creativity, and insight, such outcomes are educationally very important; however, frequently they are not encouraged as valid educational objectives by many teachers.

Restricts Teacher Creativity and Adaptability. Creative teachers dislike being bound to a prescribed set of objectives for all pupils. It is not realistic to believe that a teacher can accurately predict in advance the wide variety of complex behavioral changes that will occur among 25 or 30 students over a period of time, during which innumerable teacher interactions with pupils occur, as well as interactions among the students. The nature of these interactions and their outcomes as influences on changing pupil behaviors are entirely unforeseen and cannot be predicted accurately. Likewise, unexpected "teachable moments" occur periodically in any class with little or no advance indication. The alert teacher will recognize these moments and will convert them into a valuable learning experience spontaneously. Again, these moments cannot be planned in advance, nor will all the resulting behaviors and learnings be amenable to objective measurements.

Restricts Environment Potential. In essence, in a favorable instructional atmosphere there are far too many potential educational outcomes to be identified and selected for desirability in advance. Many teachers believe that objectives should always be tentative, that they are ever changing as instruction and learning proceed from day to day, and in fact, are not capable of being described and defined with a high degree of specificity prior to the teaching of a new unit. Rather, these teachers believe that instructional objectives stated in the planning stage should be regarded as "initiating cues" that give direction to instruction, particularly in the early phases of the unit. These objectives, and those that follow as the lessons progress, are subject to frequent revision. This view rejects the notion that educational objectives need to be stated precisely and in behavioral terms as a basis for the selection and organization of the subject content.

Raths[17] contributes thoughtful criticisms to proposals that all learning experiences should be evaluated on the basis of behavioral and performance objectives. He believes that students should have a major role and a high degree of self-responsibility in working with the teacher to help determine at least some of the educational activities in the classroom.

The curriculum should contain learning opportunities that involve more than rote memory and specific skill acquisition of predetermined levels of behavior. The curriculum should include problem-solving experiences in both social and personal realms. Likewise, students should have opportunities to discuss and debate controversial viewpoints; they should be encouraged to originate and formulate hypotheses or tentative explanations and trained to identify basic assumptions; and they should work on their skills to raise and clearly formulate pertinent questions about the topics under discussion.

Learning should not be so mechanical that it thwarts wholesome free expression of individual beliefs and deep human feelings and emotions. Pupils should be encouraged to express these unique feelings and emotions and to learn how to generalize their concepts and understandings from one situation to a new or novel one.

Pupils should be encouraged in the use of multi-sensory modes of learning rather than depending, as is typically the case, upon the spoken or written word of the teacher or the textbook. They should be confronted with direct learning experiences in a variety of classroom environments rather than having learning imposed upon them primarily through textbooks and teacher lectures.

Going Beyond the Objectives. Boys and girls should be urged to continue to learn beyond the achievement of the performance objectives. Students should be motivated to improve their performances with the aim of long-term retention rather than to be satisfied with immediate success and the belief that the lesson is over when the final examination has been accomplished satisfactorily. Learning opportunities should be individually related to the interests and preferences of each student. Students should be encouraged to engage in divergent and heuristic learning

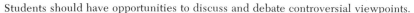
Students should have opportunities to discuss and debate controversial viewpoints.

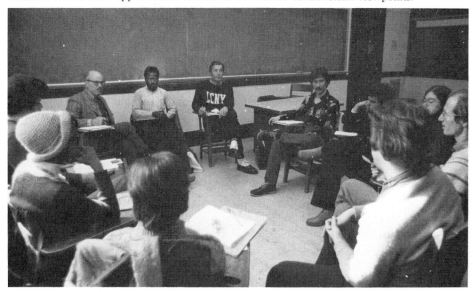

activities without fear of disappointment or criticism for failure in a given instance. The classroom atmosphere should promote the taking of calculated risks against unanticipated obstacles to learning, the acceptance of well-meant criticism, or the unexpected toll of time or energy required to see a problem to its solution. Students should have the opportunity to gamble, or take a chance, on outcomes to problematical situations. Students should have experience in, and receive reinforcement for, learning how to evaluate their own progress and the extent and type of learning they have acquired. A final caveat: it is essential to relate learning opportunities to individual student interest, ability, and preferences.

Physical education teachers and coaches should employ all of the above instructional principles, although, sadly, many do not.

Expressive objectives describe potential educational opportunities that are evocative rather than prescriptive. Terminal behaviors are not specified prior to the learning encounter, as in the case of behavioral objectives; nor are these objectives evaluated by a common standard stated in advance and applied to all members of the class. Pupils are encouraged to produce ideas, materials, emotional responses, motor movements, and other types of behaviors that are diverse and often unique; and to develop personal meanings from exposure to, and engagement in, various learning opportunities derived from a careful analysis of objectives.

Eisner[18] qualifies the nature of expressive objectives and argues eloquently for their more general use in curriculum development. They encourage the teacher and pupils to employ a variety of learning opportunities to stimulate interest and a sense of challenge.

Examples of expressive objectives are:

1. Write a poem on a subject or experience of interest to you.
2. Write a personalized interpretation of the meaning of the book *Gone with the Wind.*
3. Attend an opera and describe your emotional reactions and responses.
4. Create a new dance to music of your choice.
5. Create a novel sequence of movements in a water ballet episode involving four classmates.

Expressive objectives specify the nature of the educational opportunity to be encountered and give guidance as to the general types of motor and related responses the student should evoke, evaluate, and report upon completion to the teacher. As in aesthetic criticism, students evaluate and describe their reactions to the event and to the product, if any, in the expressive learning experiences. The inherent qualities and meanings encountered during the learning experience are described as clearly as possible. Precise behavioral criteria for evaluation are not stated in advance.

The quality of a poem or of a painting created by a pupil cannot be evaluated by available objective measures. However, the teacher may promote the objective that each pupil in the art appreciation class has an opportunity to create an original watercolor picture.

The expressive objective is also essential in the physical education program. Pupils should be encouraged to move in creative and aesthetically pleasing ways in order to express their feelings and emotions and to know the pure joy of movement. The qualitative or personal component of

Expressive Objectives

individual movement potentiality and performance needs to be encouraged and positively reinforced in all students. Unfortunately, many physical education programs lack emphasis on this essential objective.

Performance Objectives vs. Expressive Objectives. In brief, performance objectives refer to specific ("known") knowledge and skills each student is expected to acquire by the end of the learning experience; whereas expressive objectives allow the student to interpret, extend, and modify the "known" and at times provide for the creation of a novel behavior or response.

Physical education programs involve a wide variety of educational purposes. Some are readily amenable to the performance objective approach, others require the use of expressive objectives. The thoughtful physical educator is best advised to make judicious use of both types of objectives to promote optimum learning and to understand clearly the strengths and weaknesses of each approach.

Formative and Summative Objectives

Brief mention of a more recent categorization of intermediate objectives, namely formative and summative, is important. Formative objectives consist of performance schedules designed to meet both short-term and long-term educational objectives; the attending evaluation processes gauge ongoing behaviors, skills, attitudes, and other aspects of individual development in view of the objectives. The purpose of formative assessment is to inform the pupil, the teacher, and, not incidentally, the parents of the pupil's progress. Such assessment provides accurate feedback in the form of a developmental profile and also suggests which learning experiences probably are of most value and efficiency in the lessons yet to come in the course. These evaluations are not meant to be punitive, but are for counseling, guidance, motivation, accurate assessment, and feedback.

A summative objective involves a program terminating at the end of a unit, class, or any other major end point in the student's physical education curriculum and is based on announced course objectives. Summative evaluations demonstrate the pupil's behavior in terms of those objectives. One of the most obvious examples of summative evaluation is the semester report card with the letter grade the student receives in physical education. Another example is the end-of-year score made on the President's Council physical fitness test.

Teachers and coaches should emphasize the setting of formative and summative objectives, as individualized as possible, and should integrate them fully with formative and summative evaluations for each pupil. (See Chapter 11 on Evaluation and Research for further discussion.)

Competency Based Education

The concept of Competency Based Education (CBE) is now widespread in school districts, colleges, and universities throughout the United States. Many states have passed legislation requiring Competency Based Education curricula and individual pupil assessments in the public schools. Likewise, states, as well as institutions of higher education, have instrumented and given mandates for teacher education programs that are competency based.

In physical education a prestated competency level frequently is set as a standard for the achievement of specified letter grades. Sometimes a competency policy determines whether or not a student must remain in a required physical education program. Student teachers in teacher education programs must satisfactorily demonstrate teaching competencies

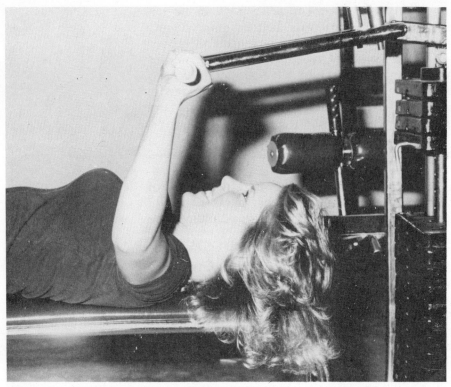

A fully "physically educated" person is the goal of competency-based education.

that can be objectively assessed as requisites for institutional recommendation and state issuance of a valid teaching credential.

There is no doubt that behavioral objectives and competency based concepts of learning and teaching now prevail in many physical education programs in the public schools and colleges of the United States. We believe that the appropriate uses of behavioral and performance objectives will be recognized and properly applied in these competency based programs. We also urge that the limitations and inappropriate uses of behavioral performance objectives be recognized by the authorities. When combined with creative, problem-solving, and novel educational opportunities, behavioral objectives in their rightful place can make important contributions to the total instructional program.

The Physically Educated Student

Certain schools, school districts, and colleges have adopted the concept of the "physically educated" student as a basis for satisfactory completion of physical education requirements in the curriculum, or even as a graduation requirement. Behaviorally stated objectives, when sufficiently and clearly developed and validated, can provide a partial description of the physically educated person, at least in certain crucial stages of progress. The students who can demonstrate, by relevant skilled performance, attitude, knowledge, and consistent behavioral patterns, that they fully meet the criteria of physically educated persons are deemed by this policy to have fulfilled the physical education requirements. They are exempt from physical education from that time on.

Student Goal Setting

Some educators hold that, while it is the primary responsibility of the teacher to develop and state the instructional objectives of the class, there should be opportunity for pupil discussion and suggestions in the formulation of these objectives. There is some difference of opinion among

CHAPTER TWO

teachers as to the extent of agreement that should exist between explicit statements of objectives formulated by teachers and the goals expressed by students when given the opportunity. However the class objectives are selected, the effective teacher will help students to clarify thoroughly the course and unit objectives. By sound motivational and explanatory techniques the teacher strives to achieve maximum understanding and acceptance of those objectives.

A second approach now coming into practice is for teachers to encourage and guide each pupil in setting personal goals within the instructional unit. Pupils select their goals in terms of performance expectations to be achieved by the end of the unit. These goals are discussed with the teacher, with classmates, and with parents if it seems desirable. The pupil writes down these personal goals on a physical education class cumulative record form, which is continually available throughout the instructional unit. Notations of progress are written on the pupil's cumulative record form and periodically pupil progress relative to the explicitly stated goals is assessed by both student and teacher. This type of pupil goal setting, based on interaction with teachers and classmates, stimulates individual responsibility for educational planning and provides opportunity for steadily increasing self-reliance and self-monitoring in achieving personal goals that are important and meaningful to the student.

Periodically the pupil is provided the opportunity to revise and reformulate these personal goals relative to the progress made to date. Students should not become too discouraged because of failure to accomplish goals set at a previous time; on the other hand, they should be encouraged to proceed at a faster learning pace than the original goals predicted if they demonstrate this capability. These goals are tentative, flexible, and, in a sense, an expression of the student's *level of aspiration*. Research has shown that most students learn more effectively when they aspire to learning goals that are within their potential. They are neither too easy to attain nor so difficult that they may be beyond the performance capability of the student.

"Hidden Objectives." Some physical educators believe that not all teacher objectives need be explicitly shared with the students. If the teacher of a basketball class has as an objective the "development of an attitude of fair play in basketball," and in any other sport contest, the skillful teacher need not state explicitly that fair play is an important objective of the class. The teacher need only encourage the pupils to develop a strong interest in, and liking for, the game, a desire to play it with others, and perhaps an ambition to "make the team" if there is an interscholastic or intramural competitive opportunity available to them. Given these conditions, the perceptive teacher can help students learn fairness with little conscious effort on their parts.

Practically all students have certain goals in mind as they participate in the school physical education program. These goals may differ considerably among individual pupils. It seems self-evident that the teacher must be fully informed of the goals held by the members of the class if optimal learning opportunities are to be provided on an individual basis. The teacher who does not provide favorable opportunities for expression of these goals, orally, in writing, or both, will not be certain which goals have the most significance for each member of the class.

Communication of Teacher and Pupil Objectives. Perhaps the question of relationship and congruence between teacher and pupil objectives is made more confusing by differences in language used by teachers and

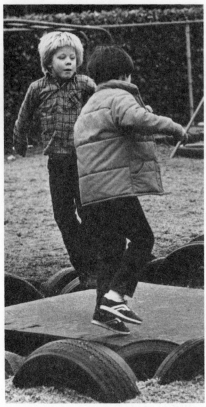

"Having fun" is a normal and natural physical education goal of children.

pupils to describe these objectives. Usually, the teacher and the administrator who prepare curriculum guides and lesson plans use educational jargon to state objectives. This language does not always communicate clearly to students and to parents. Pupils, when given the opportunity, write or speak in their natural idiom. Thus, there often appears to be a greater difference between teachers' objectives and the pupils' goals than actually is the case. In any event, it is fundamentally important to take conscientiously stated pupil and teacher objectives into consideration in developing and stating course and unit purposes.

Probably the normal and natural physical education goals of boys and girls include the following:

> To have fun
> To enjoy the company of friends
> To develop strength and endurance
> To make the team
> To develop a better physique, to be better looking
> To experience relief from the confinement associated with study
>   and attendance in academic classes

A physical educator should be pleased with students who hold such goals. The teacher should plan carefully to merge the students' goals with his or her own objectives to provide for the sincere, thoughtful agreement and understanding of the purposes of the unit or program.

Not only are today's teachers encouraging students to set their own goals in physical education classes, but also they are aiding pupils to evaluate personal progress toward the realization of individualized goals. Teachers provide helpful guidance as the need is perceived, but students are urged to take increasing responsibility for this function as they demonstrate their self-reliance to do so. This procedure helps boys and girls to develop a realistic self-concept and self-confidence. Another promising trend is to facilitate *peer evaluation* among students. Again, providing guidance and training in this skill is an important role for the perceptive teacher to play.

In recent years investigators have developed categorical models for the purpose of identifying, stating, and organizing educational objectives. Bloom and colleagues[19] created a taxonomy for educational objectives in the cognitive domain. Krathwohl and coauthors[20] built a taxonomy for objectives in the affective domain. Objectives that involve voluntary, purposeful, skillful movements have been classified in the psychomotor domain. We prefer the term motor domain, since all three domains have a psychological component. These three categories of educational objectives by and large encompass most of the educational objectives for which American schools and colleges generally are responsible.

PHYSICAL EDUCATION TAXONOMIES

Several taxonomies of interest to physical educators have been developed in recent years to classify motor objectives. Physical education teachers are using these taxonomies, along with ideas from the Bloom and Krathwohl taxonomies, as a basis for stating the objectives of physical education curricula at all educational levels.

The Simpson Classification. One of the early classification systems for the motor domain was developed by Simpson,[21] a home economist. The Simpson classification has five major categories: (a) perception, (b) set, (c) guided response, (d) mechanism, and (e) complex overt response. Each major category is divided into subcategories. Clein and Stone[22] have extended the Simpson classification to illustrate physical education objectives from the viewpoint of a student attempting to learn a specific motor skill.

The Harrow[23] Classification. This model, intended to "help behavioral objectives writers and curriculum developers classify student learning experiences and to define objectives as meaningful descriptions of student behaviors," serves "as a guide for educators concerned with preparing a meaningful sequential curriculum utilizing appropriate instructional strategies, and selecting relevant measurement techniques. Working with this type of a framework, educators will be able to make possible more meaningful experiences focused upon improved psychomotor development of children."

The basic categories in this taxonomy are:

1.00 Reflex Movements
2.00 Basic-Fundamental Movements
3.00 Perceptual Abilities
4.00 Physical Abilities
5.00 Skilled Movements
6.00 Non-discursive Communication

Harrow's excellent pioneer study and taxonomy provides a model "which can be utilized by educators to assist them in becoming more efficient in organizing their instructional goals and to better evaluate achievement of learning concerned with cognitive, affective, and psycho-motor behaviors."[24]

The PPCF Movement Process Category System. Jewett and Mullan[25] reported a monumental study under the auspices of the AAHPERD to further develop and refine curriculum theory in physical education. The study resulted in the development of the Purpose Process Curriculum Framework, a conceptual framework for physical education curricular decision making. The project moves the discipline and the profession of physical education closer to more sophisticated theory building while at the same time improving day-to-day teaching-learning experiences in physical education programs at all educational levels through the integration of purpose and process components.

The PPCF provides guidelines for curricular decision making in two major dimensions. The purpose dimension is used primarily to define the scope of the physical education program and to select program content. Purposes are based on a logical, philosophical analysis of the common human purposes for moving.

The process dimension offers a taxonomy for the motor domain. The movement process category system can be utilized in defining educational objectives, in sequencing learning materials, in providing augmented feedback to learners, and in evaluating student progress. The process dimension has been developed in the form of a classification scheme for identifying major types of movement operations, by describing seven processes through which a human being learns movement:

1. Perceiving
2. Patterning
3. Adapting
4. Refining
5. Varying
6. Improvising
7. Composing

Both the purpose concepts and the movement process categories are defined and presented in greater detail in Chapter 7.

MISCONCEPTIONS

Throughout this book runs the persistent theme that physical education is (1) a unique academic discipline with its own body of knowledge and learning opportunities, and (2) a professional field of human activity involving teaching, coaching, administration, and evaluation. In one way or another physical education touches the lives of the majority of citizens in America. The subdisciplines of physical education as an area of academic study and research are proliferating at a rapid rate. New programs continue to develop and expand and novel activities of a physical education nature are being invented continuously. It is probable that no one knows exactly the extent to which the American public is engaged in one form or another of physical education. Because of its great diversity, rapid growth, and heterogeneity of sponsorship, it is not surprising that there are many differences of judgments and perceptions concerning the nature of this field, its definition, its scope, its purposes, and other aspects of its total composition.

Likewise, we are witnessing a rapid accumulation of literature of all types, from scholarly textbooks to popular magazines with appeal to the

CHAPTER TWO

masses of people of all ages. Television and radio continue to broaden their coverage of physical education activities and programs, frequently on a worldwide basis. Billions of dollars throughout the world are being expended for physical education facilities, equipment, and supplies. Thousands of instructors with varying degrees of background and competence, serving thousands of organizations or operating independently, are engaged in instructing others in some activity in the physical education spectrum. Millions of individuals engage in physical education activities of one form or another.

In view of these facts, it is little wonder that there are a variety of views and misconceptions about physical education. There are diverse interpretations concerning the purpose of physical education, its nature, scope, and objectives. Lay members of school boards, government officials, owners and administrators of private organizations providing physical education services and programs, parents, participants, and representative political and educational leaders who must advise and make policies that govern the conduct and the financing of physical education programs are subjected to a constant barrage of assertions about the nature and purposes of the programs under their jurisdiction. This confusion and controversy at various levels of decision-making contribute to programs that, in many cases, are detrimental to the well-being of the participants or have elements of danger that need not be present.

Even physical educators and coaches who have received professional preparation in accredited colleges and universities find themselves in heated disagreement with each other about objectives, suitable programs, teaching and coaching methods, desirable principles of organization and administration, and appropriate strategies and techniques for program and pupil evaluations.

Eight of these major misconceptions are discussed in the following paragraphs. It is urged that every physical educator become aware of these misconceptions and of the fallacies therein. Nothing is more important than accurate, validated interpretation of the nature and purposes of physical education programs if they are to receive appropriate financial, legal, and educational support.

It is frequently asserted by school board members, legislators, parents, newspaper editors, teachers, and others in positions of public leadership that the primary purpose of the school is to "train the mind." It is even more startling to hear physical educators speak of their mission as "training the body." Both by implication and by direct statement, there is frequent assertion that the school child is biologically composed of an anatomical entity known as "the mind" housed in a physical body. This scientifically false dichotomy does more to diminish or obstruct a proper understanding of the contribution of physical education to total education than any other notion. It is particularly damaging to hear physical educators perpetuating this myth in their own public statements. (For further discussion on the mind-body dichotomy, or dualism, see Chapter 3.)

There is no anatomical entity called "the mind." It is a well verified scientific fact that the "whole child goes to school." Many important concepts are best learned through non-verbal activities that require skilled movements. All of the sensory systems of the human organism receive stimuli called "sensations" from the external and internal environment. The central nervous system rapidly converts sensations into

"Physical Education Is Concerned Only with the Body." (Mind-Body Dichotomy)

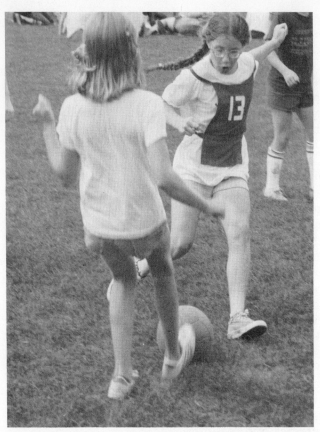

Physical education experiences contribute significantly to intellectual, emotional, and social growth and development.

perceptions, which are stored in the central nervous system for subsequent recall and use. Perceptions are the building blocks of concepts, which classify human knowledge. (The sensory systems are described briefly in Chapter 6).

The sense of kinesthesis (the sensation of movement and position) is largely overlooked in the educational literature dealing with learning. Many of our most significant concepts are learned through nonverbal modes rather than from the printed page. Physical education experiences can and do contribute significantly to human intellectual, emotional, and social growth and development. Students participating in programs of sport, dance, and healthful exercise under the leadership of qualified and perceptive teachers are engaged in a large number of significant learning experiences, many of which will be retained for a lifetime.

Physical education and physical fitness are *not* synonymous concepts. Physical fitness is one of the major objectives of physical education. It should not be regarded as the ultimate aim of physical education, although some physical education leaders today are giving it major emphasis in their programs. There is no doubt that physical fitness is an essential ingredient in the overall health status of the individual. The programs and pronouncements of the President's Council on Physical Fitness and Sport are indeed noteworthy in this respect. All physical educators should be aware of these programs and the literature that describes and publicizes them. Many exercise programs advocated in the

"Physical Education and Physical Fitness Are Identical."

name of physical fitness really are physical training, not physical education. Oberteuffer[28] and Brackenbury[29] clearly describe the difference between these two concepts.

The present-day emphasis on physical fitness in school programs tends to confuse the essential differences between physical education, physical fitness, and physical performance. Too often these terms are used synonymously. Newspaper articles and magazine stories in particular often seem to present an uninformed viewpoint concerning the crucial differentiation of these terms. Physical educators and coaches constantly should interpret these terms properly to their public.

Another false view of physical education occurs, particularly in elementary schools, when it is asserted that children need an activity period in order to "blow off steam" or to release tensions that have been built up in the academic classroom. This implies that physical education does not possess educational potentialities but rather is regarded as a catharsis or a relief from the "more serious emotionally and intellectually demanding" formal learning activities of the school. Physical education is regarded as synonymous with "recess." The fact that many elementary classroom teachers no longer attempt to conduct formal instruction in allotted physical education time further strengthens the belief that the subject is unimportant in the curriculum. The unfortunate fact that many school district budgets throughout the United States are being trimmed by eliminating specially trained elementary school physical education teachers and coordinators proves that the physical education profession has failed to interpret the nature, scope, and value of this educational discipline. The result is that elementary school teachers and administrators and parents continue to hold faulty and misguided understandings of the aim and purposes of instructional physical education.

"A Primary Role of Physical Education Class Is as a Catharsis."

In the early part of the twentieth century one of the major purposes of physical education was believed to be "body building." This notion was stimulated by Charles Atlas through physical culture advertisements in popular magazines and was abetted by Bob Hoffman and other professional weightlifters who commercialized this activity by making health studios available to the public for a fee. However, body building as a legitimate educational aim was never fully accepted by the physical education profession because it lacked scientific evidence to support its claims.

"Body Building Is a Primary Objective of Physical Education."

In contrast, weight training has become a major aspect of physical education programs in recent years, gaining respectability through the support of medical judgment and scientific evidence. When properly applied, weight training contributes to the improvement of general health status and has special benefit for athletes in various sports. It is administered under the direct supervision and prescription of coaches, athletes, physical educators, team physicians, and athletic trainers, so it is now accepted as a legitimate phase of the physical education and athletic program, and a very popular one, too.

Persuasive evidence and experience have accumulated in recent years to indicate that properly conducted weight training can significantly improve strength and promote general physical conditioning, which in turn facilitates improved athletic performance in a variety of sports. Also, boys and girls in physical education classes, and many adults as well, now realize the value of general conditioning regimens properly suited to the

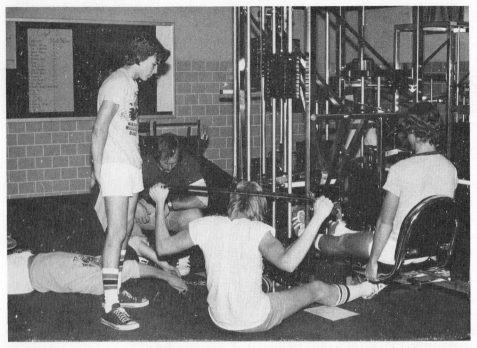

Weight training is now accepted as a legitimate phase of physical education and athletics.

individual's health status, with well-conducted weight training playing an important role.

It is not the primary purpose of weight training to build large muscles, nor to attempt to develop the "body beautiful." The idea that increased strength and muscular development per se are somehow vital indices of good health and body efficiency is fallacious and is not sustained by scientific evidence.

It is clear that increased muscular strength and power can result from appropriate physical education activities. Increased strength attained through proper programs of weight training can be an asset to improved performance in sport activities in which strength is a significant factor. Also, it has been demonstrated that weight training can be carried on satisfactorily not only during the "off season" of a sport, but also in moderate amounts during the sport season. Weight-training regimens are now designed with specific reference to the skilled movements and strength requirements of the athlete in a given sport and even in a particular position on a team.

Weight training is beneficial for girls and women when properly adapted to each individual and when conducted by highly qualified physical educators and athletic trainers. The cultural bias against this activity for females gradually is being overcome as its benefits become more fully recognized and scientifically verified.

In summary, body building per se is not a legitimate objective of physical education; weight training, properly prescribed and administered, is an acceptable phase of the physical education program; and, finally, weight training in and of itself should not be regarded as a broad aim of physical education.

Physical educators historically believed that each individual, through the fortunes of heredity and life experiences, possessed a general quality of neuromuscular coordination that contributed to varying degrees of "gracefulness" or "physical efficiency" as the individual performed endless varieties of movement tasks requiring neuromuscular skills. Thus, some physical education authorities advocated general motor ability as the main purpose of physical education.

In the past 20 years considerable evidence has been derived from research in physical education and psychology to overturn this theory of general neuromuscular coordination. The investigations of Henry,[30] Cratty,[31] Fleishman[32] and other respected researchers have negated the old theory of a general quality of coordination and have replaced it with new theories emphasizing motor task specificity. It is now believed that each individual possesses many specific abilities that contribute in varying degrees to a wide range of skilled movement performances. All physical educators should be well acquainted with the literature reporting this research, which is leading to a significant change in modern theoretical insight into the nature of skilled human performances.

Fleishman's research studies have identified nine components of *physical proficiency*.[33] These components are (1) extant flexibility, (2) dynamic flexibility, (3) explosive strength, (4) static strength, (5) dynamic strength, (6) trunk strength, (7) gross body coordination, (8) gross body equilibrium, and (9) stamina. Fleishman's main conclusion from his studies is that physical proficiency and skill consist of several relatively independent factors that are grouped together in various combinations in any one individual performer. He relates the above nine factors to physical fitness by saying that as an individual scores higher on a greater number of these factors, he or she becomes more physically fit.

Cratty,[34] a noted researcher in motor learning, strongly supports the theory of specificity of learning sports and other movement skills. He postulates from recent research that several specific abilities underlie skilled motor performance, such as (1) ability to utilize space efficiently during accurate movement; (2) ability to mobilize and to produce speed and maximum force at the precise crucial moment during a skilled movement (called summation of forces); (3) ability to think about and logically analyze the complex motor tasks to be performed; and (4) ability to relax while performing the motor skill. It is theorized that these abilities, which are of a higher order than specific skills, are relatively stable, constitutional traits that are determined in any one individual by a fortuitous combination of hereditary predispositions, basic organic structure, and physiological functioning.

Abilities and Ability Traits. Cratty also describes *ability traits*, which contribute to optimum motor performance, including agility, body equilibrium, flexibility, speed of limb movement, static and dynamic strength, explosive strength, trunk strength, and the ability to manipulate weights with both the feet and the arms. McCloy, Guilford, Fleishman, and other investigators have identified additional ability traits that could be appended to this list.

Cratty's theory also includes what he calls "personal equations," which differentially contribute to the quality of each physical performance. Examples are the preference of the individual for the efficient use of space to accomplish the purpose of the performance, an individualized sense of the most effective rhythm and tempo at which the movement is performed, the individual's ability to persist in the task even though it may be painful or uncomfortable, and the unique way in which the person employs forces most economically and efficiently to accomplish the purpose.

Occasionally, a proponent of physical education claims that its chief purpose is to promote good citizenship. Even more frequently heard is the claim that physical education develops sportsmanship. The aim of good citizenship may apply to all of education if we think of one who attains and maintains a full measure of personal development and efficiency, physically, mentally, and socially. But as a statement of the aim of physical education, these claims are too vague and require extensive explanation and justification. Furthermore, there is no scientific evidence to support the contention that good citizenship is promoted directly because of physical education experiences. In fact, there are critics who would assert that the coach of an athletic team may be teaching "bad citizenship" and "bad sportsmanship" owing to the desire to win. So there remains only supposition to support this contention. Also, if some students are in fact receiving valuable citizenship training in physical education, it is dubious that these behaviors will carry over into adult life in years ahead or will transfer to other life situations such as in social circles, in business enterprises, and in political activities. We suggest that this aim be discarded by physical education proponents.

"Good Citizenship Is the Aim of Physical Education."

The claim that the main purpose of physical education is to correct physical defects or assist students to adapt their movements to such defects was more prominent in the past than it is today. Now there is a greater understanding of the role of the school and the specialized medical services available to assist students with serious health problems. However, in many schools there still exists considerable controversy concerning the place of corrective physical education in the physical education program and in the school curriculum. Also, there are questions concerning the roles of physical education teachers in such a program and the types of corrective training they are qualified to prescribe and direct, as well as those they should avoid because they lack proper qualifications. Referral to appropriate medical authorities is the course of action to be taken by physical educators and school administrators in any case of doubt.

"The Main Purpose of Physical Education Is to Correct Physical Defects."

It is well known that certain physical defects are amenable to improvement or correction through appropriate muscular activity based on the diagnosis and prescription of qualified medical authorities. Physical educators frequently weaken their positions and interfere with the ultimate solution of problems by attempting to perform the functions of medical specialists. A majority of defects require the services of the family physician, orthopedist, surgeon, dietician, dentist, oculist, physical therapist, or school nurse, rather than the assistance of the teacher.

Health Screening. All teachers should perform a daily health screening function. They should be constantly alert to, and aware of, any type of significant health problem any child appears to have or of preliminary indications that such a problem is developing. As soon as the teacher is convinced a child may have a health problem, the teacher should refer the child to established school administrative channels, including the administrator and the school nurse, and the family should be contacted with the recommendation to seek appropriate medical aid.

Once a pupil is under the supervision of a physician, the physical education teacher can help and instruct the student in medically prescribed physical activities on an individual basis. A careful distinction of roles and responsibilities, and a full understanding and agreement among the parents, the child, the administration, the physician, and the physical education teachers at the school, can make a significant contribution to many students. If at all possible, students' continued schooling and pursuit of their regular curriculum should be encouraged and facilitated. Schools employing a nurse are in an even more fortuitous situation to carry out such a coordinated plan.

The previous suggestions indicate that physical education should be regarded as a fundamental form of general education and not as a therapeutic agency. Physical education is interested in desirable changes in individuals that can be promoted through formal educational procedures. It should not attempt to invade the fields of medicine, surgery, or nursing. A background of study in kinesiology and anatomy, along with one or more courses in adapted physical education involving observational and laboratory experiences in public school programs, should be a requirement in the professional preparation of all prospective physical educators.

Historically, faulty or lack of physical education was mistakenly blamed for the large number of young draftees rejected from military service, based on medical examinations that identified a variety of health defects. To place major responsibility upon physical education for these medical problems leading to draft rejection is muddled thinking.

The most prevalent physical defect in school children is dental decay. Defective sight and hearing are also common. To say that these defects and other types of health problems are the fault of the physical educator and were caused by participation in poor physical education programs is erroneous. Likewise, the physical educator should not be required to attempt to prevent or correct the occurrence of these health problems. Major health problems of the citizens of the United States present situations that challenge the entire social order. It is a problem area that should not be lightly passed over or referred only to a particular group of educators.

For many years schools and colleges across the nation have organized classes in "adapted physical education" for handicapped pupils. Several state legislatures have passed laws providing state financial aid to local school districts to pay the excess cost of such programs. These laws provide medical and educational guidelines for the selection and special education of pupils who qualify for specific medical or educational opportunities.

In the past, schools have generally identified handicapped children by various educational and medical criteria and, if the health problem was serious, these students were placed in a segregated, special education class. In other words, they were excluded from the regular classroom.

People gradually realized that such treatment is dehumanizing and that handicapped children were being isolated from the *mainstream* of the society at large. In fact, such segregation led to even greater handicaps with respect to ultimate rehabilitation and adjustment within existing personal limitations.

Now the trend has been reversed and there is a significant national movement to assign handicapped pupils to the least restrictive education-

"Handicapped Students Should Be Excluded from Regular Physical Education Classes."

al environment consistent with their health problems and their personal and educational needs and goals. It is now realized that the regular classroom is, after all, the most appropriate setting for these children. Likewise, the trend is toward giving the regular teacher primary responsibility for the education of the handicapped child, in cooperation with the school nurse and in accordance with specialized advice and assistance provided by the school and the family.

The Congress of the United States recently recognized the necessity of a massive, federally aided program for handicapped children across this nation. Public Law 94–142, the Education for All Handicapped Children Act, was passed in 1975 and is now being implemented. This law requires that handicapped pupils be removed from restrictive environments such as special classes and be assigned to regular classrooms whenever possible. Also, each handicapped child will be provided with an individualized educational program.

Because the aim of this law is to provide handicapped children with programs that will enhance their opportunities to become as self-responsible as possible so that they may return to the mainstream of American life, the term mainstreaming is now prominent in schools across the country.

There are arguments pro and con about this new law and public policy. All teachers should take courses in special education in order to become knowledgeable about how to carry out their responsibilities to handicapped children effectively.

The physical education department can, and should, play a vital role in this over-all program. It can make significant contributions to the improved health and rehabilitation of many, if not all, of the pupils identified as handicapped.

PHYSICAL EDUCATION SERVES THE FUTURE

Physical educators, both individually and through their professional organizations, have worked diligently for many years to promote a clearer understanding and rationale concerning the purposes of this field, based on the most valid evidence available. Many statements and publications from individuals and from professional and academic organizations provide detailed interpretations of these purposes for the edification and understanding of the lay public as well as for members of the physical education profession and other educators and administrators.

In recent years, the American Alliance for Health, Physical Education, Recreation, and Dance has intensified efforts on many fronts to describe the nature and purposes of physical education. In 1972, the Alliance published *Tones of Theory — A Theoretical Structure for Physical Education, a Tentative Perspective,* by Celeste Ulrich and John E. Nixon,[35] Project Primary Co-Investigators, which summarized the work of several Alliance committees and interested individuals over a ten-year period. National and regional conferences involving many representatives of the Alliance were sponsored by the AAHPERD to promote this project.

In 1965, the Alliance published *This is Physical Education,*[36] under the leadership of an editorial committee chaired by Professor Eleanor Metheny. This publication provides a succinct, dynamic, and clear exposition of the present-day interpretation of physical education through its description of "broader and deeper understandings." It explains the major objectives of physical education applicable to all educational levels and describes the major curricular elements recommended for each level. Stressing the necessity of basing the selection of educational opportunities for students on individual needs assessments, the work also emphasizes the roles of continuous feedback and evaluation in curriculum and instructional processes. The statement, although relatively brief, is delineated in a practical educational philosophy that stimulates and challenges the physical educator to broaden personal and professional aspirations and urges the improvement of the quality of services rendered to the American public. The message in this publication is as valid today as when it was originally written.

Physical education has been evaluated and reappraised, and has been subjected to constant scrutiny, both from within and outside its professional boundaries. All Presidents of the United States since 1956, and several of them prior to that time, have demonstrated a direct, personal interest in and concern for the physical fitness of the citizens of this country. Since 1956, each has given strong support and advocacy to the work of the President's Council on Physical Fitness and Sport.

Perceptual-motor training and movement education have come into widespread acceptance and are fundamental programs in many elementary schools throughout the country. From the early 1960s there has been a continual interest, not only by physical educators but by pediatricians, psychologists, primary grade teachers and administrators, ophthalmologists, and other specialists, in hereditary and environmental factors that inhibit or give support to general verbal and non-verbal educational development.

The movement education program emphasizes self-discovery, problem-solving, and inquiry development through participation in a variety of novel movement experiences. American physical educators eventually recognized the potential contributions this type of physical education offers, as demonstrated with great success in countries such as West Germany, England, Austria, and others in past years.

Perceptual-motor learning experiences are being emphasized in self-contained classrooms in primary grades as well as in physical education classes in upper elementary school grades. Educational consultants, classroom teachers, physical educators, reading consultants, school physicians, and other specialists have become acquainted with the studies and clinical experiences of cognitive and developmental psychologists and the work of medical specialists concerning the neurological bases of human movement and kinesthesis.

Rapid advances in the adaptation and utilization of instructional technology for the improvement of teaching and learning have caused many physical educators and administrators to rethink the physical education program and the ways it can be organized and conducted. For example, modular scheduling, made possible by computer technology, provides a method for planning and scheduling an individualized program of study for each pupil, based on interests and abilities. It has opened up new opportunities for independent study and practice in physical education in an "open laboratory" setting and in physical education resource centers.

In some experimental schools, new findings and ongoing experiences concerning differentiated duties and assignments of teachers provide viable opportunities for planning and conducting physical education programs of higher quality and greater breadth of content and experience, while taking advantage of each teacher's special expertise.

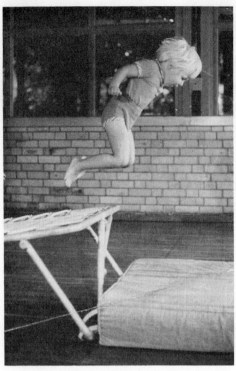

Movement education emphasizes self-discovery, problem-solving, and inquiry development.

Professor Ann Jewett was the Director of a national project of the American Alliance for Health, Physical Education, Recreation, and Dance, which developed a conceptual framework for curricular decision making. The report of this project[37] was published in 1977; the project is continuing to provide new ideas and practical curriculum suggestions that are being adapted across the country at various educational levels.

All the factors and influences described in this and other chapters have caused many individuals and organizations to review and clarify the purposes of physical education in schools and in other societal agencies. Physical educators, other teachers, administrators, school board members, parents, and taxpayers at times raise critical questions about one or more of the asserted purposes of physical education in their schools.

CONCLUSION

Basically, we believe that physical education is a fundamental subject in the school curriculum from the kindergarten through the college and university. This conclusion is strongly supported by a variety of research conclusions and by judgments of trained, experienced specialists in a variety of professional and academic fields associated with public education. At the same time, there are valid criticisms to be made of specific school programs of physical education. All criticisms, as well as positive suggestions for significant changes, are based on the conceptions one holds about what the basic purposes of the physical education program should be for each student in each educational institution.

SUMMARY

The aim of organized physical education programs is to create an environment that stimulates selected movement experiences, resulting in desirable responses that contribute to the optimal development of the individual's potentialities in all phases of life.

The personal needs of students are defined as relatively stable dispositions or tendencies that are amenable to specific types of motivation and instruction.

The general objectives of physical education are as follows: to develop the movement potentialities of each individual to an optimal level; to develop a basic understanding and appreciation of human movement; to develop and maintain optimal individual muscular strength, muscular endurance, and cardiovascular endurance; to develop skills, knowledge, and attitudes basic to voluntary participation in satisfying and enjoyable physical recreation experiences; and to develop personally rewarding and socially acceptable behaviors through participation in enjoyable movement activities.

Instructional, behavioral, and performance objectives serve the purpose of converting objectives into teaching, learning, and evaluating processes.

The physical education teacher should plan carefully to merge students' goals with the instructor's objectives in order to provide for thoughtful agreement and understanding concerning the purposes of the physical education unit or program.

Physical education is a fundamental subject in the school curriculum from kindergarten through the college and university undergraduate curriculum.

FOOTNOTES

[1]William C. Sheppard and Robert H. Willoughby, *Child Behaviors: Learning and Development.* Chicago: Rand McNally, 1975, p. 582.

[2]Frederick J. McDonald, *Educational Psychology* (2nd ed.). Belmont, CA: Wadsworth Publishing Company, 1965, p. 152.

[3]Ernest R. Hilgard, Richard C. Atkinson, and Rita L. Atkinson, *Introduction to Psychology* (6th ed.). New York: Harcourt, Brace, Jovanovich, Inc., 1975, pp. 503, 504.

[4]Ibid., pp. 330, 331.

[5]Abraham H. Maslow, *Motivation and Personality.* New York: Harper and Row, 1970.

[6]Richard B. Alderman, *Psychological Behavior in Sport.* Philadelphia: W. B. Saunders Company, 1974.

[7]Ibid., p. 160.

[8]Ibid., pp. 166, 168.

[9]Abraham H. Maslow, op. cit.

[10]Richard B. Alderman, op. cit., p. 168.

[11]The term "organic" refers to the cardiovascular system, digestive system, nervous system, and muscular system. These systems can be exercised, developed, or trained only through regular muscular activity. While muscular power is no longer directly important for the social and economic success of a majority of the population, it is indirectly so because of the dependence of organic function upon muscular activity, and because of the stress placed upon the vital organs by modern conditions of life.

[12]W. James Popham, "Instructional Objectives — A Dialog with Researcher, Supervisor, and Teacher," *Educational Researcher,* 1:8–12 (September, 1972), p. 11.

[13]Ibid.

[14]Robert F. Mager, *Preparing Instructional Objectives.* Palo Alto, CA: Fearon Publishers, 1962, p. 29. (Previously published as *Preparing Objectives for Programmed Instructions.* Fearon Publishers, 1961.)

[15]W. James Popham, "Focus on Outcomes — A Guiding Theme of ES '70 Schools," *Phi Delta Kappan,* 51:208 (December, 1969).

[16]Elliot W. Eisner, "Instructional and Expressive Educational Objectives: Their Formulation and Use in Curriculum," AERA Monograph Series on Curriculum Evaluation, No. 3. Chicago: Rand McNally, 1969, p. 15.

[17]James D. Raths, "Teaching without Specific Objectives," *Educational Leadership,* 28:714–720 (April, 1971).

[18]Elliot W. Eisner, op. cit.

[19]Benjamin S. Bloom, Max D. Engelhart, Walker H. Hill, Edward J. Furst, and David R. Krathwohl, *Taxonomy of Educational Objectives: The Classification of Educational Goals.* New York: David McKay Company, Inc., 1956.

[20]David R. Krathwohl, Benjamin S. Bloom, and Bertram B. Masia, *Taxonomy of Educational Objectives, Handbook II: The Affective Domain.* New York: David McKay Company, Inc., 1956.

[21]Elizabeth J. Simpson, "The Classification of Educational Objectives: Psycho-motor Domain," Vocational and Technical Education Grant Contract No. OE–85–104. Washington, D.C.: U.S. Department HEW, 1966.

[22]Marvin L. Clein and William J. Stone, "Physical Education and the Classification of Educational Objectives: Psychomotor Domain," *The Physical Educator,* 27:27–34 (March, 1970).

[23]Anita J. Harrow, *A Taxonomy of the Psychomotor Domain: A Guide for Developing Behavioral Objectives.* New York: David McKay Company, Inc., 1972, p. vii.

[24]Ibid.

[25]Ann E. Jewett and Marie R. Mullan, *Curriculum Design: Purposes and Processes in Physical Education Teaching-Learning.* Washington, D.C.: American Alliance for Health, Physical Education, Recreation, 1977.

[26]Ibid., p. vii.

[27]Ibid., p. 2.

[28]Delbert Oberteuffer, "The Role of Physical Education in Health and Fitness," *American Journal of Public Health,* 52:1155–1160 (July, 1962).

[29]Robert L. Brackenbury, "Physical Education: An Intellectual Emphasis?" *Quest,* I:3–6 (December, 1963).

[30]Franklin M. Henry, "Specificity vs. Generality in Learning Motor Skills," *Proc. Coll. Phys. Educ. Assoc.,* 1958, pp. 126–128.

[31]Bryant J. Cratty, *Movement Behavior and Motor Learning* (3rd ed.). Philadelphia: Lea & Febiger, 1973.

[32]Edward A. Fleishman, *The Structure and Measurement of Physical Fitness.* Englewood Cliffs, NJ: Prentice-Hall, Inc., 1964.

[33]Ibid.

[34]Bryant J. Cratty, op. cit.

[35]Celeste Ulrich and John E. Nixon, *Tones of Theory—A Theoretical Structure for Physical Education, A Tentative Perspective.* Washington, D.C. American Association for Health, Physical Education, Recreation, 1972.

[36]*This Is Physical Education.* Washington, D.C.: American Association for Health, Physical Education and Recreation, 1965.

[37]Ann E. Jewett and Marie R. Mullan, op. cit.

SELECTED REFERENCES

Annarino, Anthony A., "Physical Education Objectives: Traditional vs. Developmental." *Journal of Physical Education and Recreation,* October 1977, 22–23.

Baley, James and Field, David A., *Physical Education and the Physical Educator* (2nd Ed.). Boston: Allyn and Bacon, Inc., 1976.

Bandura, Albert, *Social Learning Theory.* Englewood-Cliffs, N.J.: Prentice-Hall, 1977.

Barrow, Harold M., *Man and Movement — Principles of Physical Education* (2nd Ed.). Philadelphia: Lea & Febiger, 1977.

Brown, Camille and Cassidy, Rosalind, *Theory in Physical Education: A Guide to Program Change.* Philadelphia: Lea & Febiger, 1963.

Freeman, William H., *Physical Education in a Changing Society.* Boston: Houghton-Mifflin, 1977.

Frost, Reuben, *Physical Education: Foundations, Practices, Principles,* Reading, MA: Addison-Wesley Publishing Co., Inc., 1975.

Goodlad, John I. and Golub, John S. (Eds.), *Facing the Future: Issues in Education and Schooling.* New York: McGraw Hill, 1977.

Hetherington, Clark W., *School Program in Physical Education.* Yonkers, N.Y.: World Book Company, 1922.

Jewett, Ann E., "Relationships in Physical Education: A Curriculum Viewpoint." *The Academy Papers,* No. 11. Washington, D.C.: The American Academy of Physical Education, 1977, pp. 87–97.

Jewett, Ann E., Jones, L. Sue, Luneke, Sheryl M., and Robinson, Sarah M., "Educational Change Through a Taxonomy for Writing Physical Education Objectives." *Quest,* XV:32–38 (January 1971).

Johnson, Warren R., and Buskirk E. R. (Eds.), *Science and Medicine of Exercise and Sports* (2nd Ed.). New York: Harper and Row, 1974.

Larson, Leonard A., *Foundations of Physical Activity.* Riverside, N.J.: Macmillan Publishing Company, Inc. 1976.

Mager, Robert, "Humanistic Education and Behavioral Objectives: Opposing Theories of Education and Science." *School Review,* 85:376–194 (May 1977).

Metheny, Eleanor, "Physical Education as an Area of Study and Research." *Quest*, IX:73–78 (December 1967).

Nash, Jay B., *Physical Education: Interpretations and Objectives* (Rev. Ed.). Dubuque, Iowa: William C. Brown and Company, 1963.

Popham, W. James, *Educational Evaluation*. Englewood Cliffs, N.J.: Prentice-Hall Publishing Company, 1975.

Popham, W. James, "Competency-based High School Completion Program." *NASSP Bulletin*, 101–5 (February 1978).

Popham, W. James, *Criterion-referenced Measurement*. Englewood Cliffs, N.J.: Prentice-Hall Publishing Company, 1978.

Rivenes, Richard S., *Foundations of Physical Education: A Scientific Approach*. Boston, MA: Houghton-Mifflin, 1978.

The School Program in Health, Physical Education, and Recreation: A Statement of Basic Beliefs. Kensington, Md: Society of State Directors of Health, Physical Education and Recreation, 1972.

Siedentop, Daryl, *Physical Education: Introductory Analysis* (2nd Ed.). Dubuque, Iowa: Wm. C. Brown Company, 1976.

Singer, Robert N. (Ed.), *Physical Education: Foundations*. New York: Holt, Rinehart and Winston, 1976.

Spitzer, Dean R., *Concept Formation and Learning in Early Childhood*. Columbus, Ohio: Merrill, 1977.

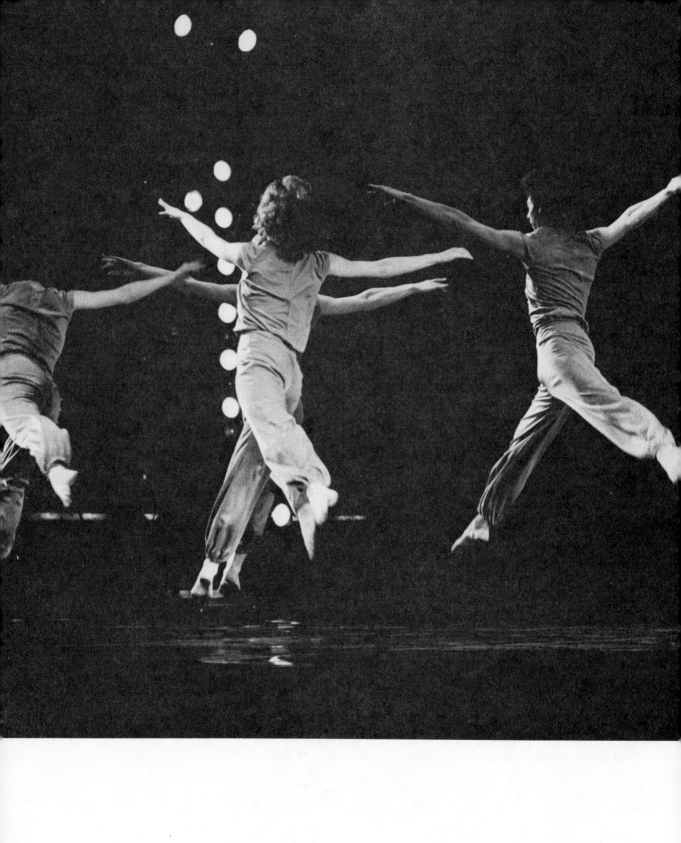

THE NORMATIVE ———— ———————— FOUNDATIONS OF PHYSICAL EDUCATION ————

The term "normative" refers to the standard, or normal, patterns of goals, speech, values, and so on, characterizing the members of a social organization. Philosophy, history, and comparative education are *normative* studies because they aim to identify, define, and describe the goals and educational activities that are highly valued by a society. According to philosophers, norms consist of an expected set of behaviors that the primary social group values strongly and seeks to inculcate in its members. Basic concepts from the philosophy and history of physical education, and from comparative physical education, specify cultural expectations and teach the basic value systems held by the social groups whose members are participants in and supporters of physical education programs.

This chapter briefly discusses (1) the roles of philosophy and educational philosophy, and the philosophy of physical education; (2) the major historical influences in the development of organized programs of physical education in America; and (3) methods of cross-cultural examination and analysis of differences and similarities between major components of systems of physical education.

With a clear understanding of the normative foundations of physical education, teachers can more clearly understand their own value system, and that of the institution in which they teach, and the values of the societal agencies which control institutional programs. Thus, one can evaluate more effectively the strengths and weaknesses of the policies, principles, and practices that determine the course contents and approaches. Finally, the perceptive, thoughtful teacher can develop insights and personal and professional skills that will facilitate more effective teaching and learning conditions and thereby produce desirable changes in pupil behaviors.

Basically, philosophy refers to the organized study of human thought and conduct. It is concerned with identifying and clearly formulating laws and principles that underlie all human knowledge and understanding of reality. Thus, philosophy is used to explain the nature of the universe and our attitudes toward the direction and control of human existence. Originally the term *philosophy* referred to mankind's love of wisdom and knowledge. Zeigler[1] defines philosophy as "that branch of learning (or that science) which investigates, evaluates, and integrates knowledge of reality as best as possible into one or more systems embodying all available wisdom about the universe."

Roger Burke[2] says that

> the content of philosophy is a rational, consistent, systematic set of pervasive general principles which explain existence, perceived facts, and causations. . . . It provides a framework, a rational theory, a logical method, a penetrating explanation, and a universal guide for the problems of human existence.

Philosophical Inquiry

Since philosophers arbitrarily subdivide their field into branches or domains, there are many taxonomies of philosophy. It is standard practice to list five main branches of philosophy:

Metaphysics (the nature of reality)
Epistemology (the nature of knowledge)
Logic (the nature of relationships between ideas, both deductive and inductive)
Axiology, or ethics (the nature and sources of values)
Aesthetics (the nature of beauty and the criteria of artistic judgment)

A variety of subdivisions of the above five branches are proposed by noted philosophers. Brubacher[3] describes 11 categories of philosophy:

Pragmatic Naturalism
Reconstructionism
Romantic Naturalism
Existentialism
Organicism
Idealism
Realism
Rational Humanism
Fascism
Communism
Democracy

There is general agreement that there are four major categories of philosophical inquiry:

Speculative, which involves synthesis of facts or ideas in order to present an overview or an integrated picture. It is an attempt to fill in gaps in knowledge.

Normative, which refers to the formulation of goals, norms, and standards of behavior for individuals or groups under study. Philosophers create principles of philosophizing as guides to action, an approach commonly found in education and physical education. Physical education is particularly committed to creating principles as a basis for establishing sound procedures and practices.

Critical, which involves generating the greatest possible clarity of meaning and understanding through the careful, precise study of terms and propositions about thought and practice in all areas of human endeavor.

Analytical, which involves careful evaluation of the concepts and clichés used by others in an attempt to make the assumptions which underlie them more explicit. It is not concerned with original thought; rather, it explains, qualifies, and elucidates the ideas of philosophers, scientists, speculators, and others who make normative conclusions.[4]

In an interesting and cogent introduction to her book, Nott[5] summarizes what the study of philosophy is all about:

> The problems are still as they have been — whenever we have time or strength to consider what we mean by being human — identity, freedom, and responsibility. The first poses the question, Who am I? And also, How have I become what I am, a concrete historical individual, a person, and a mind? The other asks: How can I maintain this identity in polarity with the identity of others?
>
> For these questions there is no collectivistic or strictly scientific answer. They are questions on which we have to philosophize.

Needless to say, the physical education philosophers can and should lend their best efforts to evolving and stating clear philosophical concepts as indicated by the above quotation, with particular reference to contributions by physical education and sport to the meaning of humankind and human existence in this world.

Generally speaking, aesthetics is the branch of philosophy that is concerned with identifying and defining concepts of art. Concerned with beauty, appreciation, taste, self-expression, and personal fulfillment, it usually concentrates on historical forms of art, such as painting, literature, poetry, sculpture, dance, architecture, and music. Very seldom are sport and other physical education activities included in traditional definitions and discussions of aesthetics or of art. *Aesthetics*

It is largely in the past 20 years that American physical educators have developed a strong scholarly and interpretative interest in sport as an aesthetic experience. Dance, historically recognized as one of the major elements of physical education, also has been a component in the area of aesthetics for many centuries.

The Aesthetic Experience. Aesthetics has two major foci, one being the artist, who attempts to express feelings and attitudes through an artistic medium or form. The other is the spectator, reader, or listener who appreciates the work of artists past and present. Both undergo personal aesthetic experiences involving interpretation, understanding, and emotion: the artist in the creation of a work of art, and the audience in its appreciation.

Aesthetics and Sport. Historically, sport performances have not generally been regarded as aesthetic expressions by the athletes nor accepted as aesthetic experiences by spectators. Physical education and sport philosophers and interpreters in recent years have challenged this view. Many articles and books are now being produced emphasizing the theme of sport as art or aesthetic experience.

The individual spectator who is knowledgeable about the intricacies of individual sport performances is more able to discern when an athlete has made a particularly difficult and beautiful movement against intense opposition or while striving to control an object in pursuing a goal in the contest. One frequently hears spectators say "Wasn't that a beautiful move?"

Many art objects of great beauty and style have been produced throughout the history of mankind and can be found in museums and art galleries around the world depicting humans engaging in sport activities relevant to the time period involved. Sculptors such as Joe Brown in the United States are internationally renowned for the artistry of their work featuring sport figures. Both still and motion picture photographers have captured the essence of beautiful, aesthetic movements of talented sport performers in a variety of activities and events for the enjoyment of thousands of spectators through the media of television, magazines, and gallery displays.

Even individuals who do not regard themselves as artists in a formal sense may experience intense aesthetic satisfaction and pleasure from certain of their own movement experiences. One can feel an aesthetic sensation from certain types of spontaneous and deliberately acted out movement experiences in informal sports, novel exercise, and recreational voluntary movements, as well as in formal sport contests. Likewise, probably most of us who enjoy attending competitive sport events would be willing to testify that there are many occasions in which we, too, as spectators, would rank the aesthetic thrills we receive through observing a skillful participant to be more meaningful than the score at the end of the contest.

Moore[6] delightfully and accurately describes the aesthetic beauty of a sport performer:

> The tumbler senses something of brief snatches of freedom, something of precarious balance in unsupported space, of underlying rhythm, and of forces initiated by himself acting upon himself. He becomes sensitive to the elements of space, force, and time in his world of movement. From this viewpoint, we see that it is not just the man's body performing; it is the whole man. The total performer then becomes both artist and material. Man and his movements become the art.

Moore goes on to say:

> As the performer feels the art he is creating, so can a perceptive spectator feel this same quality, although not to the same extent. Whether intended or not, there is silent communication between the performer and the spectator. Empathy with the elements of force, space, and time in the world of the performer and his movements can account, in part at least, for the spectator interpreting the movement as meaningful and beautiful.

Through the performance the performer-artist experiences a deeply satisfying intimacy with the spectator and with the art, a feeling accompanied with strong emotions and the realization that one is moving in graceful, smoothly coordinated sequences requiring exquisite timing and self-control.

Philosophic Research Method

Morland[7] succinctly defines what he calls the *philosophic research method* as follows:

> In formal research, other than purely descriptive and historical studies, the philosophic method is the rigorous application of the principles and processes of logic, within carefully defined limits, to the analysis of nonempirical problems.

Morland goes on to say that this type of research emphasizes the question of "why," not "when" or "how." The philosopher attempts to qualify the

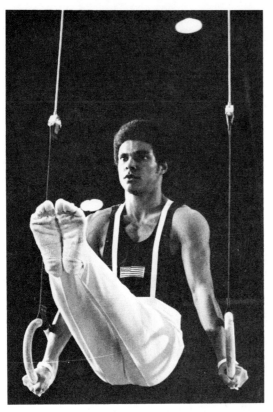
Athletics requires timing, grace, coordination, and non-verbal expression.

meaning of central ideas and to arrange them most logically in order to provide a clear understanding of concepts and ideas that bridge the gap between means and ends.

Philosophic research, according to Morland, is similar to scientific research and employs the scientific method. The researcher must be objective and free of any bias concerning the phenomenon under investigation. He indicates the following elements as central to philosophic research:[8]

> (1) the problem clearly and succinctly stated, (2) the terms defined in the context of their usage in the study, (3) the scope of the study set forth within carefully defined limits, (4) the underlying assumptions delineated, (5) the hypothesis or hypotheses stated in compositional form, (6) the rationale and significance of the problem established, (7) the pertinent literature reviewed and its relationship to the proposed study demonstrated, and (8) the procedures outlined in such a manner that the correction of the data as well as the logic of the analysis can be followed easily from the sources of the evidence through the completion of the investigation.

The major thrust of American philosophy is briefly summarized by Smith:[9]   *Summary*

> The fact is that contrary to the widespread belief that American life has no place for the life of the. mind, American philosophy in the twentieth century is the most colossal example of applied philosophy on record. Rather than keeping man's spiritual products in a museum under glass, we have sought, that is, to think of some purpose and to make purpose effective in action.

Based on the contributions of philosophy discussed above, physical educators will continually improve their abilities to make more valid and critically important professional and academic decisions concerning the importance of physical education to the lives of people. Philosophy will provide an essential, organized structure for the coherent reporting of current beliefs and values that give basic direction to physical education program activities over time.

Brumbaugh and Lawrence[10] make an interesting analysis of the foundations of philosophical thought in western civilization and apply them to a more thorough understanding of the nature and purposes of education. Two quotes are illustrative:

EDUCATIONAL PHILOSOPHY

> Unless educational theory is to be mere technology, it must examine the fundamental assumptions about the nature of man and society which underlie educational practice. Educational theory which undertakes such study is, to that extent, philosophical.
>
> A risk attaches to each of the two tendencies: technologists may plunge in, thoughtlessly, to gain some preconceived concrete end in the educational system, only to find that they have successfully accomplished a result which has not been carefully thought out in advance; philosophers of education, on the other hand, may get lost in grand abstractions filled with glittering generalities and endless debate, but with no concrete suggestions for getting the ideal job done. Neither approach, in short, can get very far without taking some counsel from the other.
>
> One of the tasks of our study of philosophies of education is to rescue the formulas and familiar notions from the sloganeers. We have undertaken to give them life and meaning to exhibit them as central in a community of ideas that make up educational philosophy. When they are presented in this way, these ideas are not easy to understand at all; they require effort and patience to be grasped in the way that the philosopher intended. The alternative to easy slogan is hard thought.

Lawrence and Brumbaugh proceed to describe the purposes of educational philosophy in the development of a viable kind of productive educational system that will best meet the American ideals.

The educational philosopher must raise basic questions and articulate them clearly. Why is required public education important? What is intelligence? How is it related to our concepts of thought, action, emotion, expression, freedom, and other important notions? What are the basic disciplines? Are non-verbal means of education (art, physical education, dance) "intellectual" or "non-intellectual"? What responsibilities does the school have for the development of ethical character? What theory of human values should be transmitted by the curriculum? What responsibility does the school have for social development, community action, state public services, and national goals? What should be the proper balance between individualism and social cohesion?

Educational philosophy is a specialized area of general philosophy that intensely investigates the aims and practices of formal and informal educational organizations. Current major educational problems and issues are the central focus of concern and initiate philosophical analysis and study. The tools of philosophical analysis are applied to these educational problems and varied practices in a search for the identification of more effective and significant strategies and methodologies for planning and governing educational enterprises.

Traditionally, educational philosophers (1) set out to describe major schools of philosophical thought and then related each to the problems, responsibilities, and challenges of educational institutions as a basis for improved practices; and (2) sought to clarify educational problems in terms of the basic tenets of the major branches of philosophy such as metaphysics, epistemology, logic, and axiology.

In recent years, the process has been reversed. Educational problems, issues, and practices have become the central focus of concern and analysis. Philosophical analyses are made of important educational problems to clarify the search for more significant and effective strategies and practices for governing and administering educational enterprises.

PHILOSOPHY OF PHYSICAL EDUCATION

Introduction

In their interesting and novel approach to the study of the philosophy of physical education, Harper, Miller, Park, and Davis[11] urge the professional student to learn how to philosophize. The first section of their book outlines the steps involved and the rationale for each of them. Their main point is that physical education students and teachers should do more than merely read and study about the major schools of philosophical thought and their tenets. In fact, such study really is not philosophic, it is educational and informative only. The student or teacher must go on and learn *how* to philosophize.

Roles of Physical Education Philosophy

In a perceptive article that launched the magazine *Quest* into the literary sea of scholarly journals in physical education, Van Dalen[12] described the roles of philosphy in physical education. Selected paraphrased concepts follow:

> Scientific findings in physical education provide quantitative descriptions of *what is,* while philosophy suggests *what should be,* the aims and purposes of physical education. Philosophy therefore interprets what is known or believed to exist by criticism, clarification, ordering, and interpretation.
>
> Philosophy continually serves as an arbitrator between the practices physical education coaches engage in and their fundamental beliefs and personal and professional biases.
>
> Philosophy will guide a continuous process of expansion, clear articulation, and order of a coherent framework of basic concepts which will give direction to ongoing physical education services and activities.

Zeigler[13] indicates the importance of the study and use of a rigorous philosophy of physical education:

> In summary, therefore, *adequately prepared* physical educators ought to be able to approach the philosophy of physical education and sport normatively and analytically and should do so increasingly in the future. The era in which the scholarly contributions to the philosophy of physical education were made by physical education leaders and administrators *with adequate backgrounds in Philosophy* is over. This is not to say that their statements will not be welcome, or that perhaps the rank and file of the profession will not pay greater heed to their words than those of the philosophy specialists, but well informed professional physical educators will be forced to take into consideration the sources and the backgrounds from which these individuals speak. In any case, there is certainly a continuing need to train physical educators systematically and thoroughly so that they may undertake normative and analytical philosophical research of high quality.

Persistent Problems Approach. Over the years, Zeigler,[14] his students, and his colleagues have developed what he calls the "persistent historical problems approach" to physical education and sport. Recently, he has adapted this approach as a basis for the philosophical analysis of 15 social forces:

1. values (aim and objectives)
2. influence of politics (or type of political state)
3. influence of nationalism
4. influence of economics
5. influence of religion
6. ecological concerns
7. professional and education concerns:
   a. relationship to the use of leisure
   b. relationship to the concept of the healthy body
   c. classification of amateurs and semi-professionalism and professionalism
   d. relationship of women to sport
   e. management theory and practice applied to sport
   f. curriculum for professional preparation and general education
   g. teaching and/or coaching methodology
   h. ethics of coaching
   i. concepts of progress in sport

Zeigler analyzes each of the 15 persistent problems beginning with the development of historical background. Following this, he indicates the philosophical position taken by experimentalists, reconstructionists, realists, idealists, and existentialists with respect to specific professional concerns. Philosophical research techniques are utilized in analyzing these particular subproblems.

Physical educators have "philosophized" about their field both orally and in writing for a long, long time. In recent years increasing numbers of young physical educators are receiving advanced training in the discipline of philosophy and are pursuing philosophical inquiry in sport and physical education. More books are being published on the subject each year, and more magazines contain philosophical articles. The *Journal of Philosophy of Sport* provides a periodic list of important, diverse articles from the philosophic perspective. College and university faculties are employing specially trained philosophers of physical education and are expanding undergraduate and graduate studies and research in this area.

The educational and personal philosophies held by the individual teacher or coach, and the pedagogical methods and curriculum designs utilized, are inseparable. All educators must realize that their teaching and coaching practices ultimately rest upon the basic philosophical beliefs and values they hold. The belief system and the value system of the individual educators seldom are explicitly organized and recorded in written form. However, it is with them always and gives continual guidance to all aspects of their teaching and coaching as they interact with each pupil.

Teachers and coaches are urged to overtly, deliberately, and conscientiously state and describe the major tenets of their personal and professional value systems. This process of thinking and reflecting on a systematic basis, at periodic intervals, will better enable the teacher and coach to think, prepare, and interact with pupils consistently and effectively. This process will sharpen one's perception of, and dedication to, the pursuit of fulfillment of the priorities and objectives that lead to the optimal educational development of each student.

Vanderzwaag[15] has created a useful and penetrating look into the philosophy of sport described around such topics as historical relationships between the concepts of sport and physical education, sport, play, games, and athletics; male and female participation in sport; the administration, organization, and teaching of sport; purposes of sport participation by the individual; the significance of group participation in sports; the proposed values of sport; and finally a scenario of what a quality program of sport should be from preschool to the Ph.D. level of education. The interested physical education teacher and athletic coach will broaden their philosophical perspectives as a basis for improved teaching and coaching practices by carefully studying this text. *Philosophy of Sport*

Philosophical Definition of Sport. Philosophers of physical education and sport join many other interested individuals in attempting to define the term sport as well as to state its purpose. For example, this application of philosophical inquiry into sport is exemplified by Fraleigh,[16] whose article builds a philosophical and logical rationale for his operational definition of sport:

> Sport is a voluntary, agreed-upon rule-bound human event in which one or more human participants opposes at least one significant human in a contest in which all participants seek the approval of the relative abilities of all to move mass in space and time by utilizing bodily moves which exhibit developed motor skills, physiological endurance and socially approved tactics and strategy.

Fraleigh[16] goes on to state what he believes to be the purpose of sport:

> The purpose of sport is to provide equitable opportunity for the mutual testing of the relative abilities of the participants to move mass in space and time within the confines prescribed by an agreed-upon set of rules.

A group of interested physical education and sport leaders with special interest in philosophy established the Philosophic Society for the Study of Sport in an initial meeting in Boston, in December, 1972. In the *Journal of the Philosophy of Sport*,[17] published by the Society, it is asserted that

> the philosophy of sport has developed in recent years toward a progressively closer association with philosophy proper. This development has served to significantly enhance our refined understanding of, and sensitivity for, sport.

Brackenbury,[18] a well-known educational philosopher at the University of Southern California, has perceptively noted what physical educators commonly fail to understand, namely, that the school program of physical education can, and should, have an intellectual emphasis. Brackenbury's article provides a compelling rationale for this belief. It is urged that all physical educators study this article and utilize the arguments at meetings where physical education curriculum objectives are *Intellectual Emphasis in Physical Education* set, programs are authorized, time allotments are assigned, and budgetary allowances are fixed. The following abstracts present the gist of Brackenbury's position:

> There is a philosophical position known as dualism which separates the intellectual from the physical, the mind from the body. . . .
>
> The dualistic physical educator is likely to stress physical fitness. The body must be kept in shape so the mind can do better its work. Since the mind and the body are two different kinds of entities, the mind need not be involved in getting the body in shape. Hence this complete separation of mind and body enables the physical educator not only to keep the "physical" in education, but to keep the "intellectual" out.
>
> Man has always been willing to sacrifice his health and longevity for pleasure. As a goal, physical fitness simply lacks sustained appeal.
>
> In seeking direction in the days ahead, physical educators might well look to the noun rather than to the adjective in their subject matter. For concentration upon the nature of "education" rather than stress upon characteristics "physical" may provide the touchstone. If all education is an intellectual undertaking, physical education must also be basically a mental undertaking — relatively sure it is one in which physical movement plays a large part. Life is a process or activity and in any process or activity both the mental and physical are present.
>
> The difference between mental and physical activity is not a difference in kind, it is a difference in degree or emphasis. Physical educators are concerned with activities and skills in which the physical plays a prominent role, but they are not activities or skills in which the mind is inactive.
>
> Physical and mental, body and mind, and matter and intelligence are useful distinctions for purposes of discussion, but we get into trouble when we push the separation too far. The mind is not one kind of entity or substance with the body another. Were this the case, the mind could never really know or understand anything about the body for they would have nothing in common. Monism, not dualism, is the philosophical thesis that may save physical education, for it provides the basis whereby physical education can legitimately make a claim to academic respectability.
>
> To the enrichment of life, physical education can make a significant contribution, if it sublimates the physical to education.[18]

In a penetrating philosophical inquiry into the age-old controversy about the mind and body and their interrelationships, and the alternative holistic view of man, Meier[19] summarizes his investigations based on philosophical research methods:

> Rather than continued repetition and support of hierarchical mind over body conceptions of interaction (positing the mind to be totally dominant over the simple, objectified, and mechanical body), it appears to be more fruitful to transcend some notions and orientations. If mental and physical polarities are eliminated and reductive orientations altered, it is possible to accord the physical aspects of man due respect for integral facets of man's nature and subsequently rejoice in a total respect of a conscious body. Merleau-Ponty's description of the body as a work of art provides an appropriate summary of this orientation:
>
>> *A novel, poem, picture or musical work are individuals, that is, beings in which the expression is indistinguishable from the thing expressed, their meaning, accessible only through direct contact, being radiated with no change of their temporal and spatial situation. It is in this sense that our body is comparable to a work of art. It is a focal point of living meanings, not the function of a certain number of mutually variable terms.*

If such a characterization is accepted, the distinctive potentialities of man's participation in sport may be vigorously explored. Rather than concentrating solely on the objectified, treadmill image of sport, predominantly centered upon the development and attainment of physical strength, motor skills, and technical efficiency, it appears legitimate and fruitful to focus upon the full and meaningfully lived experience of sport.

Through free, creative, and personally significant movement and meaning-bestowing bodily expression in sport, man asserts his uniqueness and affirms himself. Man's actions in sport represent, express, and identify his powers, intentionality and being. In sum, sport may be characterized as the celebration of man as an open and expressive embodied being.[19]

The physical educator does a disservice to his field to use Plato's historical dualistic conception of mind and body as justification for today's physical education programs.

Clark[20] succinctly states the basic purpose of history:

HISTORY OF PHYSICAL EDUCATION

> The criticism of history can, so I believe, be of value in a number of ways, but its primary object must be to get nearer the truth that lies behind any historic opinion that is worth considering.... History can serve a number of purposes. It can amuse, it can instruct, it can warn, it can encourage, it can provide the data for important decisions and it can help in the analysis of society. But it can do none of these things if it is not conscientiously aimed at the truth, for in that case it is not history but a fraud.

Clark then summarizes the purpose of history and historical criticism:

> Historical criticism is offered as an instrument formed to enable human beings to get nearer the truth. It does this by attempting to test the relationship between what purports to be history and the truth which lies behind it. It probes the evidence which is claimed to be the link between an historical opinion and reality. It promotes an analysis of the conception in which an historical opinion is expressed and draws attention to the significance of the personality of the historian. The results may be to confirm what is already believed, or to produce something which is altogether more coherent and convincing, or it may be to destroy altogether anything that seemed to be certain or made sense. Even so, it will have value for it may be that the only knowledge that can at the moment be trusted on a particular subject is that nothing is known about it, and possibly that, as far as can be foreseen, nothing more coherent or certain will ever be known about it.

Humans living prior to 6000 B.C. have been described as primitive. The first social groupings were tribal and familial. Children learned directly from their parents and from other adults and children. An informal system of cultural transmission was the earliest form of education. Youth were instructed by their parents and other adults in a form of apprenticeship. Many of life's responsibilities involved *physical* activities.

BEGINNINGS

Primitive Human Beings

From primitive times, youth have always had natural play urges, exemplified by games of war and games of chase and tag. Also, young people have been required at an early age to learn self-preservation skills. Dancing and other forms of rhythmic activity, generally related to religious beliefs, were predominant in early childhood as well as adult life.

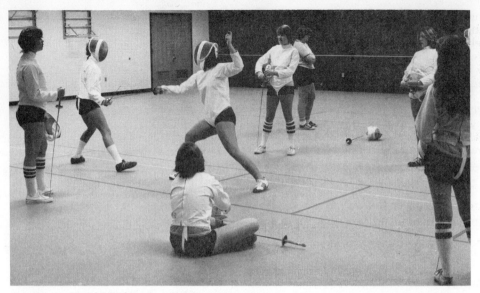
Fencing developed from early self-defense activities.

In primitive cultures the men undertook to instruct their young in various physical activities involved in the everyday struggle to maintain their existence, including self-defense, procuring food, and providing for shelter against the elements. Children also engaged in wrestling, tag games, hiding-and-finding each other, and varieties of ball games. Archery, a popular activity in today's physical education program, was taught tens of thousands of years ago, when the bow and arrow were primarily hunting weapons. The modern sport of fencing developed from early self-defense activities (Fig. 3–2).

Artifacts and ruins brought to light by archaeology, history, and anthropology clearly demonstrate that games, sports, festivals, and dances, along with the endless play of children, have created cultural patterns inseparably woven into the history of human beings whenever and wherever they have lived. Thus, the presence of fundamental elements of physical education programs began with the first family groupings and continued unabated throughout all cultures to the present time. This section provides a brief review of significant contributions to the development of physical education in various historical eras.

Early historic societies evolved in various areas in the world — Egypt, Babylon, Assyria, Palestine, China, India, Iran, and Crete. Elements of physical education were present in all of these cultures. The historian interested in various sports in early societies must possess interdisciplinary scholarly and research skills based on ancient history, art history, anthropology, archaeology, art history, and sociology, along with intensive familiarity with sports and games. The earliest evidence of sports and games in any culture is in the era of 3000 to 1500 B.C., in the region between the Tigris and Euphrates Rivers. Major activities included combat sports, such as boxing and wrestling, and dancing.

Evidence points toward sport and game participation in Egypt, be- *Egypt* tween 3000 and 1100 B.C., by the upper classes. They engaged in acrobatics and tumbling, dancing, body exercises, yoga, jumping and kicking games, ball games, and others. Egyptian history also records archery, lion hunting, swimming, equestrian contests, wrestling, foot racing, and juggling.

In ancient Egypt, dance was a major religious activity. Hunting, fowling, and fishing not only were major sports but also were necessities for obtaining food daily for survival. Archaeologists have found play equipment for various games using balls, blocks, marbles, and other objects. Stick fighting was prominent. Strength and skill in self-defense were emphasized. Later, bull fights, archery, running, swimming, horseback riding, military activities, and other forms of sport and games were developed.

In ancient China between 1700 and 800 B.C., physical education *China* primarily consisted of military training. Hunting, shooting with the bow, horseback riding, and other military arts were stressed. The dance, "Wu Yung," was one very important aspect of the six arts. Light exercises, Chinese football, and the throwing of darts at targets were popular. Ancient Chinese philosophers held varying views about the role of physical education activities in the different eras. School physical education was popularized between the 11th century and the 8th century B.C. Later, physical education was dropped from Chinese school curricula.

Ancient Greek concepts and practices have had a significant and **GREECE** lasting impact on physical education theories, programs, and practices around the world. The ancient Greeks believed strongly in the contribution of physical education to the development of mind, body, and spirit. The Golden Era of Greece reached its zenith in the sixth century B.C. Greece was not a unified nation at this time, but rather was a collection of city-states, political units consisting of a city and its surrounding area. Each city-state had its own government and military force supported by a devoted citizenry. Sparta was famed as a strong military power; Athens developed into a cultural and intellectual center; and Corinth became a noted business center. Thus, specific schools of physical education were differentiated in each Greek city-state in accordance with the prevailing values of that region. Physical education historians conclude that the Greek city-states of Athens and Sparta seem to have provided the strongest influences on the theory and practice of physical education that prevailed through centuries, even to the present time — a conclusion supported by available records and the interpretations of historians and philosophers.

Athens. According to leading historians, Athens, a small city-state composed of several thousand free citizens, spawned more brilliant leaders of highest rank in a variety of human endeavors than were ever produced elsewhere in an equal period of time. Indeed, it is doubtful whether the brilliance of Greek philosophy, literature, and art in this time period has been equalled in any other age by any nation or peoples.

Athenian boys were educated in four main areas: mathematics, literature, gymnastics, and music. A knowledgeable grammarian taught literature. Gymnastics teachers provided instruction in a wide range of physical education activities that included wrestling, jumping, running, throwing the discus and the javelin, and free play, or what we now call recess. The word "music" was broadly interpreted to include not only music per se, but also various art forms and literary modes. Music and gymnastics occupied significant roles in the educational curriculum; art, music, and physical education teachers today desire to emulate the example of the Athenian Greeks with regard to planning the school curriculum to be more equally represented by these fundamental subjects.

The Greeks saw that muscular activity developed not only the beauty of the human body, but also understanding and appreciation for the physical figure. While this naturally appealed to their sense of the artistic, it furthermore provided a strong foundation for health and respect for the human form. They did not regard physical education as a recreational release to counteract intensive mental effort, as do many modern educators. The Greeks recognized the value of physical education programs in the development of such character and personality traits as self-confidence, self-control, poise, and courage. Plato summarized this philosophy when he said that music and gymnastics are designed for the improvement of the soul.

Plato and Mind-Body Dualism. The present-day physical educator must be cautious about citing isolated quotes from Plato or other Greek philosophers in support of the retention of physical education in today's school curriculum. Plato's philosophy was a dichotomous one which we hear paraphrased frequently today as "the sound mind in the sound body." Plato considered the body and soul to be separate entities: the body was mortal and therefore inferior to the soul, which was immortal. He stated that the two purposes of physical training were (1) military preparation to protect the city-state, and (2) development of a healthy body as a receptacle for the soul. This interpretation is no longer valid because of well-established scientific evidence concerning the integrated nature of man. There is no anatomical entity in the human being known as "the mind," nor is there a physical "soul." The detailed study of anatomy and physiology will easily dispose of this invalid misconception.

Sparta. Boys were educated in the home through the age of six. They then were assigned to "packs" organized by the state, in which they remained until age fourteen. Physical fitness and military skills were emphasized in the daily training activities for the boys in the packs.

All Spartan boys were trained for military servitude from ages fourteen to twenty. They were on call for participation in any military campaign when needed from that time on throughout their life.

Spartan Girls and Physical Education. Spartan rulers believed that physical education had a vital role to play in the education and development of girls as well as boys. Although girls did not attend formal Spartan schools, the state provided supervised physical education programs that included ball games, mountain climbing, discus and javelin throwing, running, jumping, and dancing. Girls were forbidden to become overweight. Because of this restriction and the regularity and intensity of the physical education programs over a number of years, a majority of girls developed attractive and strong bodies. Physical fitness as preparation for motherhood was also stressed. Not surprisingly, these young women came to be admired for their physical beauty, general fitness, and clear complexion.

Music and Dance. Music and dance were fundamental forms of communication and expression for the youth of Sparta. Songs were a basic educational medium: through traditional hymns Spartan children learned about the valiant exploits of their war heroes; and even the laws of the state were adapted to a musical score. Children marched and exercised to the beat of martial music. Dance was instrumental in communicating the glory of state victories in battle during wartime. While the youth of Sparta enjoyed dancing for its own sake, the men related dance to warfare and developed dance forms that symbolized the warriors in heated battle, to the point of wearing the actual raiments of war.

Sparta succeeded in developing strong, healthy young men and women who were the envy of the other city-states of Greece. Spartan athletes were dominant in the Olympic Games and in lesser athletic contests throughout the land for centuries. However, this educational system gradually failed because it did not produce well-rounded citizens who knew how to lead a civilized life of peace.

According to historical tradition, Romulus and Remus founded Rome in 753 B.C. In 27 B.C., Augustus became the first Roman emperor. The last Roman emperor was Romulus Augustus, whose reign ended in A.D. 476. At its zenith, the Roman Empire included most of Europe, the Middle East, and the northern coastal areas of Africa.

ROMAN EMPIRE

Roman governmental principles, which endure today, included justice, tolerance, and a desire for peace. Romans were educated in the qualities of (1) a sense of duty, (2) a seriousness of purpose, and (3) a sense of personal worth, all of which exist now as ideals for persons in most parts of the world. But Roman governmental control of thought and custom greatly weakened the Greek ideals of the complete, harmonious development of the individual. The Romans did not develop a philosophy of education that emphasized the all-around development of the human being.

The Baths. The Romans did perform in a variety of physical activities, but their attitudes and dedication to sport were not as positive as those of the Greeks. The Greek gymnasia (or palaestra) were replaced by the Roman baths (or thermae). Available to rich and poor alike, the baths consisted of bathing compartments that were sometimes heated and often richly decorated. Water, brought in by aqueduct, was also heated and distributed to the compartments by a system of pipes. Associated with the baths were open-air swimming pools and rooms for refreshment; weight training, massage, and other related activities were also available.

The city of Rome was plagued with a lack of space and facilities for physical recreation, exercise, and sport. One and a half million citizens were crowded into an area less than twelve miles in circumference. This probably accounts for the great popularity of the baths and related activities.

Games and Sports. Many Roman leaders, such as Julius Caesar, demonstrated a high degree of skill in horsemanship and fighting and were in excellent physical condition, thus serving as models for the young men of the country. Popular sports included ball games, running, jumping, wrestling, boxing, throwing the javelin and the discus, weight lifting, hunting , fishing, swimming, boating, acrobatics, juggling, tight-rope walking, bull wrestling, hoop play, net games, and board games.

Although a variety of sports activities were available, they were not engaged in by a majority of the population; most Romans participated in sport only as spectators. Professional sports and gladiatorial combat held the citizens' attention.

At the peak of the Roman era, 31 B.C. to A.D. 68, Roman games were staged in the Circus Maximus, drawing as many as 250,000 spectators, particularly for the chariot and horse races. Wagering on the races was encouraged. In the Coliseum, gladiators fought each other as well as wild beasts. Some observers of modern American life claim to see in our enthusiasm for professional football, baseball, basketball, and other sports a development of spectator interest similar to that of ancient Rome. These critics warn that the passivity of spectators and the commercialization of college sports (another throwback to the Roman era) bode ill for America in the future.

Over time, the Romans' philosophical attitude toward physical exercise became more and more positive. A noted Greek author and physician of the period, Galen, wrote about the values of exercise and its relationship to good health, thus spreading the message.

Recently discovered historical and archaeological evidence indicates more governmental interest and encouragement concerning exercise, physical recreation, and sport in the later years of the Roman ascendancy than has been previously attributed to this era by many historians.

THE MIDDLE AGES

The Middle Ages, or the Medieval era, denotes the period beginning during the fourth century A.D. with the fall of the Roman Empire and lasting approximately a thousand years, to the 14th century A.D. No longer could the people of the country depend upon the protection of the emperor and his armies. Therefore, small groups of families joined with nearby noblemen for mutual protection, thus developing many small, independent living units. These lords created small armies. Individual tenants on the adjacent farm lands had to fight in the armies of their lords when necessary. This system was called feudalism.

Feudalism. One characteristic of the Middle Ages was the flowering of the feudal system. Selected young men were trained in chivalry as they earned the right to knighthood. They were intensely indoctrinated into a system of customs and ethics involving religion, warfare, and personal demeanor and manners. While being thoroughly trained in horsemanship, fighting on horseback, and other areas of self-defense and attack, these youth learned an array of social customs and graces appropriate to their status as "gentlemen." Placed under the influence of the Christian Church, they were expected to exemplify the Christian virtues of mercy, loyalty, and concern for the weak and the poor. They served successively as a page and a squire before becoming a knight.

The knights comprised the noble class headed by the lords. The most valued characteristic of the knight was his physical prowess. Knights were taught to be superb horsemen, to swim and dive, to shoot accurately with hand- and crossbows, to climb rapidly on ladders, to fight and tilt in tournaments, to wrestle, fence and long jump, to dance gracefully, to play the popular board games of the era, and always to display courtly manners. In a manner of speaking, physical education was the main element in the training of the knight.

The age of chivalry reached its zenith in this era. Courtesy, loyalty, generosity, and physical excellence prevailed; and it was through the practice of these ideals that selected young men progressed into the upper class and into the established system of the feudal aristocracy. Paradoxically, although physical exercise and physical skills were emphasized throughout the development of these youth and during their service as knights, at the same time church elders generally discouraged participation in dance and sport because of their recollection of the undesirable types of sport promoted by the Romans and the use of these sports as pagan ceremonies.

The Teutonic Invasions. The invasion by barbarian tribes in the 11th century was another major influence on physical education history during the Middle Ages. Physically vigorous and hardy, the Teutons possessed traits of character that made them morally superior to the decadent Romans whom they conquered. Inured to an outdoor life, these and other barbarians brought to the civilized world new vitality with different customs.

During this era the works of the Greeks and the Romans were largely forgotten. Formal education was not only neglected, but also frequently despised. It is true that the lamp of learning was kept aflame in the medieval monasteries and universities, but organized education in the modern sense was practically nonexistent.

England. The development of sports in England during the Middle Ages was one of the most specific of all historical influences on American physical education. Our heritage of sports, now a significant feature of American life, comes almost entirely from the English people. The Middle Ages in England saw the development of such sports as archery, football, tennis, and many others commonly practiced today. This English love of sport, brought to America by the colonists, has been a major historical influence in the development of modern programs of sport and physical education in the United States.

Asceticism

The philosophy of asceticism originated in the early Christian era as a revolt against the sensuality of the decadent Romans. During this time, hermits increased in number. Religious converts lived a philosophical life of extreme self-denial and self-discipline in the monasteries. Later, the Puritans developed an ascetic philosophy of life which emphasized a harsh and joyless existence of self-deprivation. Out of asceticism have come expressions such as "the flesh and the Devil" to represent the prevailing negative attitude toward the physical aspects of life; practitioners of asceticism considered play to be childish, foolish, or vicious, and happiness to be prima facie evidence of sinfulness. Asceticism, in its pure form, was unable to recognize the value of joyousness, or to tolerate freedom of expression, or to appreciate physical striving and development. Even today this spirit of ascetism manifests itself from time to time in individuals and groups who oppose the expenditure of time and money to support and conduct programs of physical education and sport for the young. Physical educators and coaches must engage in a continual program of public education to overcome these inaccurate stereotypes and prejudices.

Scholasticism

Scholasticism developed from the study of the writings of early Christian scholars and the rediscovery of Aristotle's works, signalling the general appreciation for learning that was to lead to the Renaissance. Unfortunately, perhaps in reaction to the brutal ignorance of the times, scholars tended to emphasize the importance of the mind to the neglect of the body, at times to an extreme.

Traits of this attitude can still be discerned today among college and university faculties. Mental life and achievements are glorified while physical skills and performances are degraded, or at least are awarded less important status in the college curriculum. It is disconcerting that this view prevails as strongly as it does today when its tenets are contrary to modern scientific discoveries that verify that the human organism is a biological unity and that there can be no successful physical separation of mind, body, and spirit. Sometimes the "scholastic" professor accepts physical education in the school curriculum as merely a palliative or as a disciplinary agent, at best, or as a necessary evil that he or she does not have the power to eliminate, at worst. This attitude is gradually being changed, but it still constitutes an important challenge that physical educators must meet through effective dissemination and interpretation of the latest scientific evidence about the organismic unity of the human being.

The period beginning in the late 1200s and lasting through the Reformation of the 1500s is usually called the Renaissance; however, Renaissance, a French word meaning "rebirth," is misleading. Contrary to popular belief, the Middle Ages was not entirely stagnant — indeed, great advances in learning and social and economic development were seen during that period. In view of this, one can say that the Renaissance marked a change in emphasis rather than a rebirth of culture per se; that is, the religious emphasis of the Middle Ages gave way to a secular, or worldly, view of literature, art, government, and so on. The central interest of philosophy became humankind rather than God, and this new perspective was designated *humanism*.

The Renaissance placed less emphasis upon supremacy of religion in society and more reliance on the classical cultures of ancient Greece and Rome. This phase of the Renaissance is called *classicism*. Interest was revived in geography and in world exploration. There was a new growth of cities and a dedication to new freedom for the common person. Modern science also had its beginnings in this era and sought to overthrow superstition. New religious beliefs evolved exhibiting less reliance on the authority of the church and its headquarters in Rome. The invention of the printing press speeded up the transmission of new ideas and developed language systems throughout Europe. Students revived ancient Greek and Roman forms of art and methods of analysis in the great centers of learning. It was an era in which universities were established, including several of the greatest in Europe.

The Renaissance educators no longer followed the tenets of authoritarianism and scholasticism promoted in medieval times. Instead, they developed new programs of liberal, humanistic education that included a prominent place for physical training as well as education in personal manners and moral standards. Physical education owes much to the pioneer educator of the period of the Renaissance, and to an unbroken line of successors leading to the present day, for the measure of acceptance, understanding, and appreciation physical education has attained in today's world.

Humanism and Physical Education. The Athenian ideal of the harmonious development of the mind and the body was rekindled. Increased attention was given to health education and particularly to the importance of physical exercise. Young men were trained in all types of exercises as well as instructed in the skills of weaponry. The graceful coordinated body was stressed more than pure strength. Fencing, archery, sport tournaments, and other rugged war-like activities were popular, as were ballets, dancing, bowling, and tennis. As the new humanistic ideal of education and physical education gained prominence, the concept of the "whole man" was conceived and adopted as a guiding principle.

Girls and women were urged to participate in certain aspects of

CHAPTER THREE

physical education, including horseback riding and dance. They were not encouraged to engage in sporting games; however, they were urged to be spectators so that they could understand them and be able to discuss them intelligently with the men.

Some authorities contend that Italy originated and developed new physical education practices and ideas during the era of the Renaissance. Neighboring countries took their lead from the Italians, and they too gradually developed the types of physical education programs described above.

The previous sections of this chapter have described major influences from selected major historical eras and regions of the world, which have contributed significantly to the development of physical education and sport not only in the United States but also in many other countries. The purpose of the following section is to discuss the more immediate influence upon the development and expansion of organized physical education in America, and to indicate America's integration into the world picture of physical education. Three countries that have provided influential leadership in the development of physical education, not only within their own borders but also by extending their influence around the world, are Great Britain, Germany, and Sweden.

British Influence.   The Pilgrim colonists who settled in America were largely of British ancestry. They brought with them an age-old tradition of sports. From the time of their arrival to the present day, sports in one way or another have been a major element in American culture and tradition. Early threats of scholastic and puritanical control or abolition were never able to obliterate the love of sports and physical recreation held by the majority of the citizens of the United States.

During the Renaissance, leaders in England recognized the therapeutic value of physical education, and its contributions to the overall development of young men became more appreciated. Exercise was recognized as a necessary basis for good health. Books were written and distributed on this topic throughout the medical profession as well as in the educational system.

Leaders such as Erasmus did not agree with this new emphasis of the humanistic approach to physical education and spoke avidly against it. Erasmus' influence was so strong that physical education played little or no part in the curricula of schools and colleges established during the 16th century in England, where asceticism and Plato's concept of mind-body dualism were still perpetuated.

The value of physical education was debated between Church representatives and national government leaders, the latter group holding a positive view toward the role of physical education in the total education of youth. However, physical education and sport were not encouraged in the prestigious universities of Cambridge and Oxford and, in general, physical education was held in low esteem among scholars in the universities.

The conflict concerning the methods of educating young gentlemen in England, and the appropriate role of physical education in that education, continued to the period when the early settlers made their dramatic voyages to the United States. It is interesting to note that sports and games were forbidden to the students in certain institutions of higher education in early America, the overseers regarding these activities as undignified and detrimental to an atmosphere of scholarly endeavor. They did not recognize physical education and sport as being educational in any way. However, the strong heritage of British sports prevailed over the obstacles in higher education in the United States. The present acceptance and fully recognized status of sport and physical education programs in American education, at all levels, owe their very existence to the powerful heritage of British sports brought here by the first settlers.

German Influence. In Germany during the 1700s, a strong religious influence permeated the educational system. Also, there was an emphasis on scientific endeavors and on literary contributions, present and past. Although Germany was not yet a nation proper, a strong spirit of nationalism was taking hold of the German people, and in certain states, such as Prussia, the government was exercising increasing control over education and other major societal functions.

In 1774, at Dessau, Johann Bernhard Basdow established the first physical training program on a daily basis in a German school. A year later, Johann Guts Muth became the leader of this program and opened the program to all levels of society. Thus, Guts Muth has been regarded as one of the most important pioneers of modern physical education, and is famous in Europe and in American history for his contribution. He published many books which are still praised for their perceptive outlook. Many of his ideas were brought by German immigrants to America and were established in early American schools.

Swedish Influence. Sweden established one of the earliest institutes for the training of physical education teachers, the Royal Central Institute of Gymnastics in Stockholm, in 1814. The first director was Per Henrik Ling. Ling, who had visited the newly established gymnasiums in Germany, was a master fencer and also an established poet. His main contribution was to begin the search for a scientific basis to gymnastics or what we now call physical education. The Central Institute is still one of the most famous physical education institutes in the world.

In Sweden the basic concepts of physical education at the time of the discovery of America had a scientific basis in studies of human anatomy. This was in contrast to German gymnastics systems, which centered on spontaneous human growth, development, and maturation. The Swedish system, with a scientific base, challenged the German gymnastics programs and a controversy arose throughout Europe and the United States concerning the relative merits of the two systems, a debate that continued for several decades. The Swedish system was reinforced by the research studies conducted by Ling at the Royal Central Institute of Gymnastics in Stockholm.

As a result of this controversy, American schools took an eclectic position of compromise, borrowing and adapting major features of both the Swedish and German systems. The American school and college gymnasiums of the early 1900s commonly employed apparatus such as the Swedish climbing ladders, stall bars, poles, booms, balance boards, and incline ropes. Light apparatus such as dumbells, wands, and Indian clubs were also in popular use. In contrast, other gymnasia were equipped with German side-horses, parallel and horizontal bars, and bucks and similar heavy apparatuses which required a major emphasis on gymnastic feats of power and strength rather than skill, finesse, and grace.

During the era of 1890 to approximately 1915, American leaders in physical education sought to import the best features of the British, German, and Swedish systems of physical education and to adapt them to the developing American educational system. The heritage from these three countries emphasized a disciplined approach and the virtues of hard work and long practice. They required training in special techniques under the tutelage of expert coaches. Daily practice was advocated, except on Sunday. Swedish calisthenics had the added advantage of economy of time and money; it required no heavy apparatus. The Swedish "day's order" provided a balanced exercise workout in a brief time period. Traces of the influences of these three systems still can be seen in older American universities and in traditional secondary schools.

"The Battle of the Systems." Although American physical education, under the influence of imported systems, continued to place special emphasis on gymnastics, a trend gradually developed in which changes and innovations were introduced by American educators seeking a more nationally oriented program. Other physical educators, however, were reluctant to give up those aspects of the adopted systems, in particular those of Germany and Sweden, feeling them to be adequately suited to the nation's students. This conflict between physical education leaders came to be known as "the battle of the systems." Eventually, the original appeal of formal systems of gymnastics dwindled, partly because the authoritarian nature of the systems was incompatible with the American ideals of democracy and self-responsibility in an individualistic and competitive society, but also because of the growing appeal of active, out-of-doors recreation and sport activities which were made possible by the abundance of open spaces and new forms of rapid transportation.

It is emphasized that this historical account is not intended to indict gymnastics as a non-essential element in the modern school program of physical education. On the contrary, we, and virtually all teachers and leaders of physical education in this country, agree that modern gymnastics programs are essential in physical education at all educational levels. The American physical education curriculum today includes three major categories of activities, namely, sports, dance, and gymnastic exercises, and provides opportunities for widespread participation in a variety of activities under each of these categories. Likewise, in the organized physical education class, the major activity should be intensive instruction in skill development in these activities.

Gradually, the American system has increased the study of the foundational fields of physical education, such as sociology, biology, history, philosophy, physiology, and psychology, because of their acknowledged contributions to our greater understanding of the concepts and processes of human growth and development related to physical education participation, practice, and performance. In the twentieth century authorities in education and psychology alike realize that *play* is an important aspect of the educational process and an essential facet of human life.

Physical educators have long sought methods of integrating the school curriculum with the student's out-of-school physical recreation and voluntary competitive activities, with the aim of inculcating skill and enthusiasm for these activities in youngsters. The *community-school* concept, successfully exemplified by the Mott Program in Flint, Michigan, is being adopted by many schools and communities throughout the United States. Physical educators should exert leadership to develop local community school programs.

The twentieth century has seen a rapid development of school and community programs of physical education, physical recreation, sport, dance, and exercises. This text can only give examples of influential historical segments of this movement.

Rapid Growth of Physical Education. The Annual Report for 1899 of the Commissioner of Education, a publication of the United States Bureau of Education, contained a section on physical training. In the portion of the report devoted to "athletics," it was stated that the best interests of rational and effectual physical training have suffered from the undue prominence accorded to college athletic contests and contestants by "an uncritical public and an injudicious press."

Two years later, the *Review* reported that physical training was established in some form or other in 270 colleges and universities; 98 were doing organized work, 72 required physical exercises, and 24 gave credit for physical training in courses that counted toward a diploma.

The American Association for the Advancement of Physical Education was fifteen years old in 1900, and had published a magazine for four years. The National Executive Council of the Association consisted of nine individuals, six of whom were medical doctors.

Vacation schools and playgrounds in New York City opened in the summer of 1900 with 5,000 children enrolled. In Philadelphia, 28 playgrounds and five vacation schools were operating. For the first time in the history of vacation schools in Buffalo, the city bore the expense with teachers volunteering their services. In Chicago, four vacation schools had operated during the previous summer of 1899. Three outdoor gymnasiums were open for summer use in Boston.

In the year 1900, a written examination for applicants for licensure to teach physical training in any or all of the boroughs of the City of New York was announced. By 1903, there were 52 normal schools offering courses to prepare for teaching gymnastics in the public schools, even though the teaching of physical education was required by law in only a few of the states.

In 1903, the City of Chicago passed a $5,500,000 bond issue for the establishment of additional parks and the erection of field houses in the South Park System. The following year, the City of Los Angeles set up a board of playground commissioners.

In 1905, the results of a questionnaire to which 555 cities responded revealed that only 128 cities employed teachers of physical training, of whom 102 were men and 189 were women. Of the 555 cities, 125, or 23 per cent, had one or more high school gymnasiums. Swedish gymnastics was the most frequently used method of instruction in this program. Competitive athletics in high school were approved by 115 of the 128 cities with special teachers, and by 323 of the 427 cities without special teachers. Incidentally, 243 of the 427 cities without special teachers of physical education *did* have high school athletic organizations.

Research in physical education began in the early years of the twentieth century. It was predominantly medical in focus and much of it was conducted by physicians.

Wartime Influences. Not unexpectedly, American involvement in wars always provokes an intensified interest in and attention to physical education, physical training, and physical fitness. During World War I, physical education programs were accelerated throughout the public schools of the country with strong emphasis on physical training.

The dramatic increases in physical fitness, easily demonstrable

CHAPTER THREE

through intensified exercise programs conducted by all of the armed services, along with shocking draft statistics revealing a high percentage of medical rejections among drafted young men, prompted professional leaders in education and physical education, and medical authorities, to exert pressure upon state legislatures to pass laws requiring mandatory attendance in public school physical education programs. In many cases this legislation covered the gamut from grade one through grade twelve. Likewise, four-year colleges and universities jumped on the band wagon and instituted mandatory two- to four-year programs for all students in the 1920s. To a large extent, these legislative mandates were justified on a health basis. The erroneous idea that physical education alone could make people healthy gave the program an impetus and public support that it undoubtedly could not have gained in any other way. The physical fitness objective is still the most prominent argument advanced today for retention of required programs in schools and colleges.

Playgrounds. Following World War I, the playground movement in America expanded rapidly. Voluntary sports and other play activities predominated. Many youngsters were able to take advantage of these free facilities and programs, and thus became motivated toward further participation in a variety of physical education activities. The games program readily expanded from the playground into school physical education and recreation programs. Playground programs can be credited with the general strengthening of programs of physical education in schools across the nation.

During the depression years of the 1930s, the Federal Government, through Work Projects Administration (WPA) and Public Works Administration (PWA) programs and funds, constructed many school sport facilities, such as gymnasiums, athletic fields, swimming pools, and tennis courts. By 1937, it was estimated that $75 million had been spent on such projects.

Many community governments allocated funds to build public facilities for swimming, tennis, golf, badminton, and other popular sports. Eventually, school districts contracted with communities to utilize these facilities for instructional purposes during school hours. Thus, both school physical education programs and community-based recreation programs benefited from increased participation and facility utilization.

Leisure Education. In 1918, the famous Seven Cardinal Principles of education were published. They had a marked influence on the development and change in school curricula. One of the seven cardinal principles was that of "the worthy use of leisure." Physical educators were alerted and stimulated to organize and expand their programs to meet this important objective. Likewise, it boosted their morale and provided great satisfaction with the realization that physical education was a fundamental subject in the mandatory curriculum of the public schools. Also, perceptive leaders of education, physical education, and recreation realized the tremendous importance of American citizens utilizing increasing amounts of leisure time in helpful, beneficial, and positive ways. This prognostication has, indeed, come true and use of leisure is now one of the major practical and philosophical dilemmas of American society. Physical education has an essential role to play in effecting viable programs for all American citizens as they seek "the worthy use of leisure."

Not only have school programs provided leadership in leisure activities, but also many private, semi-private, and public agencies have provided significant programs, in sports as well as other related youth and adult activities. Such organizations as the Boy Scouts, the Girl Scouts, the Young Men's and Women's Christian Associations (YMCA, YWCA), Boys' Clubs, fraternal organizations, and church groups of all denominations have provided vigorous leadership and excellent facilities for programs of physical and other recreation.

Other agencies have emphasized sports programs, such as police departments with their boys' clubs, the American Red Cross through its intensive campaigns in swimming and water safety instruction, the Boys' and Fathers' Clubs sponsored by national service clubs. Similar organizations have contributed to the continual expansion of sport and fitness opportunities for youth and adults in this country over the years.

Professional Certification. Since World War I, each of the 50 states has instituted legal requirements for the certification of teachers of physical education in order to ensure that teachers and coaches will be properly qualified. This movement has forced colleges and universities to provide comprehensive and high quality professional preparation programs for neophyte teachers and coaches. Therefore, the overall quality of professional leadership in physical education and sport has steadily improved over the years and this trend continues today.

In the period immediately following World War II, there was a rapid increase in the number of young families and a subsequent increase in numbers of children attending schools, which caused a school population explosion through the late 1960s. One outcome of the rapid expansion of new schools and the enrollment of thousands of new students in many communities was the necessity of employing additional physical education teachers with less than standard credentials. States passed emergency laws permitting schools to employ minimally qualified teachers on "emergency" credentials. In too many cases, the result was a decline in the quality of instruction provided.

Decline in School Enrollment. In recent years there has been a decline in school enrollment with the attendant closing of schools in many communities. Employment opportunities for new teachers have markedly decreased, since experienced teachers are more likely to remain in their current positions than they are to transfer or to retire. One positive effect of this movement is that there is no longer the necessity to employ less than fully qualified "emergency" credentialed teachers, but a growing problem is the lack of "new blood" because of the limited employment opportunities for highly qualified, bright, young teachers.

Coaching Credential. Another milestone in the raising of standards in physical education was the recent introduction of the "coaching credential." In some states, would-be coaches in public schools must now attain the special coaching credential before the school can assign them to coaching positions in particular sports. Many colleges and universities are now offering minor programs in coaching.

Equality for Women. During the early 1970s, passage of landmark federal and state legislation has required equal treatment of women teachers and coaches with respect to employment opportunity and assignments in sports and physical education; equal pay for equal services in teaching and coaching; and equal educational opportunity for all

Current Trends

female students in all phases of the physical education and sport programs under the jurisdiction of the schools and colleges. Chapter 7 expands on this topic.

There has been a continual evolution of attitudes with respect to the roles of girls and women in the twentieth century, which in turn has influenced school and college programs of physical education and sport. Schools and colleges have not taken the lead, as perhaps they should have, but most are now moving quickly toward establishing equal freedom and opportunities for all students.

In many localities in the United States it is obvious that more funds are spent, more time devoted, and more facilities provided for the physical education of boys and men than of girls and women. The disparity is gradually diminishing. Most educators today appreciate the importance educationally, as well as legally, of providing the same variety and quality of opportunities for participation, excellent programs of instruction, and adequate facilities for girls as for boys. One of the most encouraging aspects of the new recognition of equality for women in physical education and sport is the inclusion of girls and boys on the same teams, participating against each other on a coeducational basis. The gradual abolition of the taboo of women coaching male sport teams is laudable.

The first woman president of the American Physical Education Association, Mabel Lee, was elected in 1930. Within two years, the National Section on Women's Athletics became a recognized part of the Association. Since that time women have been elected to more and higher offices in the various professional associations of physical education and sport. In general, girls' and women's sports are now accepted as an integral part of the educational experience and of American life.

Growth of Competitive Sports. Schools and colleges continue to extend the types and varieties of sport in their programs within their financial limitations. The expansion of competitive sport has had a positive influence on the physical education curriculum. Some high schools now have as many as 30 or more sports available to all students, boys and girls alike. The design and construction of gymnasiums, swimming pools, tennis courts, and playing fields have been directly influenced by the incorporation of these activities into the total program. These facilities are now used for class instruction, intramural participation, interscholastic competition, and, frequently, for community recreation during non-school hours.

Extramural Sport for Children. Sport programs under non-school auspices are increasing at a rapid rate in the United States. In fact, this movement is among the prominent developments in the history of American sport. Countless thousands of boys and girls are now competing in Pop Warner football, Iddy Biddy basketball, Babe Ruth baseball, age-group swimming, youth tennis, soccer, and many other types of sport activities. Such programs, however, are being increasingly scrutinized, as highly competitive sports for elementary school children sponsored by agencies and organizations which are not school- or community-based become the subject of debate.

Criticism and Debate. It has been charged, for example, that the widespread popularity of Little League baseball, Pop Warner football, and similar youth programs is due to the failure of the schools and community recreation agencies to provide suitable sport opportunities for these youngsters. The tremendous participation figures, which total

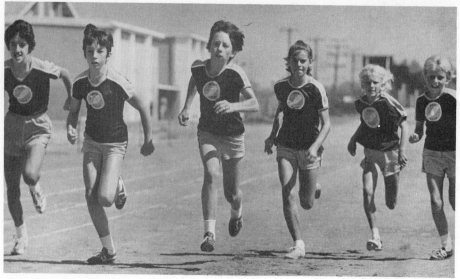

The effect of highly competitive athletic participation upon young children is a controversial issue.

in the millions in this and other countries, are direct evidence of the popularity of these sport programs, many of which are administered and conducted by adult volunteers and even teenagers, most of whom lack proper professional preparation in education, sport, and basic first aid and medical care.

Major issues involved in the controversy about the values and the potential dangers in these programs include (1) the safety and sanitary conditions under which these contests are conducted; (2) the qualifications and motives of the sponsoring and coaching adult leaders; (3) the possibilities of serious physical injury; (4) the intense emotional pressure that can be exerted on very young children by enthusiastic parents and coaches who strive to win the league championship, the city playoff, or the regional, state, and national championship; (5) the psychological effects of questionable values resulting from over-emphasis on winning at such an early age; and (6) the large amounts of money, equipment, facilities, and attention heaped on a relatively small percentage of highly skilled youngsters.

Medical and other organizations and committees have published official statements of standards, suggested rules for the conduct of the sport under safe conditions, and other educational materials in an attempt to direct the promotion and conduct of these sport programs in the safest possible manner with optimal educational outcomes. Many individuals who are professionally prepared in education, sport, and medicine are volunteering their services to local sponsoring agencies in order to communicate professional standards, educational principles, and research findings, and to provide education and guidance to the adult leaders so that the recommended standards will be adopted and used.

Increased Emphasis on Research. There is proliferation of research in various aspects of physical education and sport. More and more persons are being trained in research concepts and methodologies with respect to specialized phases of physical education on the graduate level. Major

CHAPTER THREE

universities and colleges are providing larger research facilities and more sophisticated research instrumentation to facilitate the investigations of these young scholars. In fact, the development of specialties in physical education and sport research borders on the incredible. More specialized journals are becoming available for the reporting of research findings and more cooperative research is being undertaken with colleagues in other disciplines.

Pure research and applied research are receiving increased attention. Attempts are being made to translate research findings into principles to be followed by teachers and coaches in the teaching of athletes, in the care and prevention of injuries, and in athletic training in general. As more research evidence is produced, the physical educator can more accurately assess the extent to which educational aims and objectives are being realized. Research findings give us the "final answer," and their accretion over time should provide us with a gradually improving basis for faith in the efficacy of our efforts to educate American youth.

All of the subdisciplinary areas of physical education have attracted well-trained, intelligent researchers who are now gaining collegial acceptance in the circles of academic sponsorship. Physical education practitioners should study continuously to improve their understanding and utilization of research findings to direct their everyday responsibilities of administration, program planning, teaching and coaching, and student and program evaluation.

SUMMARY

As is obvious by the length of this chapter, a review of major aspects of the history of physical education is a vast project. In addition to the standard history books in physical education listed in the references at the end of the chapter, attention is invited to other recent publications.

The North American Society for Sport History provides a source for the study of the ever evolving collection of interesting historical research reports about sport and physical education. The *Proceedings* are published yearly and contain abstracts of presentations made at the annual Society conference. The diversity and scope of the topics being studied by sport historians are impressive. The publication also provides the most inclusive and extensive listing of references and brief summaries of historical research in sport available in this country. Many of the articles are instructive and of benefit to the practicing teacher, coach, or researcher.

Another publication of particular value is *A History of Sport and Physical Education to 1900*, edited by Earle F. Zeigler.[21] It contains scholarly contributions from noted historical researchers in physical education on a wide array of interesting topics throughout human existence on this earth.

Many myths concerning sport are being overturned or modified by recent rigorous investigations. A solid knowledge of the historical background of sport and physical education serves as a platform for understanding principles and practices and applying them to the ongoing improvement of programs in this phase of American education. Also, through these materials the young physical education major can become acquainted with another area of potential study and employment in the vast and complex field of physical education and sport.

Purposes. Comparative education is one of the subdivisions of the theory of education. This special field of education concentrates on the investigation and interpretation of educational policies and practices in various cultures and countries throughout the world.

Bereday[22] says

> Comparative education seeks to make sense out of the similarities and differences among educational systems. It catalogs educational methods across national frontiers; and in this catalog each country appears as one variant of the total score of mankind's educational experience. If well set off, the like and the contrasting colors of the world perspective will make each country a potential beneficiary of the lessons thus received.

The result of these investigations and analyses is a set of general principles that provides guidance to policy-makers, administrators, and other active participants in the conduct and direction of educational systems.

At the theoretical level, comparative education is considered to be a general social science that employs theories, hypotheses, models, and laws to clarify the fundamental processes of education. Important relevant data collected by the formal research methods can be categorized and their functional interrelationships can be examined. The hypotheses of the theoretical comparative educational scientist can be tested in the crucible of experience. This field is coming to be recognized as a discipline in its own right.

Educators with a more practical slant employ comparative education processes and information as they seek new ways to improve the administration and conduct of the schools, and, ultimately, to contribute to the more effective learning of the students. Practical reform in education is their purpose.

Lauwerys[23] summarizes the values of comparative studies and research:

> Even when adaptation and adoption are impossible, the fruits of comparative study have value. Through contrast and comparison, we are led to a better and deeper understanding of what we ourselves do. And sometimes we learn that practices and arrangements which we thought were based upon reason and experience are, in fact, based only on prejudice or on an unreasoning reverence for tradition.

Research. With improved research methodology, a trend has developed toward using the phrase "international studies in education" interchangeably with the old term "comparative education." Comparative education seeks to solve educational problems primarily with research methodologies from political science and sociology. Development education uses research methods of economics. International education uses research techniques from anthropology. Some overlap in these categories is impossible to prevent.

The research procedures involved in comparative education studies are location, retrieval, and classification of information, both quantitative and descriptive, concerning schools, school systems, the administration of schools, their financial bases, pupils and instructors, teaching methods, curriculum designs, legal bases, and other relevant considerations. Information and data concerning these topics are analyzed in relation to the historical background of the development of the educational systems under scrutiny. The researcher determines the extent to which the evidence gathered has been influenced by, and is related to, philosophical, social, religious, technological, and economic factors, along with national and racial prejudices and value systems.

Eckstein and Noah[24] state that in recent years the methodology of research in comparative education has changed from emphasis on philosophical and historical tradition to the use of techniques from the social sciences. The mere collection of facts has little or no meaning unless facts are placed in the context of explanation. The new research tests hypotheses that have been developed from the most recent theoretical propositions. Pure theory is of little use unless it is tested empirically. Therefore, recent research is scientific, empirical, and uses cross-national data.

It is now customary for investigators to consider the relationship between selected areas of education and one or more specific aspects of society, such as its cultural beliefs, its economic system, or its political and social structures. Such research collects, compares, and reports data from at least two national polities or from subnational units. Some studies employ global data drawn from all of the countries being studied.

Simultaneous Comparison. Simultaneous comparison is one of the major research methodologies. It has two steps: The first step is juxtaposition, which Eckstein and Noah[25] define as " the preliminary matching of data from different countries to prepare them for comparison." Also involved is the development of one or more hypotheses, which are devised on the probability that the collected data will tell something about them.

There are two forms of juxtaposition — tabular and vertical. The latter is more popular although either method facilitates comparison. After setting up one or the other type, hypotheses are developed to define tentatively a relation between the data.

The investigator tries to make a balanced comparison. When this is not possible, what is called "illustrative" comparison may be utilized. The educational practices of various countries are selected randomly as illustrations of comparative points suggested by the data. In this process no generalizations can be drawn and thus no laws can be deduced. Thus it is an inferior type of comparison.

Some authorities are encouraging a more empirical approach to research in comparative education and the collection of better data. This aim is being carried out by a closer integration between education and the social sciences in order to make systematic comparisons with a greater degree of rigor. Arnold Anderson[26] says, "In its broadest sense, comparative education might be defined as cross-cultural comparison of the structure, operation, aims, methods, and achievements of various educational systems, and the societal correlates of these educational systems and their elements."

Two Conceptions of Comparative Educational Research. There are two major conceptions of comparative educational research. In the first, investigators deal mainly with educational data as though education were an autonomous social system. They relate or find correlations between two or more variables within an educational system. In this way educational systems between nations can be compared with reference to specific variables.

The second approach to comparative educational research is to relate traits of educational systems to other important aspects of the society. Obviously, this technique emphasizes the larger social context within which education operates. For example, there is a strong interest now in studying the relevance of education for economic development. Some political scientists are studying the influence of political socialization and the importance of schooling in developing ruling elites. In all of these ways, basically, comparative education has the aim of developing and understanding the effects of causation.

Types of Research Studies. Jones[27] gives an interesting brief description of several types of comparative research studies.

1. *The "Package Tour."* The investigator, going from one country to the next, has a check-list of topics and processes to observe and describe. Obviously, this method is largely descriptive in nature. Some investigators regard it as sufficiently interesting in itself to be valuable. It is the most superficial of the several methods described. It is not very rigorous nor scientific and has been long criticized for these reasons.

2. *The Academic Approach.* Interested scholars study educational systems of different countries primarily because they are intellectually curious about them. An ever greater mass of subject matter and knowledge is being collected. It is constantly being ordered and reorganized, and more attempts are made to analyze it and to manipulate it by increasingly rigorous scientific techniques from the social science fields. This approach goes far beyond reliance on the descriptive methods. This type of rigorous analysis is intellectually worthy on its own merits.

3. *Comparative Education as a Useful Study.* This type of research is conducted by specialists working with state or other national governments to assist in solving some of the major educational problems. Learning from and adapting successful operations and experiences from their own countries and others enables these experts to make viable recommendations to the national government with which they are working.

4. *Increased Data Availability.* Comparative education studies are increasing rapidly, and the detail and sophistication of the methodology is likewise moving rapidly. More international organizations are giving support. There is increased opportunity now for scholars and interested observers to travel to other countries on educational research assignments. More books, magazines, and research articles are being made available worldwide; and printed material is becoming more accessible through the speed-up in technological equipment that facilitates exchange of information around the world.

5. *Comparative and International Education.* In the 1960s, the Comparative Education Society changed its name to include the word International, thus reflecting a concern for the practical outcomes of education, particularly in developing countries where acute problems are faced daily. It is hoped that strong educational intervention will help to alleviate them.

6. *Purposes in Comparative Education.* Many authorities agree that there is a greater need for careful, detailed planning in the educational sector of developing countries. Such countries are reluctant to foster experimentation in schools. They seek available scientific knowledge on which to base their planning. Planning involves formulation of objectives, identification and use of relevant facts, establishment of priorities, and identification of means and procedures for achieving the objectives most efficiently. The destiny of millions of citizens may well depend upon the quality of the planning. Planners from several academ-

ic disciplines are necessary. The role of educational planners is crucial; they are vital members of this interdisciplinary planning team.

International education involves some of the procedures and methodologies of comparative education. However, in addition, it concentrates on cross-national relationships, mutual cooperation, and exchange of educational leaders. International relations and mutual cooperation are emphasized through the exchange of teachers, students, educational materials, financial aid, and instructional technology.

Another objective of international education is cross-national and international mutual understanding and good will. For example, American physical educators and sport leaders are involved in international education as Fulbright scholars and as consultants appointed by the United States Department of State to be advisors or to serve in exchange roles with colleagues from educational institutions, physical education and sport colleges, and similar institutions abroad. The many international conferences and congresses in physical education and sport discussed elsewhere in this chapter also are prime examples of international education.

Sport and physical education are major instruments in the struggle between national and political ideologies throughout the world. The American public, through Congress, gave the State Department a mandate to conduct an educational exchange program with the free countries of the world in order to develop more friendly relations and better understanding.

Noted athletes and coaches, physical education teachers, professors, scholars, and graduate students are involved in these exchange programs. The State Department understands the necessity of presenting a balanced picture of American culture in the exchange programs; when Supreme Court Chief Justice Warren, poet Robert Frost, and author William Faulkner were delegated to represent America abroad, noted sport figures such as Jesse Owens, Sammy Lee, and Bob Mathias were

International Education

West German children enjoy active participation in physical education.

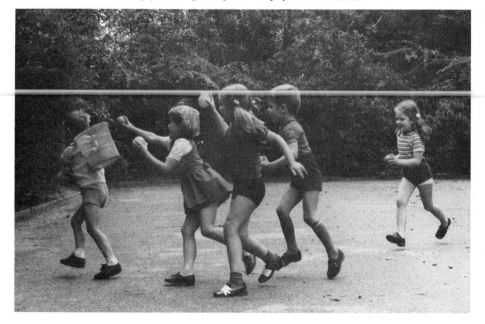

also commissioned to visit foreign countries as emissaries of the United States, thus presenting a balanced picture of the American scene.

In Soviet Russia and other countries in the Eastern European bloc sport is seen as a tool of propaganda and an instrument of national policy, one of the means for strengthening the party line of Soviet authority.

Research. Research in development education involves the study of patterns of interactions between a nation's educational system and its environment, with particular attention to those interactions which promote modernization and development. Indeed, a basic and natural assumption of this research is that education systems and processes aid in the development of the economic, political, social, and cultural life of a country. Guided by theories about development taken from other sciences, as well as from education itself, development education analyzes the results of innovations in educational systems and evaluates alternative solutions for various problems. The ultimate goal of such studies is to aid in the evolution of better government policy- and decision-making procedures, thereby contributing to the welfare of the people of the country.

To avoid confusion between the studies of comparative versus development education, some authorities claim that development education emphasizes the *dynamics* (i.e., processes, influences, and interactions) of education, while comparative education studies primarily the *statics* (or descriptive elements) of education.

Projects. Development education replaced the earlier "fundamental education" and Point Four programs of the 1950s. At that time the United States Government had committed vast quantities of financial and personnel aid to lesser developed countries in many fields, including agriculture, economics, education, and sport. Community and personal health programs were stressed, as was fundamental or literacy education, but physical education and sport played a relatively minor role in these programs. Whereas other countries, such as England, East and West Germany, and Russia, have recognized the importance of sport and physical education assistance to new nations and poor countries around the world, the United States only recently implemented such programs as the Peace Corps in these areas as part of overall development education projects.

International Development Education (IDE) is pursued within an explicit cross-national and cross-cultural framework, which permits one's analysis to escape the limitations of a given economic or ecologic setting, sociopolitical structure, or culturally given cognitive or value heritage. Each national (or subnational) system, at a given point in time, represents a certain stage of development as reflected by the output of its economic system, the extent of individual autonomy in its political system, the degree of specialization and differentiation of its social system, or the secularization of its value system.

We are now becoming aware of the major impact that aid through sport and physical education can make on the people and the governments of lesser developed countries. For example, upon the request of foreign countries, the President's Council on Physical Fitness and Sport provides consultants in sport and physical education to render expert

Development Education

assistance and advice. The State Department, also upon request, assigns selected individuals to missions that provide leadership in the development of sport and physical education programs in host countries. More and more countries are taking the initiative to invite noted leaders of sport and physical education from America to serve as consultants, instructors, coaches, and professors in national sport institutes, in national universities, and in sport medicine institutes.

Similarly, American colleges, universities, state departments of education, and other public and private educational sport organizations are inviting distinguished foreign colleagues in sport and physical education to spend time in this country in consultant and academic roles. Some institutions, such as Stanford University, request Visiting Scholars in sport and physical education to join the faculty for an academic year and to work closely with their American colleagues on projects of mutual cross-cultural interest.

INTERNATIONAL PHYSICAL EDUCATION

In recent years large numbers of physical educators from the United States have visited other countries either on a formal educational assignment or informally as interested tourists. They have attended international conferences and visited schools, sport clubs, and international sporting events. Also, they have served as visiting instructors and research specialists in response to formal invitations from physical education institutes or national governments. The *Journal of Physical Education and Recreation*, the *Physical Educator*, and other professional publications contain numerous reports of the experiences and reactions of American physical educators in various countries around the world. As a result of these stimulating and thrilling experiences, a strong interest in *international physical education* has developed, particularly in the colleges and universities in this country. Every year more institutions initiate courses in this area. Sometimes such a course is required in the physical education major program, while in other instances it is provided on an elective basis.

Research

Physical educators in America have contributed few significant, formal comparative and international research studies. It is true that physical educators in America, as well as in other countries, have written many articles and monographs describing systems of physical education and sport in their countries. But this endeavor cannot be classified as comparative research.

A recent book by Bennett, Howell, and Simri[28] is a modest beginning, offering well-reasoned comparisons of specific aspects of sport in eleven selected countries. Vendien and Nixon[29] made an early contribution with a descriptive approach utilizing national leaders in selected countries to describe major elements of health, physical education, and recreation programs in their respective countries, following a common outline in each chapter. Thus, the interested reader could develop informal comparisons between countries.

The Phi Epsilon Kappa fraternity series of monographs, *Physical Education Around the World*, edited by William Johnson,[30] also provides descriptive information about physical education and sport in selected countries. The references at the end of this chapter indicate other sources of information concerning sport and physical education in various countries throughout the world.

D. W. J. Anthony[31] states his position concerning the objectives of comparative and international research in physical education and sport:

1. To establish reliable data on each country and system, separately and collectively.
2. To analyze differences and similarities with particular attention to the relation of theory to practice.
3. To try to understand the past, to predict future trends, and to assist in the formulation of policy.
4. To examine the need for the reform of one's own methods and systems, and to contribute to a universal improvement of standards and knowledge.
5. To relate what we know about sport and physical education to our knowledge of all other relevant disciplines.

The value of study and research in comparative physical education is indicated by Vendien and Nixon:[32]

> All students are enlightened by exposure to other cultural concepts and social systems. The comparative approach is educative in providing information about the unknown, in clarifying aims and practices taken for granted but little understood in one's own culture, in stimulating insights regarding program improvements, and in encouraging international professional collaboration.
>
> The comparative education approach involves the hypothesis that: (a) Any educational system or part thereof is partially patterned by the traditional values and practices in the culture. (b) Any educational system within a former colonial country is more strongly patterned by the cultural traditions of the colonial power than by its own traditions, these foreign traditions usually being disfunctional but in many ways permanently influential. (c) Any educational system in a developing nation is subject to the danger of a sustained colonial pattern or a hastily copied Western pattern. Rationale and results should be examined, then adjusted or changed according to conscious choice. (d) Any educational system in a so-called developed nation is subject to the danger of assumed excellence. Thus obsolescence becomes a possibility. Again, the rationale and results should be examined, then adjusted or changed according to conscious choice.
>
> Any program of health, physical education, and recreation is part of the total educational system, and as such has responsibilities both to the total system and to its specific portion.

Bennett, Howell, and Simri[33] have edited the most complete book yet available on comparative and international physical education and sport. Readers interested in this topic will find valuable information about 35 selected countries. As the authors state,

> This book cannot provide the answers to questions or the solution of problems of particular countries. But it is an attempt to study in some depth sport and physical education in 35 selected countries, to gather data, and to present them in a manner which will be of optimal functional use to the reader. The authors sincerely hope that this procedure will then contribute to a better understanding of physical

education and sport which will help individual teachers, coaches, students, inspectors, administrators, and other involved people to work more effectively and rationally with programs in their own lands.

The methodological approach in this book provides useful information on a comparative basis for a wide array of fundamental topics in sport and physical education. The authors note that this methodology is a "second level step above the country-by-country analysis," and claim that a new milestone in physical education and sport comparative research is thus exemplified.

Bennett, Howell, and Simri outline methodological components essential to the comparative study of physical education and sport. Most studies in physical education and sport can be categorized methodologically as historical-descriptive. Conceptual frameworks have been created by some authors in an attempt to report and compare major features of physical education programs in two or more countries. The "Framework for Physical Education and Sport" by Reet Nurmberg and M. L. Howell, reported in the Bennett, Howell, and Simri book (pp. 33–34), is an excellent example for interested physical education scholars and researchers. Other physical education frameworks are discussed by Bennett, Howell, and Simri.

Dr. Lynn Vendien,[34] of the University of Massachusetts, compared physical education and sport in eleven countries. She reviewed demographic materials, cultural variables, economic elements, geographical descriptions, comparisons of national educational systems, agricultural resources, objectives of physical education programs, requirements in physical education programs, physical education and sport facilities, types of examinations and syllabi available in physical education and sport, levels and types of competitive sports in educational institutions, teacher and coach preparation and status, and prevailing problems and trends. Vendien's analysis qualifies as basic research in comparative physical education and provides a prototype that, when expanded, will result in significant research data and conclusions.

A review of recent articles in the *Journal of Physical Education and Recreation* and the *Research Quarterly* and of masters' and doctoral theses and dissertations in the microform catalogues fails to identify any studies that can be accurately classified as rigorous comparative physical education research. Also, seldom if ever does the physical education and sport literature contain articles that take the international educational or development educational approach in the pure sense described above.

The available American literature on comparative and international physical education and sport consists mainly of articles and books describing the visits of American physical educators to other countries, reporting on such topics as the people, programs, and facilities observed in sport and physical education contexts. Occasionally, statements of personal reaction or impressions are included.

Textbooks on comparative physical education still are scarce. The major texts now available in the United States, as cited in the footnotes at the end of the chapter, are Bennett, Howell, and Simri,[35] Vendien and Nixon,[36] Johnson,[37] Kolatch,[38] Van Dalen and Bennett[39] and Zeigler, Howell, and Trekell.[40]

Semotiuk[41] provides a provocative statement on theoretical and methodological research considerations concerning comparative and international sport and physical education:

> Because of the close relationship between physical education and education, it is quite conceivable that useful information and frameworks derived from comparative education could be applied to comparative physical education. Because of the recent emphasis on the development of classification techniques and application of techniques from related social sciences, comparative education can be very helpful in stimulating a more rapid creation of mature methodology in comparative physical education. It should be pointed out that most studies of comparative education make very little mention about physical education. The neglected treatment accorded physical education by comparative educators defies logical explanation.
>
> What seems to be urgently needed at present is a critical examination and enlargement of the current body of comparative physical educational theory; a broader, more valid and realistic formulation of aims, values, and techniques on the basis of new knowledge and contemporary problems and practices. The adoption of an interdisciplinary approach utilizing concepts and methods from several fields of inquiry exemplifies the eclectic nature that comparative physical education must assume in the future.

Physical education in the United States is in an early stage of growth in comparative, international, and developmental research. The future holds much promise for interested, bright, young scholars who qualify themselves for the research roles described above.

Organizations Concerned with International Relations in Health, Physical Education, and Recreation

1. United Nations Educational, Scientific and Cultural Organization, 19 Avenue Kleber, Paris-16e, France.

2. International Council on Health, Physical Education, and Recreation of the World Confederation of Organizations in the Teaching Profession (129-member organization in 73 countries).

3. American Alliance for Health, Physical Education, Recreation, and Dance, International Council. 1201 16th Street, N.W., Washington, D. C. 20036.

4. People-to-People Sports Committee, 20 Exchange Place, New York, New York 10005.

5. National Education Association, Committee on International Relations, Washington, D. C. 20036.

6. The Peace Corps, Washington, D. C. 20025.

7. Teacher Exchange Section, Office of Education, Department of Health, Education and Welfare, Washington, D. C. 20025. (Teaching positions in elementary and secondary schools in national and American-sponsored schools abroad.)

8. Institute of International Education, Information and Counseling Division, 800 Second Avenue at 42nd Street, New York, New York 10017.

9. Agency for International Development, Personnel Office, Washington, D. C. 20025.

10. U.S. Information Agency, Chief, Employment Branch, Personnel Division, Washington, D. C. 20025.

11. International Schools Foundation, Inc., Personnel Services, 147 East 50th Street, New York, New York 10022.

12. Asia Foundation, 550 Kearny Street, San Francisco, California 94108.

13. International Recreation Association, 345 East 46th Street, United Nations Plaza, New York, New York 10017.

14. American Overseas Educators Organization, Inc., 725 So. Division, Ann Arbor, Michigan 48103.

15. Conference Board of Associated Research Councils, Committee on International Exchange of Persons, 2101 Constitution Avenue, N. W., Washington, D. C. 20025. (Fulbright Grants; Smith-Mundt Awards.)

International Movements Art Center, Inc. The International Movements Art Center is another recent organization of interest to physical educators. It was founded in 1976, and its address is P.O. Box 0, Stanford, California 94305. Its purposes are to explore the historical, cultural, psychological, and philosophical aspects of the traditional martial arts and their derivatives. The Center also developed a martial arts-based movement education program for elementary schools. This curriculum can be adapted for use at the college level and in adult education classes. The Center endeavors to inform the public about the broad scope and rich heritage of the martial arts, and their application as gentle ways of being in the world.

International Sport and Physical Education Data System (ISPEDS). The International Sport and Physical Education Data System was founded in 1977 at the University of California, Santa Barbara, California 93106. The System provides centralized, continuously updated access to information on international and national events. It is intended to serve as a clearinghouse for information for the purpose of organizational forecasting, planning, budgeting, and participation. The System consists of a current data base of worldwide sport and physical education events as they happen. It is designed for retrieval of historical information as well as to project future events and activities within the framework of world sport and physical education.

Center for the Study of Instructional Sport and Physical Education. Another example of increasing emphasis on international sport and physical education studies is the Center for the Study of International Sport and Physical Education, at the California State University, Long Beach, founded in 1973. The syllabus from the Center indicates that "sport and physical education is a vehicle by which the oneness and the diversity of mankind may be developed, practiced and preserved in an atmosphere of trust and growth."

The Center provides an interdisciplinary curriculum, available to both undergraduates and graduates. Programs are highly individualized. Guest faculty members who are noted leaders in other countries are invited to the Center for short-term assignments. Students and faculty members interested in international education attend the Center from numerous countries around the world as well as the United States.

Study tours are conducted in the summers to selected historical sport sites in other countries. Sport teams from other countries are invited to come to the United States on tour to compete against teams of several colleges and universities. The Center also emphasizes research on many aspects of international sport in various countries.

The International Olympic Academy. The Academy was formally organized in 1961 under the sponsorship of the Hellenic Olympic Committee and the auspices of the International Olympic Committee. The proposal for the establishment of the Academy was first made in 1949 to the International Olympic Committee in Rome. The Academy occupies 100 acres in Olympia, Greece, sponsored by the national government, and is located near the famous ancient Olympic stadium.

The purpose of the Academy is to promote, maintain, and interpret the Olympic spirit and ideals. Many concerned sport leaders and educators fear that the original Olympic spirit has been lost or perverted in recent years. The Academy sponsors studies, analyses, and interpretations of the true Olympic ideal and attempts to interest individuals and groups around the world in this pursuit. For approximately two weeks each summer, the Academy conducts an international program attended by representatives of many countries. The agenda includes discussions of the ideals of the Games, the development of spiritual and moral values of sport, the evolution of theory and techniques of coaching of various sports, and the scientific foundations of training and coaching. The National Olympic Committee of each country nominates participants. The executive staff of the Academy invites noted sport authorities to give major addresses. A yearly report is published and distributed worldwide by the Hellenic Olympic Committee.

The Peace Corps. The Congress of the United States authorized the formation of the Peace Corps in September, 1961. The major purpose of the Peace Corps is to assist developing countries, upon request, in areas of fundamental education, agriculture, economics, and health. The overall theme is "to promote world peace and friendship." The Peace Corps has been highly successful; developing nations all over the world request its services. High among the specialists invited by recipient countries are sport specialists and physical education teachers. Many governments recognize that these programs are influential in helping youth develop personal pride, a sense of national prestige, and an interest in international competition in sport.

People-to-People Sports Committee. At a White House Conference in 1956, establishment of this Committee was recommended. Its general purpose is to provide an organization in which private citizens can volunteer their services and support governmental agencies in an effort to broaden friendship and understanding between American citizens and the people of other nations. It is a joint project of the American government and interested private citizens and clubs.

The Committee is responsible for organizing and sponsoring American sport teams to visit other countries for friendly competition and to give clinics in sport skills. For example, a junior baseball team went on a three-weeks' tour of Japan and Korea. The Committee hosted a cricket team from Pakistan in the United States. The Committee has provided sports equipment and training materials to sports clubs and other organizations in Brazil, Italy, Spain, Thailand, Rhodesia, and other countries around the world. The activities of the Committee are much broader and more numerous than can be enumerated here. The idea of interested private citizens and local groups joining with the United States Government in the promotion of international goodwill through sport is the key concept of this Committee.

International Council on Health, Physical Education, and Recreation. The Council, known as ICHPER, has met regularly since 1957 on a rotating basis in major cities throughout the world. It is an international member of the World Confederation of Organizations of the Teaching Profession. The Congress provides a forum for the exchange of ideas, development of professional and personal acquaintanceships, research reports and other relevant studies in the area of comparative physical education, and informal visitation of educational programs in the host country. A theme of interest to physical educators around the world is selected. The ICHPER Congresses continue to attract physical education and sport leaders and enthusiasts internationally because of the high quality of programs.

The Congress publishes its proceedings, e.g., *ICHPER 18, The 18th International Congress of the International Council of Health, Physical Education and Recreation.* The *ICHPER Proceedings* are a valuable educational resource for students and physical education and sport professional leaders.

International Congress on Physical Education and Sport for Girls and Women. This Congress meets every four years and was last held in August 1977. Approximately 700 delegates from 40 countries attended. The Congress provides an excellent forum for the exchange of personal and professional views and information on major topics of common interest to women physical educators and sport leaders.

First International Conference for Ministers and Senior Officials Responsible for Physical Education and Sport in the Education of Youth. The first International Conference of this organization was held in 1976, under the sponsorship of UNESCO. Senior physical education officials from many countries sent representatives to this Conference. Each country presented a written report of recent trends and developments in physical education. The conferees recommended that a similar conference be sponsored by UNESCO every three to five years. It is obvious that this conference is another important medium for fostering international understanding through programs of sport and physical education.

Scientific Congress "Sports in the Modern World — Changes and Problems." West Germany's Organizing Committee for the XXth Olympic Games sponsored this international congress in August 1972, just prior to the Olympic Games, in Munich. The aim of the Congress was to contribute to a greater understanding of sport science through lectures, discussions, publications, and audio-visual programs concerning questions and problems of major importance in the vast field of sport. Opportunities were provided for experts in various phases of sport and physical education, representing the different scientific and humanistic disciplines, to come together to hear addresses and to debate the issues and directions of modern sport science. Another purpose of the Congress was to provide an academic, cultural, and artistic setting within which to frame and conduct the magnficent spectacle of the XXth Olympic Games. The Congress was indeed a feature of these Games.

More than 2,000 delegates from approximately 100 countries attended the Congress. A majority of the conferees were appointed to be delegates by their national governments. Interested individuals also were invited to attend. Approximately 120 scholars, each a national or international expert in his or her specialization, presented major addresses. The Congress probably was unique in the history of international meetings on sport because of its emphasis on interdisciplinary analyses and critiques engaged in by so many noted experts from around the world, before a vast international audience of men and women who were engaged daily in carrying out their professional leadership roles in the field of sport and physical education.

Many programs provide for the international exchange of athletes competing in a variety of sporting activities. The list is too long to recount here. Vendien and Nixon[42] describe a variety of international competitions in more detail. Brief mention of selected events follows. *International Sports Competitions*

The Olympic Games. From their beginning in 1896 in Athens, Greece, the modern Olympic Games have promoted interest in sport around the world. Each year the number of participating countries has increased. However, following the recent action of some governments to withhold their athletes from competition in the Games as a form of political sanction, the number of athletes and countries represented is not as large as it might otherwise be.

The Games are spectacularly staged and are accessible to viewing by millions of people in many countries through international television channels. Host countries build magnificent sport facilities for both the summer and winter Games. Usually, the cost of these facilities exceeds the original planning estimate by millions of dollars. As a result, many countries now believe they are unable financially to sponsor future Olympic Games. Proposals are being considered for dividing the Games into segments to be held in various countries in different months of the Olympic year. Overall interest in the Games has not subsided. However, their organization and administration are so complicated now that new formats probably will have to be developed for their financing, scheduling, and staging.

Two problems associated directly with the Games are the tendency toward exhibitions of excessive nationalism by some and the complex issue of eligibility of professional sportsmen as participants in the Games, which historically have been reserved for the amateur athlete.

World Championships. A large number of international sports federations exist, each of which represents and controls the administration of a particular amateur sport worldwide. These federations sponsor world championships. It is customary for the site of a world championship in a sport to be rotated to various cities and countries for each event. There is no consistent pattern among the sports as to the frequency of meeting, selection of host countries, or even eligibility of participants on the basis of the amateur rules that govern in each federation.

Regional Championships. Contiguous countries in various areas of the world hold regional sport competitions. The Asian Games are an example; there are Commonwealth Games, Pan-American Games, and others. The intent and scope of these games are shown by the titles.

Other Competitions. Examples of other programs of sport competition between two or more countries are numerous. Of particular import and interest was the initial visit of the United States Table Tennis Team to Mainland China in 1972. In this case, sport was used deliberately as an instrument of national policy and was a highly symbolic gesture by China and the United States as the opening move by these nations to develop diplomatic relations with each other. President Nixon's historic visit to China followed soon thereafter. This unique sport and political episode is now referred to as "Ping Pong diplomacy."

Even earlier, the United States and the U.S.S.R. joined in an agreement in January, 1958, providing for exchanges in cultural, educational, and technical fields of human endeavor. The United States and the U.S.S.R. have since organized exchanges of sport teams, particularly in basketball and gymnastics. Thus, sport is used to intensify diplomatic relations between these two countries.

The Ryder Cup challenge in men's amateur golf between the United States and Great Britain and the Wightman Cup tennis competition, involving American and British women, are of similar international significance. The Wimbledon tennis tournament and the International Davis Cup matches in tennis bring together outstanding players from many nations to compete in the friendly arena of sport. The diplomatic and political benefits of these sport contests are not to be underestimated.

The decision of top government officials to use sport as a vehicle of national policy for the improvement of international political relationships is indeed a noteworthy phenomenon. It is not only of popular interest to American citizens and citizens of other countries, but it also merits close scholarly study by political scientists, sport leaders, and other interested scholars. Lucius D. Battle,[43] a former Assistant Secretary of Educational and Cultural Affairs, writing in the Department of State Bulletin in 1962, made this cogent statement, which is still relevant:

> When we come to communication between people, however, we want more than a formal dialogue. It is for this reason that our government's programs in education and the arts have come to play a more and more significant role in contributing to the attainment of the United States foreign policy objectives, often producing results that cannot be achieved in any other way. For they provide direct access to people — people who are glad to purvey as an illumination of the quality of our lives and an enrichment of their own. . . . In the long run they can create a world-wide common market of ideas, cultural attainment, and human discourse. . . . By arising above ideological differences, education and the arts make possible intuitive contacts that can ripen into mutual trust and understanding and enduring friendship.

It is obvious that international exchange programs in sport sponsored on such a large scale by the United States Government are a fundamental portion of a policy of the United States as enunciated by Lucius D. Battle.

Although comparative, international, and development education *Conclusions* have been included in this chapter, "The Normative Foundations of Physical Education," in one sense, at least, a portion of its content really is not "normative" in the formal definition of the term. In other words, the results of comparative studies do not result in specific recommendations as to exactly what the schools should do, what the curriculum should be, or how teachers should teach. Comparative education does not stipulate what educational programs should consist of and how they should be conducted. It does attempt to understand what is transpiring in the educational system and the factors and reasons why it is progressing and developing as it is. History and philosophy do meet the formal criteria of normative disciplines.

SUMMARY

Philosophy, history, and comparative education are described as *normative* studies because they continuously aim to clearly identify, define, and describe the goals and educational activities that are highly valued by a society.

Philosophy is the organized study of human thought and conduct. It is concerned with identifying and clearly formulating laws and principles which underlie knowledge and understanding of reality.

Educational philosophy is a specialized area of general philosophy that intensively investigates the aims and practices of formal and informal educational organization.

Van Dalen described the roles of philosophy in physical education by stating that scientific findings in physical education provide quantitative descriptions of *what is,* while philosophy suggests *what should be,* the aims and purposes of physical education.

Evidence from archaeology, history, and, anthropology clearly demonstrates that games, sport, festivals, and dances, along with the endless play of children, have created cultural patterns inseparably woven into the history of humans whenever and wherever they have lived.

In Egypt, between 3000 and 1100 B.C., evidence points toward sport and game participation by the upper classes.

The development of sport in England during the Middle Ages was one of the most specific of all historical influences on American physical education.

In Sweden the basic concept of physical education had a scientific basis in studies of human anatomy. The Swedish system challenged the German gymnastics system. This debate was carried on for several decades. American schools took an eclectic position of compromise and adopted and adapted major features of both systems.

American involvement in wars always provokes an intensified interest in and attention to physical education, physical training, and physical fitness.

The *Proceedings* of the North American Society for Sport History are published yearly. The publication provides the most inclusive and extensive listing of references and brief summaries of historical research in sport available in this country.

Comparative education seeks to solve educational problems primarily with research methodologies from political science and sociology. Development education uses research methods of economics. International education uses research techniques from anthropology.

As a result of ongoing exchange programs involving physical educators from different countries, a strong interest in international physical education has developed in this country, particularly in the colleges and universities.

[1]Earle F. Zeigler, *Philosophical Foundations for Physical, Health, and Recreation Education*. Englewood Cliffs, N. J.: Prentice-Hall, Inc., 1964, p.12.

[2]Elwood C. Davis, *The Philosophic Process in Physical Education*. Philadelphia: Lea & Febiger, 1961, p. 26.

[3]John S. Brubacher, *Modern Philosophies of Education* (4th ed.). New York: McGraw Hill, 1969, p. 76.

[4]Harold J. Vanderzwaag, *Toward a Philosophy of Sport*. Reading, MA: Addison-Wesley Publishing Company, Inc., 1972, p. 10.

[5]Kathleen Nott, *Philosophy and Human Nature*. New York: New York University Press, 1971, p. 16.

[6]Linda Kay Moore, "Music, Art, Theatre, and Physical Education," *JOPER*, 43:21 (October, 1972).

[7]Richard B. Morland, "This Philosophic Method of Research," In Alfred W. Hubbard (Editor), *Research Methods in Health, Physical Education and Recreation* (3rd rev.). Washington, D.C.: American Association for Health, Physical Education, Recreation and Dance. 1973, pp. 308, 309.

[8]Ibid., p. 312

[9]John E. Smith, *The Spirit of American Philosophy*. Oxford, England: Oxford Press, 1963, p. 25.

[10]Robert S. Brumbaugh and Nathaniel M. Lawrence, *Philosophical Themes in Modern Education*. Boston: Houghton-Mifflin Co., 1973, pp. 3, 4, 6.

[11]William A. Harper, Donna Mae Miller, Roberta J. Park, and Elwood A. Davis, *The Philosophic Process in Physical Education* (3rd ed.). Philadelphia: Lea & Febiger, 1977.

[12]Deobold B. Van Dalen, "Philosophy: An Initial Consideration," *Quest*, 1:19–22 (December, 1963), pp. 19, 20, 21.

[13]Earle F. Zeigler, *Physical Education and Sport Philosophy*. Englewood Cliffs, N.J.: Prentice-Hall, Inc., 1977, p. 16.

[14]Earle F. Zeigler (Editor), *A History of Sport and Physical Education to 1900*. Champaign, Ill.: Stipes Publishing Company, 1973, pp. 3–13.

[15]Harold J. Vanderzwaag, op. cit.

[16]Warren P. Fraleigh, "Sport – Purpose," *Journal of the Philosophy of Sport*, II:74–82 (September, 1975), pp. 78, 80.

[17]*Journal of the Philosophy of Sport*, "Introduction," 1:1–5 (September, 1974).

[18]Robert L. Brackenbury, "Physical Education and Intellectual Emphasis?" *Quest*, I:3–6 (December, 1963).

[19]Klaus V. Meier, "Cartesian and Phenomological Anthropology: A Radical Shift and its Meaning for Sport," *Journal of the Philosophy of Sport*, II:51–71 (September, 1975), p. 70.

[20]G. Kitson Clark. *The Critical Historian*. New York: Basic Books, Inc., 1967, pp. 209, 210.

[21]Earle F. Zeigler (Editor), *A History of Sport and Physical Education to 1900*. Champaign, Ill.: Stipes Publishing Company, 1973.

[22]George Z. F. Bereday, *Comparative Methods in Education*. New York: Holt, Rinehart and Winston, Inc. 1964, p. 43.

[23]Joseph A. Lauwerys (Editor), *Education at Home and Abroad*. London: Rutledge and Kegan Paul, 1973, p. viii.

[24]Max A. Eckstein and Harold J. Noah (Editors), *Scientific Investigations in Comparative Education*. London: The Macmillan Company, 1969.

[25]Ibid., p. 5.

[26]Arnold Anderson, *Education and Economic Development*. Chicago: Aldine Publishing Company, 1965, p. 27.

[27]Phillip Jones, *Comparative Education: Purpose and Method*. St. Lucia, Queensland: University of Queensland Press, 1971.

[28]Bruce L. Bennett, Maxwell L. Howell, and Uriel Simri, *Comparative Physical Education and Sport*. Philadelphia: Lea & Febiger, 1975.

[29]Lynn Vendien and John E. Nixon, *The World Today and Health, Physical Education, and Recreation*. Englewood Cliffs, N. J.: Prentice-Hall, Inc., 1968.

[30]William Johnson (Editor), *Physical Education Around the World*, Monograph #1. Indianapolis, IN: Phi Epsilon Kappa Fraternity, 3747 North Linwood Avenue, 1966.

Ibid., Monograph #2. Indianapolis, IN: Phi Epsilon Kappa Fraternity, 4000 Meadows Drive, Suite L-24, 1967.

Ibid., Monograph #3. Indianapolis, IN: Phi Epsilon Kappa Fraternity, 6919 E. 10th St., Suite E-4, 1969.

Ibid., Monograph #4. Indianapolis, IN: Phi Epsilon Kappa Fraternity, 6919 E. 10th St., Suite E-4, 1970.

Ibid., Monograph #5, Washington, D.C.: AAHPER, 1971.

Ibid., Monograph #6, Washington, D.C.: AAHPER, 1972.

Ibid., Monograph #7, Washington, D.C.: AAHPER, 1973.

THE NORMATIVE FOUNDATIONS OF PHYSICAL EDUCATION

[31]D. W. J. Anthony, "Comparative Physical Education," *Physical Education*, LVIII (November, 1966), p. 73.

[32]Lynn Vendien and John E. Nixon, op. cit., p. 6.

[33]Bruce L. Bennett, Maxwell L. Howell, and Uriel Simri, op. cit., p. vii.

[34]Lynn Vendien, "A Brief Comparative Study of Eleven Countries with the U.S.A.," Unpublished manuscript, University of Massachusetts, Amherst, MA., 1969.

[35]Bruce L. Bennett, Maxwell L. Howell, and Uriel Simri, op. cit.

[36]Lynn Vendien and John E. Nixon, op. cit.

[37]William Johnson (Editor), op. cit.

[38]Jonathan Kolatch, *Sports, Politics, and Ideology in China*. New York: Jonathan David Publishers, 1972.

[39]Deobold B. Van Dalen and Bruce L. Bennett, *A World History of Physical Education*. Englewood Cliffs, N. J.: Prentice-Hall, Inc., 1961.

[40]Earle F. Zeigler, Maxwell L. Howell, and Marianna Trekell, *Research in the History, Philosophy and International Aspects of Physical Education and Sport: Bibliographies and Techniques*. Champaign, Ill.: Stipes Publishing Company, 1971.

[41]Darwin M. Semotiuk, "Theoretical and Methodological Considerations for Comparative and International Sport and Physical Education," *Gymnasion* (International Journal of Physical Education), XI:10–16 (Spring, 1974), pp. 14,15.

[42]Lynn Vendien and John E. Nixon, op. cit.

[43]Lucius D. Battle, "Cultural and Educational Affairs in International Relations," *Department of State Bulletin, XLVII*, July 9, 1962, p. 7.

SELECTED REFERENCES

Benthall, Jonathan, *The Body as a Medium of Expression*. New York: E. P. Dutton & Co., 1975.

Cassidy, Rosalind and Caldwell, Stratton, *Humanizing Physical Education* (5th Ed.). Dubuque, Iowa: Wm. C. Brown Co., 1974.

Comparative Physical Education and International Sport. Washington, D.C.: AAHPERD, 1973.

"CSU, Long Beach Goes International." *CAHPER Journal*, March/April 1976, p. 29.

Freeman, William H., *Physical Education in a Changing Society*. Boston, MA: Houghton-Mifflin, 1977.

Harper, William A., Miller, Donna M., Park, Robert J., and Davis, Elwood C., *The Philosophic Process in Physical Education* (3rd Ed.). Philadelphia: Lea & Febiger, 1977.

Johnson, William (Ed.), *Physical Education around the World*, Monograph #5, Washington, D.C.: AAHPER, 1971.

International Sport in a Social-Cultural Setting. Washington, D.C.: AAHPERD, 1975.

Kuntz, Paul G., "Aesthetics Applies to Sports as Well as to the Arts," *Journal of Philosophy of Sport*, 1:6–28 (September 1974).

Leonard, George, *The Ultimate Athlete: Re-Visioning Sports Physical Education and the Body*. New York: Viking Press, 1975.

Link, Hans, *Social Philosophy of Athletics*. Champaign, IL: Stipes Publishing Company, 1979.

Lowe, Benjamin, Kanis, David, and Strenk, Andrew (Eds.), *Sport and International Relations*. Champaign, IL: Stipes Publishing Co., 1978.

Metheny, Eleanor, *Vital Issues*. Washington, D.C.: American Alliance for Health, Physical Education and Recreation, 1977.

Nixon, John E., "Comparative International and Development Studies in Physical Education." Proceedings, National College Physical Education Association for Men, 1968.

Osterhoudt, Robert G., *An Introduction to the Philosophy of Physical Education and Sport*. Champaign, IL: Stipes Publishing Company, 1978.

Palmer, Denise, and Howell, Maxwell L., "Sport and Games in Early Civilization." In Earle F. Zeigler (Ed.), *A History of Sport and Physical Education to 1900*. Champaign, IL: Stipes Publishing Company, 1973.

People's Sports Publishing House (Ed.), *Sports in China*. Peking: Foreign Language Press, 1973.

Polidoro, J. Richard, "Professional Preparation Programs of Physical Education Teachers in Norway, Sweden, and Denmark," *Research Quarterly*, AAHPERD, 48:640–646 (October 1977).

"Political Ideology and Sport" *Arena Newsletter*, Vol. I, No. 2. Norfolk, VA: The Institute for Sport and Social Analysis, Virginia Wesleyan College, February 1977, pp 1–17.

The 1974 Proceedings of the Society on the History of Physical Education and Sport in Asia and the Pacific Area. The Wingate Institute for Physical Education and Sport, Wingate Post Office, Israel.

Renson, Roland, Leuven, Pierre-Paul, and Ostyn, Michael (Eds.), *The History, Evolution, and Diffusion of Sports and Games in Different Cultures.* Brussels, Belgium: Dienst Algemen Zaken, 1976.

Report of the United States Delegation, UNESCO Conference on Physical Education and Sport. Washington, D.C.: AAHPERD, 1977.

Riordan, James, *Sport in Soviet Society.* New York: Cambridge University Press, 1977.

Shea, Edward J., *Ethical Decisions in Physical Education and Sport.* Carbondale, IL: Southern Illinois University, 1978.

Shneidman, N. Norman, *The Soviet Road to Olympus.* Toronto, Canada: The Ontario Institute for Studies in Education, 1978.

Zeigler, Earle F., *Personalizing Physical Education and Sport Philosophy.* Champaign, IL: Stipes Publishing Co., 1976.

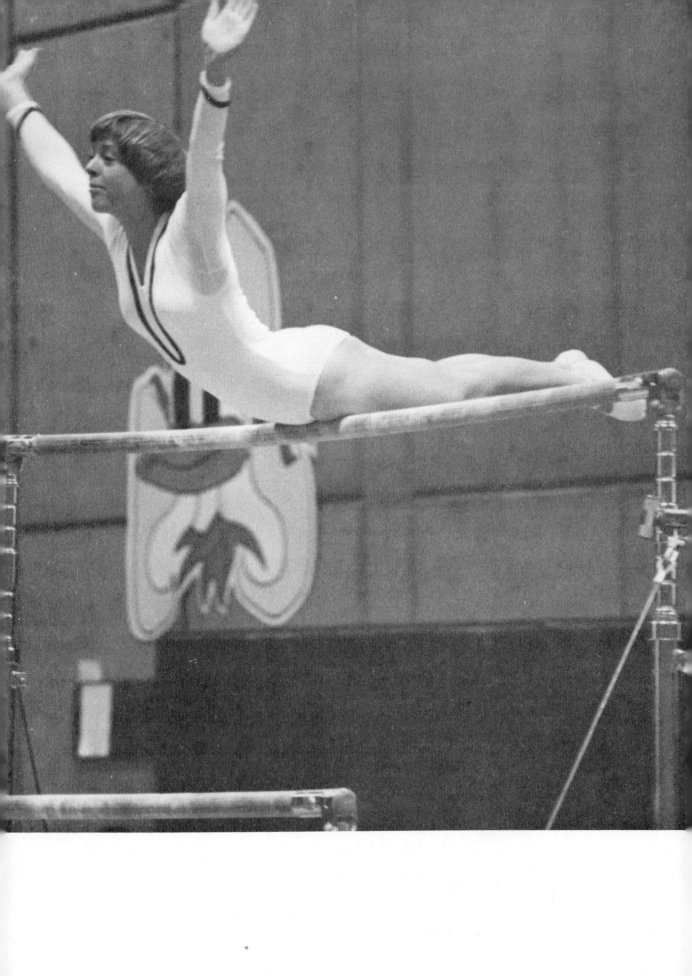

4

SOCIO-CULTURAL —— —————— FOUNDATIONS

It is common to define anthropology as a science of man, or more literally, the study of human beings. The word is a combination of the Greek words anthropos which means "man," and logos, which means "study." Anthropologists not only study humans as individuals but also compare and contrast various societies of people both contemporary and historical.

There is a close overlapping of the disciplines of anthropology and sociology; also, of course, the study of biology is highly integrated with research in these two fields. Some authorities believe that anthropology now serves as an overall synthesizing science for human beings. Two major branches of anthropology are physical anthropology and cultural anthropology; these will be discussed later.

The current view of anthropology is expressed by Pearson:[1]

> Modern evolutionary anthropologists see men as an integral part of a total life system which cannot be carelessly disrupted except at their own peril; indeed, they see the whole history of human evolution as having taken place within this ecological system, as a result of interacting biological and cultural adaptations which serve to promote the continuing survival of the species in a constantly changing environment.

Anthropologists are interested in evolution and genetics with respect to understanding the total evolutionary development of the species of living human beings. They are particularly concerned about ecology and adaptation concepts. They study the territoriality of humans and animals. They are interested in the history and concepts basic to the life and development of mammals, particularly monkeys and gorillas, the ancestors of primitive men and women. Scientific evidence of early human evolution is pursued. In tracing the history of the human race anthropologists study ontogeny, which refers to the life history of individual organisms, and phylogeny, which describes the evolutionary development of species of organisms.

Some anthropologists specialize in anthropometry, which involves

113

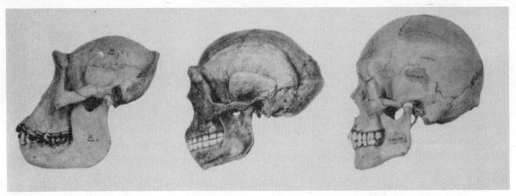

Anthropologists are particularly concerned with the total evolutionary development of the species of living organisms called man.

descriptions and measurements of the human body, with special emphasis upon skeletal dimensions and interrelationships. There are anthropologists who are interested in the biochemical makeup of the human body, and they particularly study the activities and functions of glandular secretions and moving tissues. Other anthropologists concentrate on a science called seroanthropology, which analyzes and classifies variations in the content and character of human blood.

Other major subjects in anthropology that are studied by researchers include how individuals join together in bands, tribes, and nations; the institutions of marriage and kinship; how behavior is controlled or punished or rewarded within the group, or custom and law; and economic organization, such as property, household, redistribution of ownership, slavery, commerce, and other economic influences. Other topics of interest are magic, taboo, religion, personal adornment and aesthetic values, art, archaeology (the science of ancient objects); ethnographic studies as a means for carefully analyzing a society and its culture through intensive observations within a particular group; ecological adaptation; horticulture, fishing, hunting; the rise of urban civilization; the development of civilization in recent times; peasant society; industrial society; and the development and role of language.

Basically, anthropologists study the behaviors of human beings and their interaction with their environment. They collect genealogies and censuses, transcribe languages on tapes, collect personal documents, and attempt to participate in as many of the natural aspects of the lives of the people being studied as possible, even if only marginally.

Research methods in recent years are using new techniques such as formal mathematical models; symbolic logic; microanalytic methods; proxemics (the use of space between persons in social interactions); and gestures and bodily movements (kinesics), which are forms of nonverbal communication. New and more refined methods of computerized statistical analyses are being formulated to organize and evaluate the data from various sources indicated above.

The study of anthropology usually identifies four major specialized fields of research: archaeology, linguistics, cultural anthropology, and physical and biological anthropology. All of these areas must be studied and interrelated in anthropological research.

The anthropological researcher must live with the people being studied and engage in participant-observations as well as have a detailed and precise method of recording observations and information.

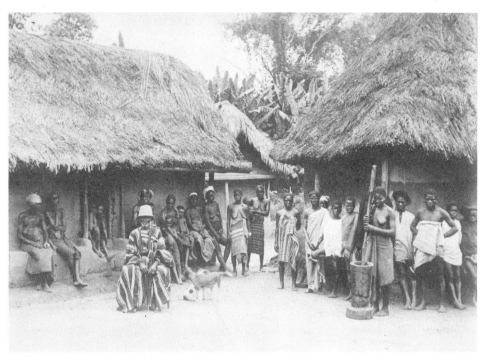

Anthropologists study the behaviors of human beings and their interaction with their environment.

The anthropologist's purpose is to examine behaviors and infer the reasons why these behaviors exist in their particular form, or for that matter why they exist at all. This type of research is called ethnography. For this purpose the anthropologist, like other scientists, needs theory, which provides the logic of inference and observation, and therefore guides interpretations of observed behaviors.

Greenwood and Stini[2] emphasize a recurrent theme found in recent anthropology textbooks, namely, that there is an inseparable relationship between culture, biology, and environment, and that there is constant interaction among these three elements. Human nature can be understood only by research efforts that combine information from various types of studies mentioned in prior paragraphs. This holistic research approach studies the continuously available evidence of the interrelationship between human culture and biology as it is traced throughout history and in as many cultural settings throughout the world as researchers can mount appropriate investigative searches.

CULTURAL ANTHROPOLOGY

One major area of specialization in the general field of anthropology is called cultural anthropology. Researchers in this field are particularly interested in human institutions, social interrelationships among human groups, and the customs and mores that are distinctive within each cultural grouping. Research focuses on similarities and differences between selected human cultures and on analysis and understanding of the processes of change through acculturation and enculturation. It also studies the behaviors humans learn and how distinctive behaviors are deliberately modified.

Definition of Culture. The term *culture* has many definitions. Most definitions seem to include the custom, knowledge, art, law, belief, and morals that any individual acquires as a member of a specific cultural group. Individuals who live with other persons are subject to strong social pressures to accept the attitude and basic beliefs of the group. The study of these phenomena is divided into folk ways and mores. The main values of a specific culture are passed along to the offspring by a process called cultural transmission. When a child or a new member of a social group acquires the culture of that society, the process is called enculturation or socialization. Acculturation is the transmission of a culture from the members of one group to another.

A. L. Kroeber and Clyde Kluckhohn[3] studied and analyzed 164 definitions of culture. Some of the common threads running among these definitions are:

> It is a set of learned behaviors rather than inherited ones; children begin to acquire and accumulate their particular cultural heritage very early in life and it is strongly reinforced throughout their youth and adult years; it strongly influences all aspects of each individual, including psychological, sociological, and physiological components; it is understood, communicated about and passed on through a system of symbols, both verbal and nonverbal; it reflects basic societal values and ideas and is organized in patterns; and, of course, it is characterized by reciprocal interacting human behaviors.
>
> The entire ever-continuing process of cultural development is typified by powerful, emotional forces. In its largest context there is a strong element of continuous unity working to consolidate and integrate all cultural influences and developments into a total cultural integration.

Cultural Universals. Scientists who compare cultures observe marked similarities and wide differences concerning various anthropological phenomena. Also, they discover what they call cultural universals, general traits that exist in every culture. In this list are found sport, dance, games, education, hygiene, and other activities fundamentally associated with physical education and physical recreation.

Culture refers to learned behaviors, a set of techniques that enable an individual to adapt to the surrounding environment. Unless the individual is in isolation there is a human group present that defines appropriate ways of responding as the learning is taking place. The term *contraculture*, or *counter-culture*, is well known to young people these days. It refers to specific groups, such as young delinquents, having a distinct set of learned behavior patterns that are not accepted by the dominant society.

Humans create that part of their environment called culture. There is a universally accepted concept of culture, and within that notion are the many specific cultures on the earth that determine all of life's activities. Human nature defines all cultural aspects, both general and specific, within the compass of the laws of nature and human biology. Culture is often described as modes of feeling, believing, and thinking, and ways of retaining and recalling them at any appropriate time in the future. Culture has a highly regulatory function operating from the instant of birth until the point of death, constantly directing the life of any one human being, either consciously or unconsciously. Cultural functions that are not practiced or repeated soon die out.

One of the major functions of culture is in providing direction to the human being and societal groups in their continuing attempts to understand themselves and their behaviors. Also, knowledge and understanding of major aspects of a culture facilitate awareness of possible actions that individuals can take in a specific culture. Finally, it must be remembered that all humans enter life in an environment with already existing cultural patterns and expectations. It is possible for human beings to develop keener insights into the dynamics of cultural processes and to predict and prepare for at least a limited degree of control over their cultural destiny.

Culture and Physical Education. The physical educator should help uninformed individuals to realize that sport, dance, exercise, and physical play are fundamental elements of the culture of the American people. Well-intended critics of public school curricula sometimes assert, either directly or by implication, that certain subjects in the school curriculum are "cultural" and that others are not. Physical education is frequently included in the latter list. Therefore, the argument goes that physical education should be dropped from the school curriculum for more "cultural" subjects. This assertion is nonsense and should be countered with effectual statements by physical educators based on relevant research and literature cited in this chapter and in the reference list at the end of the chapter. Especially recommended is the famous book *Mirror of Man*, by Clyde Kluckhohn,[4] published in 1949 by McGraw-Hill, Inc. Ultimately, a correct understanding of the concept of culture is vital for the understanding of individual persons and their behaviors.

Anthropologists sometimes specialize in a particular aspect of the life of ancient cultures. One such specialization is physical anthropology, the study of human morphology and evolution; it is also called biological anthropology. It concerns ecological and cultural influences that gradually change the composition and structure of human populations over time. The distribution of genetic characteristics within and between different racial populations is investigated, as are racial differences, constitutional variations (particularly with respect to motor capacity), and behavioral traits associated with specific body types. Physical anthropologists also conduct research to discover the physiological responses of different groups of human beings in various historical eras to exercise, altitude, nutrition, cold and hot weather, and to disease infestation. They relate the findings and variations among different human populations to interest, abilities, and performances in warfare.

PHYSICAL ANTHROPOLOGY

Physiological anthropologists study the adaptation of humans through physiological responses to environmental conditions that have strong influence on physiological functioning. Examples are the relationships of genetic variations and morphological (form and structure) features of humans to physiological processes; how individuals of various racial backgrounds respond to certain environmental stimuli such as light, heat, altitude, and psychological stresses. Are there population variations in the above physiological responses among people in various geographical parts of the world? Do disease and nutritional variations between populations have a greater influence on morphological variation than stress due to climate factors? Present evidence suggests that the answer to this last question is "yes."

Physiological, or Biological, Anthropology

Effects of Hot, Dry Climates. Selected research findings from physiological anthropology research are of interest to the physical educator. In dry, hot climates, such as on the Sahara Desert, it is fallacious to believe that an increase in the amount of water consumed will increase the rate of sweating. Neither does the sweat rate decrease markedly until a serious degree of water deficiency occurs. Therefore, drinking large amounts of water in advance with the hope of protecting against dehydration is not helpful because excess water beyond that held in the fully hydrated body cannot be stored up for use to combat later dehydration. What is the lesson here for coaches whose players compete in very hot weather? Drinking small amounts of water more often is better than ingesting large amounts infrequently, which results in considerable fluid loss through increased urination.

In addition to water loss through sweat, in hot weather the loss of salt in the body combines to cause cardiovascular problems because of extracellular dehydration. Physical performances are thus impaired because there are adverse increases in the heart rate and rectal temperature, and a reduction in intracellular fluid volume. There is also a demonstrated inverse correlation between body weight and the mean ambient temperature; thus, a loss of weight is accompanied with an increase in temperature. Also, heavier persons are more likely to suffer heatstroke. The more overweight a male is in relation to mean weight, the greater his chances of having heatstroke in hot climates. Age also is related to the tolerance level of dry heat. Very young children and older adults both react more negatively to heat exposure, probably because of lower sweating capacity, lower blood flow, and lower degree of vasodilation.

Physiological anthropologists have also discovered that hair and skin color are related to rate of heat absorption in hot desert areas. A higher rate of heat absorption accompanies darker color of hair and skin. Furthermore, the myth that black people sweat more profusely than European whites has been proved false. Women generally sweat less than men.

Effects of Cold Temperatures. Likewise, physiological anthropologists have developed the following tentative conclusions about the effects of cold temperatures upon human performances and basic physiological health. People living in colder areas of the world show genetic and natural selection adaptations that protect them with more efficient physiological extremity-warming capabilities than people living in tropical areas. Other adaptations of people living in colder climates include larger chest, shorter arms and legs, more total body weight, less body surface area per unit of weight, more rounded head, and nose that is higher and narrower.

Effects of High Altitude. Physiological anthropologists have also studied physical performance levels at various altitudes, a subject of considerable interest to physical educators and coaches. It is not surprising that the conclusion of these anthropological studies parallels that of exercise physiologists; that is, the altitude factor deleteriously affects athletic performance at progressively higher altitudes. The acceleration of decrement in performance begins at about 2,000 meters, mainly owing to a decrease in the maximal work capacity of the cardiovascular system. At 4,000 meters, there is an average decrease in maximal oxygen uptake and a 40 per cent decrease at 5,000 meters.

The examples just cited demonstrate the availability of scientific sources of research studies, findings, and conclusions that can be of immense value to physical educators, coaches, athletic trainers, dance instructors, and others who are in charge of programs of sport, dance, and exercises for people of all ages. Perhaps physiological anthropology is an area of human research and evaluation that should be explored much more intensively for its contributions to improved understanding and instructional practices in movement arts and sport sciences.

Archaeology is the anthropology of extinct cultures: a study of artifacts — such as weapons, tools, abodes, and remains of the earth's surfaces such as irrigation systems, terraces, fuels — used by early people. The purpose of research in archaeology is to learn about the culture of ancient peoples through the discovery, excavation, and reconstruction of relics, artifacts, buildings, dwellings, canals, graves, utensils, religious objects and shrines, cities, arms, and similar human remains that have potential for revealing the type of lives people led during various historical eras. Archaeological research provides information and insights into the history of sport, dance, physical education, and other forms of physical activities in earlier civilizations and is a basis for inferences and generalizations about the forms, content, and values associated with these activities.

ARCHAEOLOGY

Dr. Maxwell Howell and his wife, Dr. Reet Howell, from the California State University, San Diego, are noted historical and archaeological researchers in physical education who have visited many sites and countries of early civilizations, as well as museums and other modern sources of archaeological discovery and history. Tentative generalizations concerning the influence of sport, dance, and exercise upon the lives of people in these countries result from their investigations.

Play, Learning, and Evolution. Anthropologists have established that play had its origins in mammals many thousands of years ago. These mammals had the capacity to engage in a variety of behavioral responses to environmental stimuli; play was one major type of behavior and was believed to be highly adaptive. Through play behaviors, and other animal movements, learning was taking place. Thus, this process was crucial to the ongoing evolution of mammalians.

Physical educators rarely trace the play history of humans to mammals of an earlier historical era. However, anthropologists have verified that there is a demonstrable continuity between the play activities of mammals in which reality was simulated and the later development of problem-solving processes in human beings. It has also been verified that the play behavior of animals is basic to the utilization of physical energy that is required to establish ever-developing neurological patterns that lead to learned responses in a wide variety of situations in the environment. Thus, animals evolved up the scale of biological adaptation primarily because of the processes of learning that were engendered through play behavior that, in turn, was encouraged and protected by adults. Greenwood and Stini[5] make the assertion that the significance of play and its contribution to the learning of animals and the ultimate development of human beings cannot be overestimated.

It is interesting to note that very few physical education researchers have become specialists in the anthropological foundations of physical education, sport, dance, and fitness, an area with such rich research potential. On the other hand, many anthropologists have made intensive studies of the play and exercise habits and activities of humans.

Recently anthropologists and others have engaged in a new area of investigation called *kinesics*, or *gestural communication*. Kinesics refers to nonverbal communication that takes place in the form of highly organized structures of body movements that occur simultaneously with speaking.

KINESICS

Kinesics is a system of notation of body motions as well as an analysis of bodily movements as a mode of communication in nonverbal form. It has already been demonstrated that kinesic communication is an important concomitant of speech communication. Bodily motions interact with verbal communications either to facilitate clear verbal communication or, in some cases, to create such confusion that meaningful vocal interaction cannot continue.

Humans must learn to accurately process kinesic information and to make appropriate responses to it. We are able to process such information acutely. Body language differs from culture to culture, but most cultures do not place a high value on learning kinesic communication; in fact, they tend to resist it. This is because the philosophy of western cultures is based on a rigid separation of the body and the mind; western cultures are learned and directed almost solely by the world of the mind. Therefore, kinesics, which depends so much upon overt body movement, is rejected.

Many physical educators have given attention to body language and shown it to be one of the outcomes of educational endeavors in play, dance, sport, and fitness activities. Perhaps physical educators could exert even greater leadership and interpretative clarity concerning the validity and importance of kinesics.

Synchrony. Another aspect of communication and human movement is called synchrony and should be of interest to the physical educator. High-speed motion pictures indicate that individuals move their bodies in approximately the same ways at specific times. These movements are not responses to physical cues, but are apparently some kind of unconscious synchronization of bodily movements set off by person-to-person interaction.

Body Rhythms. Research studies indicate there are body rhythms, such as the heart beat, which also become synchronous with various processes of communication. Theories and scientific explanations are lacking for this phenomenon at the present time. In any event, it is obvious that several forms of communication pervade every human culture. Physical educators may be more influential in the communications realm than they realize.

Ethnology. The term *ethnology* refers to specialized processes of collecting anthropological evidence. Some physical education researchers are now employing ethnological methods of data collection in evaluation projects concerned with teaching effectiveness. Immers-

RESEARCH

CHAPTER FOUR

ing himself into the group being studied, the ethnologist performs formal and informal observation of behaviors; conducts interviews; compiles field notes of activities observed; and writes descriptions in anecdotal form or as impressions of what has been observed, heard, and engaged in by himself within the target group. When it is feasible the researcher uses formal research methods such as projective techniques, genealogies, censuses, tape recorders, and other useful instrumentations.

Basically, the ethnologist constructs theories of how a particular human group behaves, why it behaves that way, what the group goals are, and how well they are being achieved. It is beyond the scope of this book to describe ethnological research in greater detail. References cited at the end of this chapter elaborate these research techniques.

Ethnology, or the science of cultural description, as it is sometimes called, is emerging as a major research tool in studies of teacher and learner behaviors in classrooms. Briefly described, it is the collection of evidence and descriptions concerning all the aspects of life in the classroom. It involves several research methods such as life histories, unobtrusive measures, projective techniques, questionnaires, oral interviews, the use of portable television and tape recorders, and extensive notes by observers. This total approach is eclectic and is pursued over a long time period. Overall, it is highly intensive.

Research Methods. The major difference between research methods used by anthropologists and those of other social scientists is the former's reliance on qualitative, holistic, ecological, and naturalistic investigations and data collection. Educational researchers in curriculum development and evaluation, and in research on effective teaching, are now using these anthropological research processes to add the qualitative dimension to the quantitative evidence being collected and analyzed. Teachers and researchers are also becoming more sensitive to ethnic and linguistic diversity among students and teachers.

There is a growing realization that human behavior is fundamentally influenced by the settings in which it is occurring, and therefore, educational investigation should take place more in the classroom settings and less in the artificial laboratories of the university. We must learn how to collect direct, valid data and information from natural classroom situations indoors and out-of-doors, as in the case of physical education. Examination of learning behaviors and teaching behaviors in the total learning environment with particular reference to its specific cultural context is the new direction for educational research. An encouraging development is that improved data-based theories are emerging from these research efforts and more sophisticated analyses of resulting data. There is rigorous attention to validity, objectivity, reliability, and universalization.

Singleton and Textor[6] outline seven characteristics of an anthropological approach to educational research and practice:

1. Ethnographic observation is the most common data collection tool.
2. Data interpretation is based on the broad, environmental, social, and cultural context of events and processes.
3. Interpretation of data is comparative in both a cross-cultural and intracultural sense.

4. Consideration is not limited to one conception of reality. In other words there is more than one reality.
5. Units of analysis are considered to be significant only in their culturally specific context.
6. Education is seen broadly as a process of cultural transmission.
7. Behavior should be observed and analyzed in natural settings.

In summary, anthropology as an applied social science is being used extensively in educational research and increasingly so in physical education. Its popularity and utility undoubtedly will continue to grow in the years ahead.

It is a recurrent theme of this chapter that sport is a fundamental component of culture. Physical education activities, different sports, specific games, and dance varieties are all culturally determined. Each culture develops and perpetrates notions of individual self-concept; specifies the roles of learned movement skills that contribute to the human welfare within the society; encourages specific types of movements and discourages others as educational modes for the attainment of mastery of customs, mores, and beliefs of the culture; and in other ways contributes to the total development of the individual within the boundaries of specific cultural aims. Specified movement forms contribute to goals, economic fulfillment, political success, and educational progress within any society.

ANTHROPOLOGY AND PHYSICAL EDUCATION

Aesthetics. The term *aesthetics* refers to appreciation of the beautiful, artistic phenomena, and ability to appreciate and perceive beauty wherever one finds it. Although not strictly known as a subdivision of anthropology, it is appropriate here to note that dance, rhythmical sports, and other forms of graceful human movement are individual expressions of appreciation and enjoyment of manifestations of beauty and grace. The topic of aesthetics is becoming more and more prominent in physical education literature. Individuals participating in sport, dance, and specialized types of exercises are regarded as artists expressing beauty, emotion, feelings, and making overt, personal statements of internalized values. Many voluntary physical movements possess qualities that appeal to the emotions, sensitivity, and sense of taste, beauty, and aesthetic quality of observers and performers alike. The term *kinesthetic imagery* is used to express a feeling of deep appreciation, or sense of empathy, regarding the beautiful movements of another person, thus providing testimony that they are indeed an art form.

Certain aspects of sport can be regarded as performing art. The majority of art forms are stationary and non-living, such as paintings, sculpture, buildings, and so on. In sport, as in dance, an actual performance exists temporarily and suddenly ceases to exist. The only way it can be preserved for posterity in its active form is through the use of motion pictures, video-tapes, or television film. Some people prefer to call sports kinesthetic art. Metheny[7] summarizes this viewpoint about aesthetics succinctly: "My thesis is that the sensory experience of movement is as inherently meaningful as the sensory perception of color, design, and musical sounds."

Finally, because of the great potentiality for the development of aesthetic appreciation and values that exist in physical education,

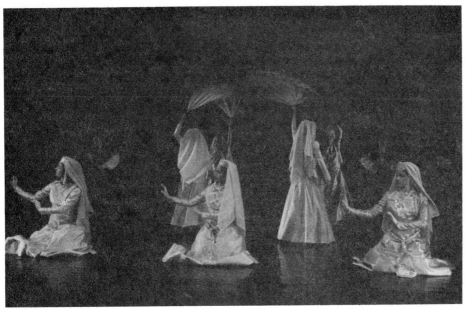

Many voluntary physical movements such as dance possess qualities of sensitivity, taste, and beauty.

sport, and dance, physical educators should include courses in fine arts, aesthetics, and philosophy in their degree programs. After all, physical education is one of the oldest of the arts of the humanities. Physical educators, dance specialists, and human movement teachers should learn and teach appropriate concepts and perspectives with regard to the fundamental aesthetic values and contributions of sport, dance, and selected exercises.

SUMMARY

The preceding comments and references, although highly selective and restrictive, are cited to illustrate the fundamental role of research findings and validated concepts from the field of anthropology as one of the essential foundations of physical education. We urge greater study in breadth and depth of relevant aspects of anthropology on the part of neophyte physical educators in their formal college and university programs as well as self-study by experienced practitioners.

Beals, Spindler, and Spindler[8] summarize the scope of anthropology as an academic discipline:

> The field of anthropology includes four major subdisciplines: cultural anthropology, physical anthropology, archaeology, and linguistics. Physical anthropology approaches the study of the human species from a biological viewpoint. It is concerned with human biological evolution, comparisons between human beings and other animals, and the nature of human biological variation. Archaeology and linguistics are, in a sense, highly specialized subdivisions of cultural anthropology, archaeology being concerned with the reconstruction of past cultures through the study of their material remains and linguistics being concerned with the development and nature of language. Cultural anthropology, because it is broadly concerned with the nature of culture, provides general understandings that are utilized by the other subdisciplines. More specifically, cultural anthropology is concerned with the description and comparison of cultures for which historical records are available or which

exist in the present and may be studied by direct observation and through the use of interviews.

Throughout the evolution of the human race, physical education and physical recreation have been essential elements in all cultures world-wide, according to scientific evidence from history, anthropology, archaeology, and sociology. Today most countries have national policies directing and encouraging the conduct and expansion of educational and recreational programs and opportunities in sport, dance, and exercises for all of the citizens, with special emphasis on formal school programs for youths. In the United States, sport permeates many important segments of the cultural life of most of the citizens. As a medium of expression, education, and appreciation, dance has dynamically expanded its activities and contributions throughout this country and the trend is for more of the same in years to come. Sport, dance, and exercise, in one form or another, exert influence on most Americans. This statement can be made about most of the other cultures of the world. This chapter presents an overview of these influences from areas of formal study, research, and empirical experience that we entitle *sociocultural foundations*.

Social scientists are interested in group processes and the roles of individuals within societies and their subgroups. Major topics of research include (a) patterns of living within the family group and within the rural, suburban, and large urban communities; (b) social class, symbols of social status, and avenues of social mobility; (c) the institutions that promote the functioning of society, such as churches, schools, labor organizations, business organizations, and governments; and (d) unifying and destructive forces relating to the stability of the structure of a given society. Sociologists explore and describe characteristics of American culture as a whole. Also, they study the many variations that characterize regional cultures and large numbers of subcultures, such as schools, minority groups within a city population, various types of workers within the labor force, and participants in various levels of organized sport.

Sociology is the academic discipline concerned with people living together in social groups and with the history, development, organization, and problems of these groups and the individuals who compose them. Major topics of interest to sociologists include the family, religion, crime, organizations, population, social stratification, institutions, education, the polity, the economy, and the status of minority groups and women.

Schools of Thought. Rose[9] indicates that sociologists can generally be classified according to different schools of thought. For example, social criticism attempts to diagnose and sometimes to prescribe corrections for social problems. Social behavior is viewed as interpersonal exchange, or the ways in which persons attempt to manipulate others with the expectation of some type of gain. Functionalism refers to careful analyses of sociological groups, societies, and communities organized as specific social systems. Conflict deals with various types of opposition that operate in human societies. Social disorganization concerns the study of malfunctioning of services for citizens in large cities. Social psychology investigates the challenges individual citizens face in coping with problems and conflicts within the community.

Methods of Research. Through a type of research called ethnomethodology scholars study social situations in an attempt to understand the dynamics of major influences upon persons involved. Other methods of research employed in sociology are experimental control, social survey, participant observation, statistical analysis, and community study. Some theoretical perspectives commonly found in sociological research include functionalism, symbolic interactionism, Marxism, phenomenology, and conflict theories.

McNall[10] believes there are three central questions around which sociological research is conducted. The first question requires analysis of the structure of an industrial society, including queries such as what are the essential elements of the society, what are their interrelationships, and how does one society differ from others in these respects? The second research question investigates the status of a particular society in human history, how is it changing today, and where does it seem to be heading? The third question concerns the nature of the people in a given society and how changes will affect them in the future. The reader is referred to McNall for a description of the use of theoretical perspectives.

Not only are social groups investigated, but also the roles and functions of individuals therein are of fundamental interest. The identification of the major values that give direction to the activities and goals of the cultures and the people who compose them is basic. Analysis of forces and influences that cause changes in values is another central research activity. Examples of sociological concerns relevant to the responsibility of physical educators and sport leaders follow.

SPORT

Only a limited number of resources are available for the study of physical education and sport in public and private agencies. Scholarly journals in sociology have been reluctant to publish articles related to the sociology of sport. Until recent years there has been no scholarly journal specifically dealing with sport phenomena. Also, traditionally, the study of sport has not been accepted as academically prestigious among sociologists and scholars in related fields. Administrators, coaches, and teachers of sport have been reluctant to permit observers and researchers to observe closely their operations and programs and to make available relevant information and data for fear of unfavorable or negative reports about various aspects of the programs.

Definition. Coakley[11] defines sport as follows;

> Sport is an institutionalized competitive activity that involves vigorous physical exertion or the use of relatively complex physical skills by individuals whose participation is motivated by a combination of the intrinsic satisfaction associated with the activity itself and the external rewards earned through participation.

Roles. Several authorities agree in their explanation of the roles of sport in society. They generally regard sport as a social institution that faithfully teaches and reinforces esteemed societal values, thereby contributing to socializing athletes into the major cultural, social, and behavioral patterns of the society in which they live. In this way sport contributes to the development, stability, and future progress of the particular society. Many industrial societies use sport to promote the development of achievement, motivation, and the desirability of a competitive activity in order to produce better products or more desirable social policies. Two other prominent themes in support of formal sport educational agenices include the development of physical fitness, mental alertness, self-control, and self-discipline, and an appropriate blend of cooperative-competitive values.

On the other hand, scholars of sport also point out that there may be negative consequences from sport programs, such as teaching young people distorted values ("winning at any cost"), being undemocratic and highly autocratic in coaching and policy control, setting groups in opposition to each other based on their affiliation with respective sport teams or organizations, and the use of sport for advocating a particular governmental or political position or goal. The accusation has also been made that sport is used by business and political leaders as a propagandistic device for promoting the values of the capitalistic system.

The roles of sport in American society in general, in addition to its roles in formal school settings, are also a subject of current interest. The extent of voluntary, active participation in sport, dance, and exercise is indeed widespread across all age levels. In fact, it is beyond the capabilities of researchers to make other than gross estimates of the extent of such participation, the financial cost, and the amount of time associated therewith in the United States. It is enough to say that sport, dance, and exercise, in one way or another, infringe upon both the work and informal leisure life of a high percentage of all Americans and constitute a pervading force in American society. Their direct influence on millions of Americans surely make them collectively one of the most potent and widespread phenomena present and available for enjoyment and consumption, in one form or another, in this country. Social scientists, economists, social psychologists, newspaper reporters and editors, magazine and book publishers, civic officials at all levels, parents, the health sciences community, and virtually every other segment of the American public in one way or another are concerned with, and participate in, some aspect of what we call the "sporting life," in its broad connotation of exercise, healthful living, creative expression, recreation fulfillment, and just plain fun!

Other ways in which sport is deeply interconnected with sociological aspects of American society have been noted. Various social classes have differing sport preferences as participants and as spectators. People in the so-called working class seem to enjoy being spectators at sports that involve physical strength, physical skills related to self defense and to mechanical manipulation, self-defense movements, the necessity for courage or "guts," ethnic pride, non-school sports, and individual sports such as bowling and racing. Spectator sports such as auto racing, motorcycle racing, demolition derby, horse racing, and others of a similar nature are appealing because they symbolize excitement, risk, rapid movements, courage, and physical skills that involve a component of strength.

Particular sport programs may not always develop in the partici-   *Values*
pants the types of values and behaviors that are described in most

statements of the goals and objectives of sport programs. Coakley[12] points out that

> organized sport programs for youngsters may not be influencing the development of participants in the ways often claimed by program supporters. Although data are scarce, those that do exist suggest that involvement in organized programs does not inevitably lead to the development of character, that is, positive personality traits. In fact, it may primarily influence youngsters to be outcome oriented rather than process oriented and may lead them to emphasize instrumental involvement in sport rather than expressive involvement.

Effect of Sport on Scholastics. Many studies have been made correlating athletic success as measured by the earning of letters, grade point averages, and other measures of educational attainment. Although any one study produces results differing from another study, the general consensus is that high school athletes achieve a higher grade point average, have more plans for college and university attendance, and, in fact, attain a higher level of education in colleges than do non-athletes.

Concerning girl athletes, Buhrman and Jarvis[13] draw the following conclusions from their study:

> Girl athletes are more popular with both male and female peers and are found more often in the social elite, according to their peers and teachers, than their non-athletic counterparts. . . . Other analyses reveal that the more a girl actively participates in athletics and the higher her measure of status with her peers, the more official

Girl athletes are often more popular than their non-athletic counterparts.

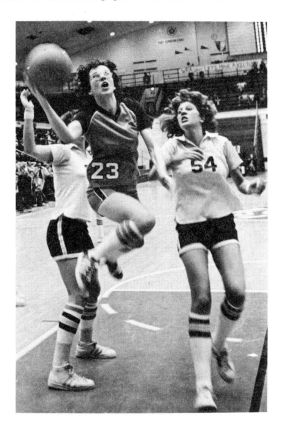

leadership positions she holds in school organizations, the more she attends girls' and boys' athletic events as a spectator, and the higher her level of scholarship.

Coakley[14] summarizes research on the relationship between participation in athletics and academic scholarship:

> there have been no studies showing that participation *causes* actual changes in the athletes of these relationships or other dimensions. On a more general level, there is no empirical evidence demonstrating that interscholastic sport programs contribute to the efficiency or success of the school in achieving educational goals.

Eitzen and Sage[15] level a serious indictment at sport:

> the prevailing form of sport — the corporate level — has corrupted the original intentions of sport. Instead of player-oriented competition (informal sport), sport has become a spectacle, big business, and the extension of power politics. Play has become work. Spontaneity has been superseded by bureaucracy. The goal of pleasure and the physical activity has been replaced by extrinsic rewards, especially money. (p. 20)

They sum up the contribution of sport to what they call American values:

> sport is a microcosm of American society. The types of sports, the way in which sport is organized, who participates and who does not, all provide clues about the nature of society. Thus, the study of sport, like the study of any institution, provides important indicators about (1) a society's values, (2) a society's social structure (social stratification and social organization), and (3) societal problems. (p. 59)

Again to quote Eitzen and Sage:

> Sport and education are inexorably intertwined in American society. (p. viii)
>
> Sport serves the following needs of the institution called "society." (1) Sport serves as a safety valve for both spectators and participants, dissipating excess energies, tensions, and hostile feelings in a socially acceptable way; (2) athletes serve as role models, possessing the proper mental and physical traits to be emulated by other members of society; and (3) sport is a secular quasireligious institution using ritual and ceremony to reinforce the values of society, and thereby regulating behavior to the channels prescribed by custom. (p. 11)

The sociology of sport is rapidly developing as a subdiscipline in physical education, as more sociologists are researching and writing interpretive articles on this specialization. Universities increasingly are emphasizing the sociology of sport at both masters and doctoral degree levels. There are new scholarly journals and new academic organizations devoted to this subject. Several new books appear each year. Conference and convention programs expand sessions for members interested in the sociology of sport.

SOCIOLOGY OF SPORT

Important variables in sport contexts have been identified such as (1) the reputation and influence of the socializer, and the social and personal characteristics of the participants; (2) the effect of voluntary or required selection and participation by individuals; (3) the degree and intensity of involvement in the sport activity by the participant; and (4) the influence of expressive or instrumental socialization relationships.

Loy[16] provides a rationale for the development of the sociology of sport and the need for critical inquiry and research in this field:

> sport is such a pervasive social phenomenon, intruding upon all aspects of daily life, that it deserves sociological attention in its own right. Sport . . . is a social institution having its own interaction, and strategic structural relationships with other significant social institutions. (p. 51)

Sport programs enable the researcher to investigate the fundamental nature of social processes and social structures such as socialization, social change, and social stratification. Other research areas of interest are sport as an institutionalized game, as a social situation, as a social institution, and sport game occurrence.

Sport sociologists are particularly interested in the nature and effects of socialization through sport and physical education participation. There is evidence to date indicating that instructional programs in physical education are not very effective in socializing participants into diffuse social roles. On the other hand, many lasting social relations occur in interscholastic and intercollegiate athletics.

The term *socialization* generally refers to the processes employed *Socialization* by a group or society to channel the development of individuals involved in socially acceptable and personally rewarding behaviors, particularly with respect to fulfilling expected roles of a social group. A person's role is the basic unit of socialization. The role consists of the activities the individual is expected to engage in because of the normative demands made by the particular society. Early in life we learn to engage in specified roles. It is through these roles that societal tasks and responsibilities are allocated and assigned to each of us. The same person engages in different roles, in different social situations, or as a member of different social groups. Different roles within a particular group are played by different individuals at different times. Overall, the learning of proper behaviors to carry on specific important roles allocated by society or its subgroups results in socialization. Physical education and sport provide specific learning situations in which students can learn various roles that later may be transferred to positions having larger responsibilities in the greater society.

Leadership. Most, if not all, groups have an appointed or self-declared leader, or one evolves over time as the group begins to function. The group holds certain expectations of the leader, whether the person is elected or appointed. Leadership is directed toward the identification and clarification of group goals, the development and maintenance of group integration to enhance the achievement of goals, and the provision of individual identity for each member. In the physical education context these leadership roles are played by the teacher, coach, team captain, game official, or squad leader.

Competitor. America is known as a competitive society as indicated by the free enterprise business system, the election of public officials by individual vote, and the prevalence of sport and game contests in many forms throughout the country. Therefore, the role of competitor is central in sport education programs in a free society such as

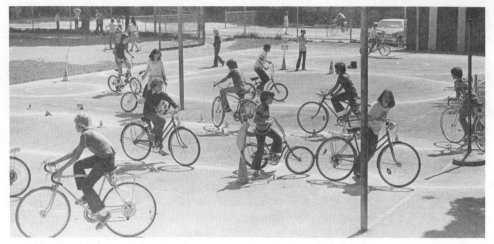

Various roles learned in physical education may later be transferred to positions having larger responsibilities in the greater society.

ours. The competitor is counted upon to meet expectations such as diligent practice to improve, to compete well, and to perform at the highest level possible, to maintain personal and emotional control, and to demonstrate respect for opponents and officials. Overall, a personal role of commitment and strong will to succeed is the hallmark of a true competitor.

Cooperator. The cooperator is another social role that is taught by various segments of the American democratic society. In sport the *teammate* is the conspicuous example of the cooperator. The cooperator learns to facilitate the achievements of teammates, to submit self for the good of the team, and to contribute as fully as possible without undue concern for personal glory or private gain.

The physical educator and the coach must understand the essential concepts of social roles. Appropriate learning environments must be provided in physical education classes and with regard to sport teams so that the important role behaviors valued by the society can be fostered and reinforced. It is essential to realize that the physical education environment has the potential for the development of undemocratic role performances if proper leadership is not exerted continuously.

Sex Roles. Another essential aspect of role expectation is that of sex differentiation. From day one, babies are taught sex-role expectations by their parents and siblings. Obviously these role expectations differ according to the mores and customs of the society in which they are being raised. School-age boys and girls experience considerable difficulty in meeting cultural expectations of femininity or masculinity. Humanists and social philosophers urge that role connotations of femininity and masculinity be abandoned because such notions are not compatible with free and equal democratic values. Rather, we should stress humanness in each individual. Therefore, it is incumbent upon physical educators to examine their responsibilities for the development of role expectations and the effect of those expectations on student growth and development. It should be remembered that social education is only one aspect of total human development and learning. Schools are social agencies in American society; they are charged with the responsibility to maintain, transmit, and improve the general social order that typifies American culture.

Because of the emphasis upon the individual and his uniqueness in a democratic society, the responsibility of the school to guide the socialization processes is enormous. The goal of self-actualization of each individual, a prominent feature of American education, makes the task particularly complex. Physical education teachers and coaches are members of an academic faculty who work together to provide an effective environment in the schools that is conducive to the legitimate socialization needs of the pupils.

It is recognized that members of the pupil's immediate family are key agents in the continual socialization process. The American public school has been charged to assist the parents, and other agencies of American society, in strengthening the values of the American democratic code. Educators in the American democratic system are responsible for fostering and reinforcing individual value systems that encourage behavior consistent with democratic values.

Another aspect of sport interest and participation that is investigated by sport sociologists has to do with the differences in status in society and the types of spectator sports attended. Upper-class individuals, who are normally in higher income brackets, attend football, basketball, and baseball contests. They belong to private sport organizations such as golf clubs, tennis clubs, swimming clubs, and racquet clubs. Some business leaders receive financial perquisites and rewards such as paid memberships in private clubs, opportunities to go duck hunting or quail hunting on private preserves, deep sea fishing on private yachts, and so on. The price of admission tickets alone can keep many middle- and lower-class individuals from attending certain elite commercial sporting events, at least on a regular basis. *Social Stratification*

Upward Social Mobility. It is interesting to note that sport participation is a route by which a few talented performers from lower income groups may move either slowly or rapidly into a higher economic status. There are notable examples of "instant millionaires" among professional players in football, baseball, and ice hockey. Competitors in professional sports such as horse racing, golf, tennis, and hockey can earn substantial sums of money, even though they are not of top championship caliber. Of course, the time period during which these high salaries are earned is quite short compared to the total life span. Also, the percentage of American society talented enough to qualify for these high incomes is minute.

A recent research study of black athletes in football and baseball regarding achievement of upward social mobility and assimilation into the general society concluded that blacks have not advanced very far in these professional sports. Apparently, blacks are treated no differently in professional sports than they are in other sectors of society. "Sport can no longer be identified as the epitome and example of racial harmony and equality."[17]

Brown[18] administered a questionnaire to 60 black and white junior class males in three public high schools in an anonymous northeastern city. The subject for investigation was the degree of participation or non-participation in interscholastic athletics. Brown's major conclusions were that the black athletes did not regard sport as a vehicle for higher education any more than did non-athletic blacks. Concerning all of the students in the survey he concluded that athletic participation does not significantly influence future educational plans of the players, black or white. He even suggested that it is possible there is a lessening effect on college continuation plans of these high school youths, race notwithstanding.

Coakley[19] has summarized available literature on the issue of upward mobility.

> The most logical conclusion emerging from this review of race and sport is that sport provides an abundance of dreams for the Black population in this country, but it provides few actual opportunities. This is not to say that opportunities do not exist, but only that the number of opportunities available are far below what is needed to bring about changes in socioeconomic conditions among Blacks. Some individuals have made it in sport, and others will make it in the future, but the role of sport in the lives of Blacks has been blown far out of proportion.

Eitzen and Sage[20] summarize their chapter, "Sport, Social Stratification, and Social Mobility," as follows

> First, sport, like the larger society, is stratified. Socioeconomic status is related to the types of sports in which one participates and watches. The lower the status, the more inclined toward contact sports and pseudo-sports such as professional wrestling and roller derby. The socioeconomic strata are segregated in sport not only by preference but also by such barriers as entrance requirements and prohibitive costs.
>
> The second theme is that sports participation has limited potential as a social mobility escalator. There is evidence that being a successful athlete enchances self-confidence and the probability of attending college. Thus, social mobility is accomplished through sport indirectly because of the increased employment potential from educational attainment. Social mobility through sport is limited, however, if one is provided an inferior education, as is often the case. It is also limited by failure to graduate, and the *very* few number of positions in professional sport. Even for those who attain major league status, the probabilities of fame and fortune are small because of the fierce competition and injuries.
>
> The myth that sport is a mobility escalator is especially dangerous for minority youth. Ghetto youngsters who devote their lives to the pursuit of atheletic stardom are, except for the fortunate few, doomed to failure — failure in sport and in the real world, for sport skills are essentially irrelevant to occupational placement and advancement.

Sport and Political Ideology

Another important phenomenon relative to sport, particularly at national and international levels, is the rapidly increasing use of sport as a vehicle for promoting self-serving goals, particularly in the areas of propaganda, national pride, and social integration. The importance placed on sport by the governments of many Communist countries is particularly evident. Very young boys and girls are identified as having potential abilities to become national and international champions, especially in those sports having competitions at the international level, such as the Olympic Games, or important regional invitational sport contests and games meetings. East Germany, Russia, and Cuba come to mind instantly as examples of countries using sport as an instrument of national policy to achieve recognition and support from peoples of other countries as well as to build prestige for and commitment to the government in its own citizens.

CHAPTER FOUR

Roles of Sport in the United States. In an unpublished study, Nixon[21] identified ten roles of sport as an instrument of national policy in the United States. Briefly these roles are:

1. Politics
2. Propaganda
3. International understanding and good will
4. Education
5. Health
6. Economics
7. Militarism
8. Crime prevention
9. Recreation
10. Ritual and ceremony

Sport and Other Political Systems. In Russia and other Communist countries sport and designed exercise are used as instruments of social control and to inculcate government goals in the people. Communist China, and other nations with similar political ideology, use sports to support their revolutionary purposes. It is well known that the Union of South Africa denies black people opportunities to compete in national sports against whites, thus giving emphasis to their political policy of separation or apartheid through sport. Many national governments have a policy of developing strong international competitors for the Olympic Games and other prestigious sporting events around the world so as to demonstrate symbolically the strengths of the national political system and to promote national propaganda and good will.

Hart[22] says:

> Communist countries have long openly regarded their sporting representatives as political emissaries who can do more than diplomats to recommend the Communist philosophy and way of life to those who have not adopted it. East and West sportsmen, whether they like it or not, are "ambassadors of good will" and are under pressure to vindicate not merely their own prowess, but the ideology of their country. There are few governments in the world which do not now accept the political importance of success in international sport.

Some countries, primarily those governed by dictatorships, require that all sport programs within the country be directed by a national political agency and guided by political ideology. It is perfectly clear in these countries that sport is used as a medium for promoting political ideology and also for unifying the masses of the population in the service and support of the government.

Racism in Sport

Racism in sport has become a popular topic in the past few years. Some advocates of educational sport proudly declare that sport is free of this prejudice, which exists in most other areas of American society. It is asserted that all players are equal in the athletic arena, but there is much evidence to refute this contention. Harry Edwards[23] and other authors and sportsmen have offered many examples of members of minority racial groups being excluded or in some way deprived of the benefits of full participation in amateur and professional sports in America.

The very slow assimilation of minority group members into professional sports is well documented in America. Likewise, it is only recently that members of minority groups, and blacks in particular, have become relatively more numerous in American collegiate athletics. Selected references at the end of this chapter provide illuminating insight into historical and current trends concerning racism in American sports, a topic that should be carefully studied by every physical education major. Both amateur and professional sports in America still are far from free of racial prejudice.

Girls and Women in Sports

The women's liberation movement was a major catalyst for more rapid development of equal opportunities for female participation in the organized sporting life of American institutions, particularly in schools and colleges. This movement was given official Federal Government sanction by the passage of Title IX, which, in essence, decrees that all physical education and sport programs conducted by public agencies will provide equal opportunity in every respect for girls and women. There are many historical influences and sources of control that contributed to long-term development of bias and prejudice against full and equal participation of girls and women in sports in American history; these are well documented in many publications, including those listed at the end of this chapter.

Although many new and revised programs and policies have recently made broader participation in sport available to girls and women, by no means has this movement yet come close to optimum fulfillment. In fact, there are complaints of "foot-dragging" and lack of full cooperation, particularly from certain males who occupy strategic leadership positions in the administration of recreation, physical education, and sport programs. On the other hand, most objective observers probably would agree there have been substantial changes in attitudes, policies, program expansion, qualified leadership, and other essential ingredients that combine to produce continuing improvements in programs of sport for girls and women. Full support must be given to the momentum currently established to continue to build these programs in the future, moving ever onward toward the ultimate goal of complete equity.

An interesting study by Bohren[24] investigated the family background of intercollegiate varsity female athletes and compared their socioeconomic status with that of a sample of nonathletes. A disproportionately large representation of such athletes came from the low socioeconomic group. The majority of fathers who participated regularly in sports had wives who were basically non-primary sports participants. On the other hand, the majority of mothers who were primary sport participants were married to men who were also primary participants. For some inexplicable reason women athletes are more likely to have an older brother who was not an athlete.

Sport and Religion

The role of sport in the assimilation of the basic creed of several religions is more prominent than most of us realize, and is another interesting topic usually included in the study and discussion of the sociology of sport. It is well known that certain religions deliberately use sport as a vehicle for attracting young people, as converts to a particular faith. Also, sport celebrities are used as exemplars of the basic principles of a particular religion by "spreading the word" to interested groups of youths and adults, thus communicating and interpreting the basic beliefs of the religion through sport. For many years various churches have had recreational rooms in the basements of their buildings, and they have sponsored volleyball and basketball teams and other forms of physical sport and recreation in an effort to attract and retain young members. The Young Men's and Young Women's Christian Association (YMCA, YWCA) the Christian Youth Organization, and other quasi-religious groups use sport, exercise, and fitness as educational modes for teaching and learning the creeds and concepts of those organizations.

Athletes have banded together to form religion-based voluntary groups primarily to work with young people. Examples are the Fellowship of Christian Athletes and Athletes in Action. These groups, composed of athletes and ex-athletes from high schools, community colleges, and universities, form teams and schedule games with schools, colleges, and other groups primarily for the purpose of developing friendships and spreading the gospels of their respective religions. Coaches are integrally involved in most of these organizations; "big name" coaches are particularly sought after because of their public appeal.

Popular magazines have published articles describing these organizations, their objectives, their services, and their programs. Hard-bound and paperback books that describe them in even more detail also are available.

Coaches and athletes use religion in various ways. Many school and college teams kneel in silent or oral prayer in the dressing room prior to coming out onto the playing field before games, or sometimes almost immediately before a contest begins. Such a prayer may appeal to "fighting a good fight," playing without serious injury, and even, on some occasions, to suggest some assistance toward winning the game. Individual players will symbolically express a personal religious value such as crossing themselves before attempting a free-throw in a basketball game.

Leisure and Work

Historically, the United States has been regarded as a work-oriented society. The "work ethic" has been a traditional American value. Our status in the hierarchy of the American social system is enhanced in proportion to our recognition as a productive, stable producer of services or goods. However, in recent years this traditional value has been eroded owing to the many complex changes that have occurred in American society. The advent of shorter working hours per week, the availability of local, state, and federal financial welfare services support to large segments of the American population, the rapidly increasing use of labor-saving devices, and the "do your own thing" motto have combined to reduce the influence of the work-oriented cultural values.

More and more leisure time is becoming available to most Americans owing to the shorter work week, more paid vacation days, and similar trends. The worthy use of leisure time thus becomes even more important than it was before. The positive use of leisure must be emphasized for individuals and for societal groups. The family, the educational system, and other social agencies should emphasize the uniqueness of each individual and urge that human capacity for the optimum use of leisure be stressed. Individual and collective capacity for positive uses of leisure and the opportunities for productive work should be accorded equal importance in the value system of the society and the individuals that compose it. Leisure and work must complement each other to sustain the creative energies of the nation that ensure continuous, genuine cultural advancement. Social science research studies have revealed significant differences in the uses and patterns of leisure time in relation to such factors as occupational status, ethnic background, and socioeconomic categories.

It is not difficult for the average citizen who reads a daily newspaper, listens to the radio, or watches television to realize that there are enormous economic and monetary implications associated with recreational, educational, and professional sports. As a result of the sports boom in America, tremendous industrial growth has developed to provide facilities, equipment, supplies, uniforms, and other accessories needed for the conduct of and participation in a wide range of sports. In fact, sports now constitute one of the largest segments of American industry. As long ago as 1972, the New York Times[25] asserted that billions of dollars were being spent in support of sport in America; this capital outlay exceeded the cost of the national defense budget at that time. Whether this generalization is true today is not known, owing to the lack of verified data. However, enormous expenditures for all aspects of sport, physical education, and exercise continue and are almost beyond comprehension.

Sport and Economics

Spectator attendance increases yearly at college and university athletic events such as football and basketball, and in professional sports throughout America and Canada. Despite the ever-increasing price of individual admission, millions of spectators from all walks of life, young and old, healthy or handicapped, somehow seem able to allocate some of their discretionary income to attendance at amateur or professional sporting events. Sport constitutes an area of human activities involving billions of dollars in the construction and operation of facilities, equipment, and supplies, the employment of sport performers, commentators and the instructional, maintenance, and service personnel required to conduct, control, and communicate the sporting events.

Sport in America is said to reflect the values of democratic capitalism. The payoff (the winning of the game or the earning of a corporate profit) depends upon the individual and collective effort of the workers (or the players), striving for a common goal, being rewarded for a successful performance, displaying habits of compliance to orders, perseverance, fighting or working hard even during times of difficulty, and being a contributing member of the "team." All of the above attributes are woven together through belief in law and order and the need for collective discipline to attain the desired end. Employers will give preference to individuals with a strong sport background, other prerequisite factors being equal, because of attitudes and behaviors learned in sport settings, which are assumed to be transferable to the world of business and economics.

Commercial Sport. Also, business and industry use sport contests as vehicles for promotion, advertisement, and corporate good will, all of which supposedly contribute to maximize profits. The profit motive applies not only to commercial ventures, but also to "big time" sports in American institutions of higher education. Gate receipts, television and radio contracts, along with ticket sales and the monetary gifts from team supporters run into millions of dollars yearly in the United States.

The remuneration of sport stars for commercial appearances on television and radio are reaching unbelievable proportions. O. J. Simpson at one time was under contract simultaneously with at least eight large American corporations to make television, radio, and magazine appearances for the promotion of the products and services.

Sport and the City.   Cities build new stadiums in efforts to attract professional sport teams to their areas. They subsidize a considerable portion of the operation expenses of the teams and provide other forms of service to the owners. In return, the cities expect to benefit enormously through increased tourist and spectator expenditures in the hotels, restaurants, department stores, night clubs, and at the sporting events themselves — generating a profit well in excess of expenditures. Likewise, the national and international publicity through radio, television, and newspapers contributes to the reputations of these cities and surroundings. Thus, these cities become internationally famous as sites for vacation visitors from around the world. International tourism is a major source of income for cities and commercial agencies in the United States. Interlacing all of these promotional efforts are big-time professional sport events, entertainment, night clubs, luxury hotels, expensive dining establishments, and other manifestations of commerce and industry that contribute to the financial health of these metropolitan areas.

Athletic Scholarships — Aid or Pay?   The controversy about criteria and enforcement of rules and regulations governing legal financial aid to bona fide student athletes in American colleges and universities is another topic of both educational and financial significance that is beyond the scope of this book. However, such controversies are commonplace in many of our American institutions of higher education, and the trend seems to be growing rather than decreasing. Students majoring in physical education should become acquainted with the available facts and the guiding concepts prevalent today in the relationship between sport and economics. Of course, many important issues are involved in this topic, such as institutional integrity, intellectual honesty, ensuring that bona fide students attend the university and earn the academic right to play on the teams, as well as other vital questions.

In the United States each of the fifty states makes legal provisions for the inclusion of sport and exercise programs as fundamental aspects of the public school curriculum. The sport program is a required part of the curriculum for all children. It is generally included in other public and private schools curricula until grade twelve, although in upper-grade levels it may become an elective subject. It is a basic component of the course of study in most American community colleges, four-year public colleges, and universities. In fact, it can be contended that in many states, physical education is one of the most required subjects in the entire curriculum by State legal mandate.

In California, for example, all students enrolled in public education from grade one through grade ten are required to be enrolled in suitable physical education classes on a regular basis throughout the school year. Physical education is an optional academic class in the eleventh and twelfth grades. In addition, interscholastic athletic programs provide a voluntary formal instructional physical education experience for as many

SPORT AND PHYSICAL EDUCATION

Sport and Formal Education

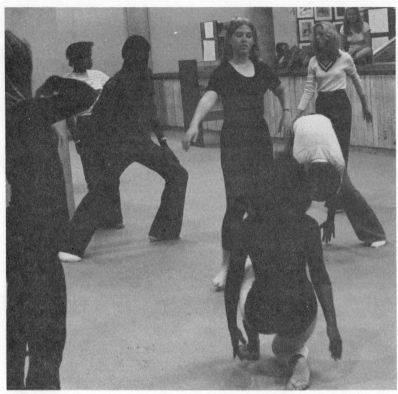

In schools, physical education, dance, and sport programs are centers of considerable social interaction.

as 40 per cent of the boys and girls in schools in an intensively motivated environment under the supervision of expertly qualified men and women coaches. Academic credit frequently is awarded for satisfactory participation. No other subject in the school curriculum comes close to being required for so many years on such a regular basis in many states.

Public School Expenditure for Physical Education. During the era of rapid expansion of public school enrollment and the consequent development of new school sites and facilities, unpublished studies by Nixon revealed that a typical four-year high school site meeting the State (California) legal requirement of 40 acres, would devote more than 50 per cent of the land area to physical education, sport, and recreation. Of the total budget for purchasing the land and building the school, approximately 25 per cent was allocated to provision of sport and physical recreation areas, facilities, and major equipment and supplies. Surely these figures demonstrate strong support by the society at large for physical education and sport as basic subjects in the school curriculum. Parents and other taxpayers exert the power of approval or disapproval of policies and budgets that provide for the educational program, staff, facilities, and supplies. Such support for physical education and sport has been strong throughout many years in most states, and this trend continues today in spite of the need for financial "belt-tightening."

Social Integration and the Physical Education Program. Social integration is another major role of the physical education program. A school is a special social system within society at large. Administrators, teachers, students, and staff members have well-defined roles within the school system. There is a continuing need to facilitate increased social integration within schools so that all individuals involved can interrelate and cooperate more effectively to achieve the goals of the organization.

In schools, physical education, dance, and sport programs are centers of considerable social interaction, often including members from society at large as well as individuals who spend the day in the schools. Physical education and sport programs can assist in this social integration process by providing interesting and helpful programs that attract people from various ethnic groups and social and economic factions in the community.

Individual social development has long been an objective in school *Social Development* physical education programs. However, there is still a paucity of validated evidence concerning the achievement of this goal in most schools. A major problem is the lack of agreement concerning the specific social behaviors that should be learned by all children. Answers need to be sought for these pertinent questions:

— Should the game really belong to those who play it?
— To what degree should the contest be directed and controlled by the teachers, coaches, and administrators, rather than by the students?
— What is a satisfactory definition of amateurism and how can the amateur status of athletes be accurately determined and assured?
— What are the bounds of fair play and good sportsmanship in a sports contest?
— Can eligibility rules be clearly written and implicitly enforced so as to provide equal opportunity for all participants?
— There are many examples of inconsistencies between the ideals and objectives of formal school physical education and sport programs and their actual conduct. If the professional leaders are unable to develop clear and meaningful interpretations of valuable educational standards in physical education and sport, how can we expect to influence the students under our direction to learn and develop in the direction of so-called desirable social standards?

Satisfactory answers to the above questions depend upon the development of more sophisticated and objective research techniques for measuring and evaluating specific aspects of social development. How can we validly assess an individual's progress in the learning of desirable socialization habits, attitudes, and behaviors? How can we determine whether or not the student is developing a positive attitude toward a sport or dance activity rather than a distaste for it as a form of drudgery or work? Is the student really learning respect for authority as represented by a humanistic teacher or coach? Or is the pupil developing an attitude of rejection of authority because of an experience with a dictatorial type of coach? Valid assessments of social behaviors of children, and their direction of change, are still in the stage of scientific improvement and refinement.

It behooves teacher educators to help preservice physical education majors, and teachers on an inservice basis, to become aware of their major responsibilities in the proper social development of children under their tutelage and to assist the children in developing in socially desirable ways through discussion and personal example. Social learning concepts developed through physical education experiences in schools must transfer to situations in other aspects of students' lives if the educational experiences are to be worth the time and money expended on them. Therefore, transfer of learning must be consciously directed toward all students in the physical education and sport programs if we are to expect pupils to learn appropriate social behaviors to carry over into areas of life outside of the school environment now and in the future.

Spectator Appreciation. School and college programs in physical education should teach "sport-spectator appreciation." All students should learn what to look for while observing athletic performances so that they can quickly recognize, for example, the execution of a perfect dive, the graceful coordination of a gymnastic routine, the intricacies of form involved in a fencing duel, or the strategic significance of a football play. All instructors should enable their students to recognize, understand, and appreciate the beauties of player movements produced spontaneously, quickly, and accurately despite human, mechanical, and time impediments. Teaching students to become "literate" in sport participation and observation is an important objective of physical education and sport programs. Students should learn to appreciate the beauty of sport.

The purposes of formal research studies in the sociology of sport are concisely stated by Yiannakis, McIntyre, Melnick, and Hart.[26]

RESEARCH AND SCHOLARSHIP

> This perspective (the sociological study of sport), in its broadest sense, employs theoretical frameworks and the empirical tools of the social sciences to aid man in better understanding human behavior in sport contests. All the research tools available to the sociologist, social psychologist, and anthropologist, can and have been used in an effort to ascertain the manifest and latent functions of sport in modern society. As in any other scientific effort, scholars with an interest in sport have also attempted to describe, discover, and explain this phenomenon with the eventual goal being the prediction of sport-related human social behavior. The study of human social behavior must be constantly aware of the fact that prediction of behavior is not absolute but is necessarily stated in probabilistic terms.

Snyder and Spreitzer[27] present a clear, detailed explanation for the need for research in sociology of sport. Extracts from their article follow:

> We suggest that as a substantive topic sport has as much claim on the sociologist's attention as the more conventional specialties of family, religion, political, and industrial sociology. Sports and games are cultural universals and basic institutions in societies, and are some of the most pervasive aspects of culture in industrialized societies. . . .
> Basically, we argue that a sociologist studies sports for the same reason as any other topic — for intrinsic interest and to impose so-

ciological frameworks as a means of constructing and refining concepts, propositions, and theories from the larger discipline. . . .

The phenomenon of sport represents one of the most pervasive social institutions in the United States. Sports permeate all levels of social reality from the societal down to the social-psychological levels. The salience of sport can be documented in terms of news coverage, financial expenditures, numbers of participants and spectators, hours consumed, and time samplings of conversations. Given the salience of sports as a social institution, a sociology of sport has emerged that attempts to go beyond the descriptive level by providing theoretically informed analyses and explanations of sports activity.

The sociology of sport has received little attention from traditional researchers in sociology in past years. Some of them regard it as frivolous or non-serious. Very few articles or research studies have been recorded in academic journals until recently. Because sport is so pervasive in American life, an assertion that can be readily demonstrated, it is essential that research studies and textbooks explaining the sociology of sport be encouraged. The editors of the *Christian Century* support this contention:

> It is because sports are so much more than simple amusement that they deserve serious attention. Sports claim high priorities in the budgets of families, schools, cities, and the media. Emotional and ethical styles, both individualistic and collective, are shaped in athletic arenas.

Reasons for Sociological Study of Sport. Coakley[28] states there are three major reasons why the sociology of sport is an important area of study and research. The first is that sport permeates American life in many significant ways.

Second, through sport programs and activities the interested researcher can study important social relationships and processes for three reasons: (a) Formal sport teams differ from other types of social organizations because they are governed by explicit rules, their size is strictly controlled, and there is an obvious relationship between the different positions occupied by individuals on the teams. (b) Because many sport contests are publicized and accurately recorded in the score book, and in the public media, there is abundant sociological evidence available at low cost. Much of it involves accurate measurements; therefore, a rich store of data is available for researchers. (c) Sport provides examples and evidence of cross-cultural and comparative participation between racial groups within a country and between national teams. There is a long history of anthropologists intensively studying the roles of games in numerous contemporary and primitive societies upon which a comparative study of sport can be undertaken.

Third, the study of sport by sociologists will provide information and suggestions for administrative and policy changes that will lead to the further development and refinement of sport activities and opportunities for the social and educational benefits of more people at the level of direct participation.

Journals. A basic scholarly journal in the socio-cultural aspects of sport is the *Journal of Sport and Social Issues*, published by ARENA, the Institute for Sport and Social Analysis. Published literature, both in magazines and in book format, is proliferating rapidly, as is indicated by the other current magazines such as the *Canadian Journal of Applied Sport Sciences; International Review of Sport Sociology; Journal of Human Movement Studies,* published in England; *Journal of Leisure Research; Journal of Sport Behavior; Journal of Sport History; Review of Sport and Leisure; Journal of Sport Psychology,* and the *Sport Sociology Bulletin.*

The ERIC (Educational Resources Information Center) Clearinghouse on Teacher Education at the University of Maryland is an excellent source of recent literature under the title of Social Sciences of Sport. SIRLS is another information retrieval system concerning the sociology of sport and leisure, published by the Faculty of Human Kinetics, University of Waterloo, Waterloo, Ontario, N2L 361, Canada. Many new books and magazines are appearing on this topic in the United States and abroad.

New professional and academic organizations are formed from time to time. One example is the North American Society for the Sociology of Sport.*

SUMMARY

The socio-cultural foundations of physical education are essentially composed of anthropology and sociology and consist of major concepts from those basic disciplines that have direct application to primary physical education concepts and applied concerns.

Briefly, anthropology can be identified as the study of the science of human beings, both historical and current. Biological and cultural adaptations of the human race throughout history are the central focus of anthropologists. Research in genetics and evolution is basic to the discovery of major anthropological generalizations.

Anthropology relates to physical education because of common interests in the evolution, growth, and development of the human organism; types of societal organizations into which humans group themselves, and the specific attributes of organized physical activities pursued in those groups; ecological development including hunting, fishing, and farming activities as essential to physical survival in early times; familial relationships; languages and non-verbal movements used to express common concepts; in general, how humans interact with each other and with the physical environments in which they live.

Cultural anthropologists study human institutions, group relationships, and customs and mores of groups. Physical anthropologists study the details of ancient cultures with particular emphasis on morphology and evolution. Sometimes this area of study is called biological anthropology and involves many fundamental concepts of primary interest to the physical educator.

Archaeology is the study of extinct cultures based on discovered artifacts, remains, relics, and other evidence that reveal how people lived in a bygone era. Sport, dance, and physical activities are fundamental categories of evidence derived by the study of archaeology.

Kinesics is an anthropological specialization within the broader area

---

*The first newsletter was published in December 1978, editor Andrew Yiannakis, Department of Sports Studies, University of Connecticut.

of anthropological study designated as linguistics, that refers to non-verbal communication through bodily movements in culture-specific environments.

Synchrony is another form of non-verbal communication involving the careful analysis of high-speed motion pictures of bodily movements engaged in as people attempt to interract with each other. Body rhythms, in a physiological sense, are part of this area of anthropology.

Ethnology is the term used to describe a major anthropological research methodology for collecting evidence about how humans live. The ethnologist works and lives as closely as possible with the group being studied, in an unobtrusive way, and makes many qualitative evaluations of his observations, as well as available quantitative measures.

Physical educators rely heavily on concepts and evidence from anthropology as guides to improved understanding of aims and objectives as well as guidance for optimal values to accrue through valid teaching-learning experiences. Aesthetics are of concern to the thoughtful physical educator. Sport as an art form, with cultural identity, and sport as kinesthetic art are examples of the application of fundamental anthropological concepts to the enlightened understanding of, and competent instruction in, physical education, sport, and dance in the life of any nation.

Sociology is the study of human social groups with interest in such areas as family, religion, crime, social organization, population trends, social stratification, education, political expression, economic aspects, and the status of minority groups.

The sociology of sport is a rapidly rising field of specialized study. Such topics as roles of sport in society, social class preferences in sport, values and behaviors reinforced by sport participation, relationship of sport to academic attainment, the pervasive nature and influence of sport in the life of a country, socialization through sport, social stratification as influenced by sport participation, upward social mobility through sport and political ideology, racism in sport, evolving roles of girls and women in sport, the relationship of sport and religious creeds, the relationship of leisure and work ethics in a culture, sport and national economy, sport and formal education, social development through sport, spectator appreciation, and research in the sociology of sport are examples of current trends in the study and exposition of the nature and purposes of the sociology of sport.

New specialized academic and professional organizations with central emphasis on the sociology of sport are developing in many countries throughout the world. Likewise, there is a continuous proliferation of academic and professional journals, books, and other publications concentrating on sociocultural aspects of sport, physical education, and dance.

FOOTNOTES

[1]Roger Pearson, *Introduction to Anthropology*. New York: Holt, Rinehart and Winston, 1974. p. vii.
[2]Davydd J. Greenwood and William A. Stini, *Nature, Culture, and Human History*. New York: Harper & Row, Publishers, 1977.
[3]Alfred L. Kroeber and Clyde Kluckhohn, *Culture: A Critical Review of Concepts and Definitions*. Cambridge, MA: The Museum, 1952.
[4]Clyde Kluckhohn, *Mirror of Man*. New York: McGraw-Hill, Inc., 1949.
[5]Davydd J. Greenwood and William A. Stini, op. cit., p. 33.

[6]John Singleton and Robert B. Textor, Unpublished working paper, Stanford University, 1975.

[7]Eleanor Metheny, *Connotations of Movement in Sport and Dance*. Dubuque, Iowa: Wm. C. Brown and Company, 1965.

[8]Alan R. Beals, George Spindler, and Louise Spindler, *Culture in Process* (2nd ed.). New York: Holt, Rinehart and Winston, 1973.

[9]Jerry D. Rose, *Introduction to Sociology* (2nd ed.). Chicago: Rand McNally College Publishing Company, 1974.

[10]Scott G. McNall, *The Sociological Perspective: Introductory Readings* (4th ed.). Boston: Little, Brown and Company, 1977.

[11]Jay J. Coakley, *Sport in Society: Issues and Controversies*. St. Louis, MO: The C. V. Mosby Company, 1978, p. 12.

[12]Ibid., p. 122.

[13]H. G. Buhrmann and M. S. Jarvis, "Athletics and Status: An Examination of the Relationships between Athletic Participation and Various Status Measures of High School Girls," *Journal of the Canadian Association for Health, Physical Education and Recreation*, January/February 1971, pp. 14–17.

[14]Jay J. Coakley, op. cit., p. 154.

[15]D. Stanley Eitzen and George H. Sage, *Sociology of American Sport*. Dubuque, Iowa: Wm. C. Brown Company Publishers, 1978, p. 20, 59, viii, 11.

[16]John W. Loy, "A Case for the Sociology of Sport," JOHPER, 43:50–53 (June 1972).

[17]Joseph Dougherty, "Race and Sport: A Follow-up Study," *Sport Sociology Bulletin*, 5:1–12 (Spring, 1976).

[18]Ronald H. Brown, "Educational Plans of Black and White Athletes and Non-Athletes," *Sport Sociology Bulletin*, 5:57–64 (Spring, 1976).

[19]Jay J. Coakley, op. cit., p. 312.

[20]D. Stanley Eitzen and George H. Sage, op. cit., p. 230.

[21]John E. Nixon, "The Roles of Sport as an Instrument of National Policy in the United States." Unpublished study, School of Education, Stanford University, 1979.

[22]Marie Hart, *Sport in the Sociocultural Process* (2nd ed.). Dubuque, Iowa: Wm. C. Brown Company, Publishers, 1976.

[23]Harry Edwards, *Sociology of Sport*. Homewood, IL: Dorsey Press, 1973.

[24]Judy M. Bohren, "The Role of the Family in the Socialization of Female Intercollegiate Athletes." Unpublished doctoral dissertation, University of Maryland, 1977.

[25]*New York Times*, December 31, 1972, p. 14.

[26]Andrew Yiannakis, Thomas D. McIntyre, Merrill J. Melnick, and Dale P. Hart, *Sport Sociology: Contemporary Themes* (2nd ed.). Dubuque, Iowa: Kendall/Hunt Publishing Company, 1979.

[27]Eldon E. Snyder and Elmer Spreitzer, *Social Aspects of Sport*. Englewood Cliffs, N.J.: Prentice-Hall Publishing Co., Inc., 1978.

[28]Jay J. Coakley, op. cit.

SELECTED REFERENCES

Allen, Dorothy J., and Fahey, Brian W., *Being Human in Sport*. Philadelphia: Lea & Febiger, 1977.

Ball, Donald. W., and Loy, John W. (Eds.), *Sport and Social Order*. Reading, MA: Addison-Wesley Publishing Company, 1975.

Best, David, *Philosophy and Human Movement*. London: George Allen and Unwin, Inc., 1978.

Brubacher, John S., *On the Philosophy of Higher Education*. San Francisco: Jossey-Bass Publishers, 1977.

Damon, Albert (Ed.), *Physiological Anthropology*. New York: Oxford Press, 1975.

Davis, Elwood C., Harper, William A., Miller, Donna Mae and Park, Roberta J., *The Philosophic Process in Physical Education*, 3rd Ed. Philadelphia: Lea & Febiger, 1977.

DuBois, Paul E., "Sport, Mobility, and the Black Athlete." *Sport Sociology Bulletin*. 3:55, 56 (Fall 1974).

Eitzen, D. Stanley, *Sport in Contemporary Society*. New York: St. Martin's Press, 1979.

Hilmi, Ibrahim, *Sport and Society: An Introduction to the Sociology of Sport*. Los Alamitos, CA: Hwong Press, 1975.

Klafs, Carl E., and Lyons, Joan, *The Female Athlete* (2nd Ed). St. Louis, MO: The C. V. Mosby Company, 1978.

Landers, Daniel M. (Ed.), *Social Problems in Athletics*. Urbana, IL: University of Illinois Press, 1976.

Landry, Fernand, and Orban, William (Eds.), *Sociology of Sport*. Miami, FL: Symposia Specialists, Inc., 1978.

Lowe, Benjamin, Kanin, David. B., and Strenk, Andrew, *Sport and International Relations*. Champaign, IL: Stipes Publishing Company, 1978.

Loy, John W., The Cultural System of Sport. *Quest*, Monograph 29:73–101 (Winter 1978).

Loy, John W., McPherson, Barry D., and Kenyon, Gerald, *Sport and Social Systems*. Reading MA: Addison-Wesley Publishing Company, 1978.

Luschen, Gunther, "Toward a Structural Analysis of Sport," *Beyond Research Solutions to Human Problems, Academy Papers, No. 10.* Louisville, KY: American Academy of Physical Education, 1976.

Malina, Robert M., "Ethnic and Cultural Factors in the Development of Motor Abilities and Strength in American Children." In G. Lawrence Rarick (Ed.), *Physical Activity, Human Growth and Development.* New York: Academic Press, 1973.

Martens, Rainier, *Social Psychology and Physical Activity.* New York: Harper & Row, 1975.

Michener, James, *Sports in America.* New York: Random House Publishers, 1976.

Nixon, Howard L., *Sport and Social Organization.* Indianapolis, IN: Bobbs-Merrill Company, 1976.

Rooney, John, *A Geography of American Sport — From Cabin Creek to Anaheim.* Reading, MA: Addison-Wesley Publishing Company, 1974.

Sage, George H. (Ed.), *Sports and American Society: Selected Readings* (2nd Ed.). Reading, MA: Addison-Wesley Publishing Company, 1974.

Spindler, George D., *Education and Cultural Processes: Toward an Anthropology of Education.* New York: Holt, Rinehart and Winston, 1974.

Stevenson, Christopher L., and Nixon, John E., "A Conceptual Scheme of the Social Functions of Sport," *Sportwissenschaft,* 2:119–132 (1972).

Zeigler, Earle F., *Physical Education and Sport Philosophy.* Englewood Cliffs, New Jersey: Prentice-Hall, Inc., 1977.

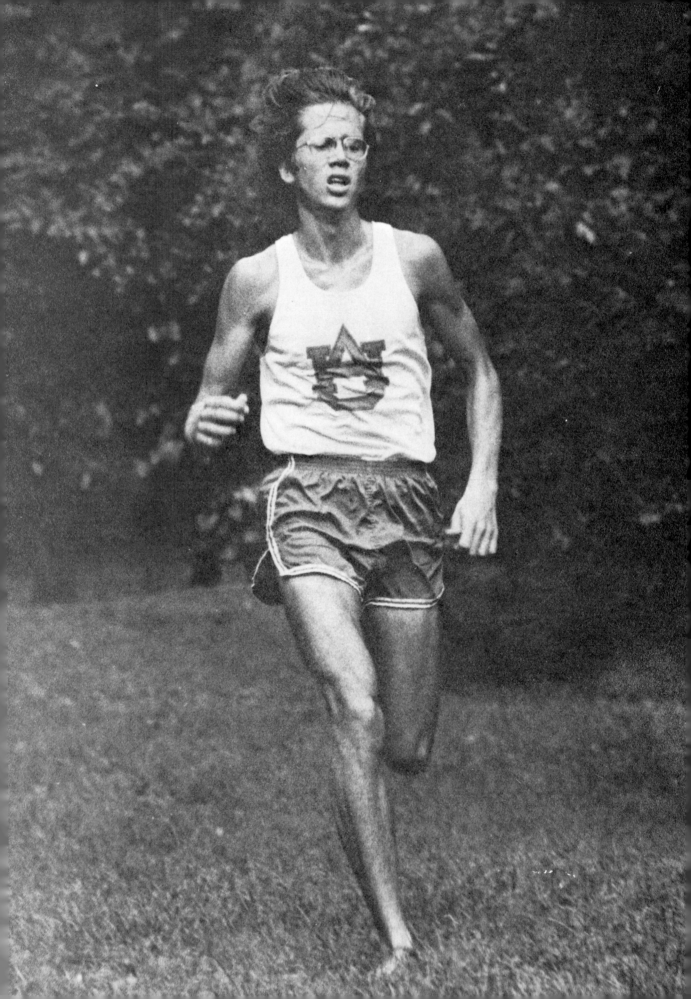

5

BIOLOGICAL ———
——— FOUNDATIONS

Introduction. Biology is defined as the science that studies energy and matter as functions of a living system. It comprises a body of knowledge about living organisms. A living organism is distinguished from inorganic matter by its ability to develop and its continual refinement of structure-function organization. Homeostasis, or continuous self-direction and maintenance, is one of the basic drives of the organism. Biologists define life according to the following characteristics: *irritability* (response to stimuli), *motility* (movement), *self-regulation* (control), and *reproductivity* (multiplication). In brief, an organism seeks to progress from its innate potentialities to a degree of self-fulfillment.

EVOLUTION

Darwinism

Darwin's theory of evolution, based upon the concepts of adaptation and natural selection, is accepted by most modern biologists as the fundamental statement on the development of life forms. Because the environment usually is changing, all living creatures must continually adapt to it or become extinct. The biological mechanisms that account for hereditary characteristics of the newborn also change over time, which leads to the evolution of animal species. Thus, it is contended that all inherited, adaptive changes in organisms are evolutionary changes.

McElroy, Swanson, and Macey[1] summarize these very complex theories and phenomena:

> *Adaptation* can be viewed as a state of being or as a process. As a state of being, adaptation is the sum total of all the characteristics — including the element of chance — that permit an organism to live and reproduce. As a process, adaptation, or *natural selection*, is the manner by which evolutionary success is achieved. Since environmental changes occur, adaptation involves a continual adjustment in organisms to the environment. The bases for adaptation are the inheritable variations in a population and the fact not all individuals in a population contribute their genes to the next generation.
>
> Change is inevitable and evolution proceeds. Therefore, all heritable adaptive changes contribute to evolution, but all evolutionary changes are not necessarily adaptive. The fossil record indicates that many species are now extinct, even though at one time these species were adaptively successful. Adaptation, consequently, is only a tempo-

147

rary success, and adaptation in one set of circumstances does not guarantee equal success under a different set of circumstances.

Darwin's theory of evolution through natural selection most satisfactorily explains the successive changes that have occurred in one generation of organisms as one generation of organisms succeeds another.

There is a competing theory that emphasizes the role of cooperation between organisms. This theory contends that cooperation is a very strong drive in a biological sense and that human development relies more heavily on this principle than on any other one, including the survival of the fittest, as a rational explanation of evolution. The principle of cooperation is asserted to be fundamental in all non-human forms of life that survive and evolve as well.

The "Cooperation Principle"

The cooperation principle explains natural selection by asserting that organisms are most likely to survive and develop in relation to their ability to work together among themselves and with their physical environment to facilitate their chances for survival. This theory is also supported by biological evidence that suggests that all forms of life, even the lowest forms, are possessed of some innate tendency toward social relationship.

Villee, Walker, and Barnes[2] allude to the phenomenon of cooperation as an element in the survival of various animal species although they do not use that term. They infer cooperation when they state

> Aggregation in clumps may increase the competition between the members of a group for food or space, but this is more than counterbalanced by the greater survival power of the group during unfavorable periods. A group of animals has much greater resistance than a single individual to adverse conditions such as desiccation, heat, cold, or poisons. The combined effect of protective mechanisms of the group is effective in countering the adverse environment, whereas that of a single individual is not.

Likewise, these authors continue,

> The concept that animals and plants live together in an orderly manner, not strewn haphazardly over the surface of the earth, is an important principle of ecology.

The Human Animal. Humans are unique among all animals because they have developed a culture, something no other living organism has accomplished. McElroy, Swanson, and Macey[3] state,

> Man is a maker and user of tools, a planner, an inventory of symbols and of spoken and written languages. Man also has a system of values. And he can do things with a purpose, not only for himself, but for future generations as well. All of these add up to a cultural inheritance, a unique phenomenon that is different from the biological inheritance common to all living things.

As humans evolved they established living groups for mutual protection and survival that we now call communities. Gradually they developed a form of written communication. Thus, it was possible from that point on for mankind to record cultural achievements and to pass them on to future generations. It also facilitated more comprehensive instruction for the young.

McElroy, Swanson, and Macey[4] summarize humankind's historical development as follows:

Man is a vertebrate mammal belonging to the Primate group, which includes the tree shrews, lemurs, tarsiers, monkeys, and apes. He is a product of evolution like any other animal, and his evolutionary history can be traced back through fossils more than one million years. As man gradually evolved he assumed an upright stature and a bipedal walk; he learned to use fire and to make tools. He was first a hunter, then a farmer, and later a builder of cities and nations. In the process he domesticated plants and animals for his use. and gained an increasing measure of control over his environment.

Among his unique features are his hands, which have opposable thumbs, his much-enlarged brain, and his use of a complex language for communication. These features have given rise to human cultures; man today is evolving more rapidly in a cultural than in a biological way.

Man is one species consisting of many races. The races arose (probably) from small isolated groups in which certain variations were affixed by natural selection. The mobility of man and continued interbreeding between races tends to break down the distinctions between races.

The human being is an animal who has evolved biologically over thousands of years. McElroy, Swanson, and Macey[5] point out, "It is as biological for man to dream, build, paint, and sing as it is for a muskrat to build a shelter of mud, sticks, and grass."

The following selected observations concerning the evolving human species are of significance to the physical educator.

CONCEPTS OF HUMAN BIOLOGY

The study of evolution suggests that humans are the dominant species on earth because they are "generalized" rather than "specialized" animals; that is, they are not confined to one particular mode of life or habitat. The primary physical asset of humans is their *erect posture,* which allows the hands freedom to manipulate objects in the environment (in contrast to animals that must walk on all fours). With this great advantage, humans evolved with a steady enlargement of brain tissue and a corresponding improvement of intellectual power. The ability to transmit knowledge through speaking and writing was later developed.

The discovery of control of fire and the development of tool-making processes enabled humankind to move further ahead of all other organisms in procuring shelter, safety, and basic needs. Finally, humans are the only organisms capable of developing and expressing spiritual beliefs that serve as a guide for conduct. Humans alone hold a belief in immortality.

Human biology teaches that human beings by nature are creatures who must have sunshine, fresh air, and frequent opportunities for stimulating physical and mental activities or failure to grow, develop, and flourish to optimal potentiality will ensue.

Humankind's physical, mental, and social progress has been primarily achieved by virtue of the continuous development of higher rational powers through thinking, memory, and communication.

Physical educators should realize that all too frequently humans have been described as weak, slow, unprotected, unable to fly by their own power, and therefore as being physically inferior to many other animals. Actually, the evidence indicates that humankind is a giant among animals. Very few species can run faster, or are larger or stronger. Humans have the capability to kill a large majority of the more than one million species of animals on this earth even without resorting to contrived weapons. Humankind's greater ability to modify and control the environment than any other animal substantiates Plato's statement of more than 2,000 years ago: "Mind is ever the ruler of the universe."

Four Principles. Physical educators and coaches should be knowledgeable about major concepts concerning the growth and development of humans from babies to young adults. Four basic principles undergird this process of growth and development.

1. There is a lawful order of human development. Specific types of human behaviors occur in the same time sequence for all children. Therefore, the development of a particular child at any point in time can be compared with the general expectations of all normal children.
2. In general, the developmental processes are continuous and gradual. Major spurts or plateaus in growth and development seldom occur with the exception of occasional periods of marked height increase.
3. Children tend to possess individual abilities and qualities that, in general, are of similar levels. Scientific evidence shows a positive (but low) correlation between these qualities and abilities.
4. Knowledge, skills, and other basic intellectual responses develop from the general to the specific. An overall conclusion from child growth and development studies is that human beings are the end products of all of the experiences they have been exposed to from time of birth, including prenatal influences.

There is considerable evidence to indicate that normal children need vigorous, daily physical activity for a period of four to six hours if optimal growth and development are to occur. These children will have less fatty tissue, stronger and more pliable musculature, and all-round stronger physiques than children who are not very active physically.

Regular physical activity contributes fundamentally to normal increase in bone density, to elasticity of connective tissue, and to increased resistance to strain or tear of these tissues. Daily, systematic exercise is essential to optimum growth, weight, vital capacity, and height of children and youth.

Overview of Physical Development. Growth is most rapid from birth to age two. It slows down for a year and then increases steadily from age three through six. From the time the child enters school until adolescence, height increases steadily, ranging from one and a half to three inches per year. The second most rapid growth then occurs — three or four inches per year for three or four years. The so-called adolescent spurt occurs in girls about age 11 and tapers off at about age 13. Boys start the "spurt" a year later, at about 12, which is why girls are generally taller than boys at that age. Boys then grow taller more quickly, from approximately age 12 or 13 until 15 or 16. By 17, most girls have reached their maximum height. The boys then pass them, although growing at a slower rate, and continue to increase in height until between ages 18 and 20. Of course, there are variations in these rates with respect to individuals. Some studies show positive relationships between height, intelligence, and academic performance.

Heredity and Environment. Children generally become taller than their parents. Heredity is involved in this but is not the only factor. Environmental factors are now recognized as having strong influence on

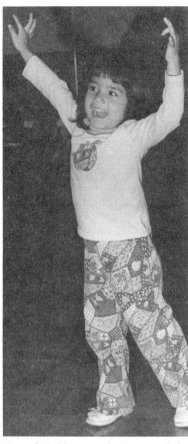

Normal children need vigorous, daily physical activity for optimal growth and development to occur.

various growth characteristics of individual children of either sex. Heredity provides the potential for growth, whereas environment may be said to develop that growth, directing what actually occurs in the child's development within the hereditary limits.

Personality Development. Researchers are uncertain as to whether psychological or personality growth and development is primarily continuous or whether there are periodic spurts. It is clear that personality development begins almost immediately after birth. Parents, other adults, and older siblings should encourage physical activity, manipulation of objects, freedom to crawl, move, turn, and so forth, within the logical limits of physical safety. Appropriate physical contact with parents and other close persons is known to contribute significantly to normal emotional and personality development. A child's basic personality pattern may be quite well established between the ages of six and ten; future behaviors can be quite reliably predicted, especially with respect to sex-role standards.

Play-Learning Experiences. Normal children are able to walk automatically (without thinking) by the age of three. From early childhood on, youngsters spend a major portion of their wakeful hours engaged in play, most of it quite active in nature. It is believed that the child's play may well be a very serious business during these early formative years. If so, it is vital that parents and guardians select appropriate equipment, toys, play materials, indoor and outdoor spaces, and a generally safe physical

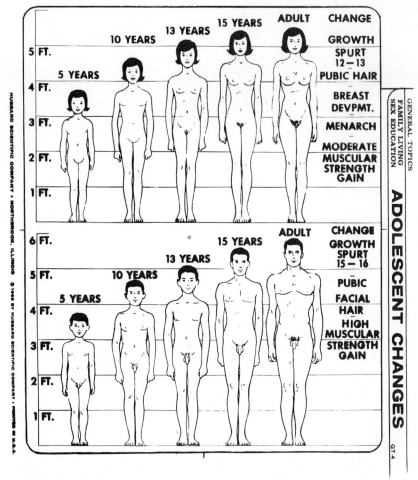

HUBBARD SCIENTIFIC COMPANY • NORTHBROOK, ILLINOIS © 1969 BY HUBBARD SCIENTIFIC COMPANY • PRINTED IN U.S.A.

GENERAL TOPICS
FAMILY LIVING
SEX EDUCATION

ADOLESCENT CHANGES

GT-4

Adolescent body development and sexual maturation in girls and boys.

environment, although not too restricted, to enable the children to play "hard" and enjoy a variety of movement experiences and challenges.

During the elementary school years (ages six to ten or twelve) physical growth tends to be steady and not too rapid, thus enabling the children to concentrate on basic skill trials, repetitions, and improvements. Adults should help these children learn to vary and to generalize these skills so they can be used in different, novel situations.

Maturational Readiness. Maturational readiness is an aspect of growth that teachers and parents should continually be aware of. A child's developmental needs and characteristics are not accurately reflected in chronological age; many children of the same age are more advanced than others in intellectual, emotional, or physical development. Taking into account children's mental and psychological ages, which may be determined by observing behavior patterns, teachers should select learning activities and encourage children to try new physical skills accordingly. No one program of physical education activities will be of equal interest or challenge to all pupils in the fifth grade, or at any other grade level; and imposing skills that may be too complex for children at their current individual stage of development may cause emotional damage.

MATURING: GIRLS VERSUS BOYS. American children are taller, heavier, and in better health today than ever before; and both boys and girls are maturing more rapidly than in previous years. Girls mature faster physically than do boys, achieving maturity about two years earlier.

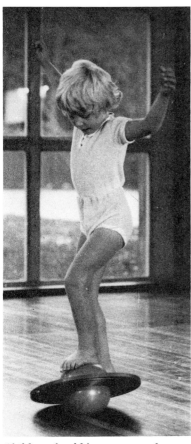

Children should be encouraged to try new physical skills.

Childhood. Elementary school age boys show significant superiority over girls in strength and in body size. Also, boys are slightly superior in running and jumping skills. Girls excel in activities requiring fine motor coordination. Obviously there are many instances of overlapping skill performances between boys and girls at any age.

Adolescence. In adolescence, the early maturing boy is more likely to succeed in physical skill performances than later maturing boys. The physical skill performances of girls tend to level off just before reaching biological maturity, which is roughly three years prior to skeletal maturity. Boys, on the other hand, seem to display continued skills development along with increased skeletal maturity over the years.

Of course, the above generalizations must be evaluated not only in terms of biological inheritance and physical growth and development potential, but also in the context of restrictive cultural influences that, in past years, have markedly inhibited girls from participating in vigorous physical activities to the same extent and with the same parental and societal sanctions as boys. With the new era of increased opportunity in physical education and sports for girls, it can be predicted that over time girls' physical skill performances will increase dramatically. No one can accurately predict the ultimate limits of skills girls and women may reach in sport and other physical performance in the years ahead, or whether they will reach parity with boys.

Adulthood and Physical Skills. In adulthood there is a general decrement in all human physical skills as the adult years pass by. However, individuals who continue to practice, participate, and train regularly in sports and exercise activities decline in skill performances at a slower rate. Also, there is strong evidence that regular exercise throughout a lifetime can contribute significantly to reduced medical problems and possibly to increase longevity. From the point of view of physical education, it is evident that persons who have learned enjoyable physical skills in sports and fitness have found pleasure and health rewards that tend to persist into adulthood and result in regular participation in pleasurable physical activities for many years.

The Infant.   From age one month to one year, the infant has a rapid *Stages of Growth* physical growth in which significant changes occur with respect to sensory-motor coordination as well as the formation of social relationships. Voluntary physical movements and actions normally begin at about seven months of age, when a child is no longer relying on simple reactions to external stimuli. According to Munsinger,[6]

> Psychologist Jerome Bruner argues that voluntary behavior requires the anticipation of a goal, the selection of a way to reach that goal, freedom from immediate sensory control, the ability to maintain a sequence of behavior, the skill to order responses, and the desired motor acts. Bruner believes that the seven-month infant can initiate and carry out voluntary acts like reaching for an object without having to see both his hands and the object.

Voluntary behavior development through play is deemed to be an important basis for later development of knowledge and understanding. It is believed that the child makes use of play to further his understanding of the world in which he lives. The cognitive theory of play supports the child-rearing principle that children should be encouraged to use toys imaginatively, to move as freely as possible in space, and to manipulate and move as many concrete objects as they are capable of managing. There is considerable evidence to indicate that children with a rich, unfettered movement involvement in the early months ultimately become more creative as adults than children who are reared in a restricted physical environment. The overall cognitive abilities of the child seem to be enhanced in such a rich play environment.

The Toddler.   Munsinger[7] labels the age range of one year to three years as the toddler. He and other authorities maintain that during this period a child learns to be independent rather than dependent and is very active and self-mobile. This ability to move freely in an independent manner is perhaps the most important aspect of all the growth development experiences undergone at this age; the toddler's expanded environment results in more rapid social, linguistic, and cognitive development. All these experiences presumably form the base of intelligence.

This time period is also one of rapid physical growth and development. Physiological maturation is accompanied by motor accessory coordination and integration. Munsinger says, "almost all theorists of development agree that the first few years of a baby's life leave permanent imprints on his perceptions, thoughts, and personality."

The newborn baby possesses a number of complex motor responses and behavior patterns. Indeed, this repertoire of motor responses should be regarded as quite amazing; it will provide the basis for continual, complex sensory-motor development and improvement for years to come. Munsinger states, "Jean Piaget, the Swiss psychologist who has done many childhood studies, believes these early sensory-motor coordinations form the basis for all later development of understanding and knowledge."[8] This very powerful generalization is worthy of intensive consideration by curriculum planners, teachers, coaches, school administrators, parents, PTA groups, and all other adults associated with planning, operation, and evaluation of school curricula and instructional methods at all levels of education. It is particularly important for the physical educator to be familiar with the work of Piaget and with the concepts and research findings on this subject so frequently reported in a variety of reputable textbooks on psychology, child development, and sensory-motor learning.

Concomitant with responding to sensory-motor impulses and environmental attractions, the toddler becomes deeply involved in the development of language and thinking. Piaget and other psychologists believe that during this period the child learns to symbolize events and activities through movement activities; he develops perceptual images and begins to learn the use of language. The toddler attempts to demonstrate his intellectual development through many types of movement activities in solving problems found in his natural environment or deliberately displayed to him by his parents or other attending adults.

The Preschool Child. The next stage in life, between three and six years, is generally called the preschool era. Now the child develops the capability that Piaget calls "concrete operational thinking." It is an age of intuitive thought. Children are now able to develop mental images. Perceptual development increases very rapidly. Cognitive abilities expand and become more acute.

Many children engage in their first formal school environment when they are sent to a playschool or a nursery school at age four. For the first time they spend a few hours several days a week away from the home environment, under the control of adults not associated with their families. Also, they learn to interact and play with other children. Thus, the development of social relationship becomes primary.

Adults have an important responsibility to guide the personality development of sensitive young children at this age level. Also, the development of moral standards is heightened at this time. Children begin to be exposed to samples of sex role differentiation in their play groups and even in some of their study groups.

These children continue to lead a very active physical life. The nursery school provides for a considerable variety of physical activities over a period of two to three hours along with so-called recess. The cognitive and attitudinal developments discussed under the section on the toddler continue with the preschool child.

Childhood. Children typically enter the first grade at age six and complete their elementary school education by progressing through grade six by age twelve. This stage of development can be labeled childhood.

Child growth and development research and literature, as well as recent physical education investigations, have clearly demonstrated the fundamental importance of unfettered, positively oriented movement experiences and challenges starting at birth and continuing throughout life. A broad repertoire of carefully selected and directed movement activities provided for babies and young children provides a solid and permanent base from which future types of learnings can be developed, thus contributing to appropriate physical, emotional, social, and intellectual growth, development, and maturation. Movement-based learning

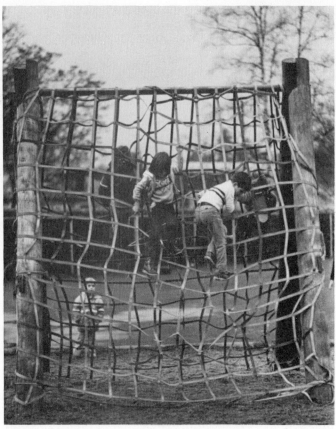

Elementary school children enjoy testing skills in novel situations.

experiences and activities contribute to the fundamental aspects of human maturation, education, and normal adjustments to internal and external environments throughout life; hence the essential role of elementary school programs of formal instruction in physical education and movement education under the supervision of well-qualified teachers and administrators.

Children spend several hours daily in various forms of vigorous physical activities. The elementary schools may organize formal physical education classes for these children but in most schools these classes soon turn into another recess or free play period. Owing to economic reasons, only a small percentage of elementary schools across the United States now employ qualified physical education teachers. Consequently, classroom teachers must be encouraged and aided to provide sound instructional physical education classes.

Childhood is a time for rapid growth and development. Muscle, bone, and other body tissues become larger and stronger, provided the child is encouraged and allowed to participate daily in appropriate physical activities. The cardiovascular system likewise grows and develops through vigorous daily activities.

Socially, this is a very important time period in the life of the child. Each boy and girl is continuously attempting to locate a comfortable place in his or her social world. Children are strongly influenced by parents, teachers, peers, and friends. Desirable socialization through properly supervised sport, rhythms, and exercise activities in elementary schools can contribute significantly to this social development.

Personal Identity Development. Each child seeks a personal identity that is unique. Sex-role determination is associated with physical growth and development. Teachers and coaches become role models whom these young children look up to and depend upon for effective counseling and guidance. Physical activity programs, when properly organized and supervised, contribute important experiences that result in desirable self-confidence, emotional control and security, and the learning of acceptable social roles and interrelationships with others, peers and older persons alike.

Fundamental motor skills are learned in these formative years, either with or without formal physical education instruction in elementary schools.

Normal perceptual-motor development is essential to proper growth and maturation. Body image, spatial awareness, directionality, time perception, and object identification while moving are fundamental processes to be developed through varied movement education experiences.

Positive Self-Concept. Perhaps the term *positive self-concept* can be stated as the overall goal of the complex processes of growth and development through which children progress in elementary school years. The self-concept refers to the child's sense of personal worth, which is a result of all of life's ongoing experiences. Properly selected and directed movement activities of a vigorous nature can make fundamental contributions to the overall development of the self-concept.

In general, the research results tend to indicate that elementary school teachers should provide well-planned and carefully directed movement education programs adapted to the needs and abilities of each child. Through this program teachers and administrators, and sometimes parents, can carefully observe the children in action and can deduce how they feel about themselves and their social relationships with others. Helpful guidance can then be provided to meet the individual needs of the children, thus enhancing development of a positive self-concept.

The Adolescent. The growth and development period from age 12 to 17 is called adolescence. Another expression is "teenager." Girls mature earlier than boys. There are significant changes in physical growth and maturation in both sexes. It is interesting to note that Munsinger[9] says, "Generally, boys who mature early are considered sociable, dominant, conforming, and secure in their vocational choice compared to males who mature later. By contrast, girls who mature late are considered more feminine and socially well-adjusted than their early maturing peers."

Cognitive Development: Formal Thought. In terms of cognitive development, Piaget believes that "formal thought" begins during adolescence. Included in this concept are the abilities to reason deductively, to devise and compare various possibilities in problem-solving, to think in abstract terms (for example, manipulating symbols), and to formulate and test different hypotheses about various aspects of the environment.

Most adolescents have a normal interest in a variety of vigorous physical activities. However, they benefit from the encouragement and instruction provided by competent teachers, coaches, recreation leaders, and peers. Some adolescents of both sexes may tend to withdraw from voluntary physical recreational activities and from opportunities to join competitive sport teams owing to a previous background of lack of success in sports and recreation in the younger years. In many schools and neighborhoods the boys and girls who excel in sports activities are highly valued by their peers. Frequently, these individuals are elected to positions of leadership in the high school by their classmates. The famous Medford studies by Clarke and his associates report findings and conclusions on this topic that should be of interest to all physical educators.

Physiological Development and Personality. Munsinger[10] emphasizes the important role that genetics and the biological bases of the individual play in the development of the child's personality. He says that personality results from a combination of "genetic predispositions, physical growth, and interaction with a social environment." Furthermore, he stresses the role of physiological growth in personality development.

> There is a close link between physiological functions and personality. If the thyroid gland secretes too little thyroxine, the active hormone of the gland, the child will exhibit a low metabolic rate, sluggish behavior, and little endurance. Too much thyroid will produce restless, nervous, frantic behavior. Hormonal secretions from the gonads, the reproductive organs of both sexes, trigger sexual growth and to some extent, sexual behavior, although human sexuality is influenced by environmental factors as well. Secondary sexual characteristics, facial hair, female breasts, for example, and body build can also exert some influence on personality development.

Hilgard[11] states,

> Late-maturing boys face a particularly difficult adjustment because of the importance of strength and physical prowess in their peer activities. During the period when they are shorter and less sturdy than their classmates, they may lose out on practice of game skills and may never catch up with the early maturers who take the lead in physical activities. Studies indicate that boys who mature late tend to be less popular than their classmates, have poorer self-concepts, and engage in more immature attention-seeking behavior. They feel rejected and dominated by their peers. The early maturers, on the other hand, tend to be more self-confident and independent. A few of these personality differences between early and later maturers persist into adulthood, long after the physical differences have disappeared.

Hilgard also discusses girls. His last conclusion differs from Munsinger's:

> The effects of rate of maturation on personality are less striking for girls. Some early-maturing girls may be at a disadvantage because they are more grown-up than their peers in the late elementary grades, but by the junior high school years the early maturers tend to have more prestige among classmates and to take leadership in school activities. At this stage the late maturing, like the boys, may have less adequate self-concepts and poor relations with their parents and peers.

The obvious implication from the above conclusions is that physical educators and coaches should be particularly sensitive to the growth and personality problems of late maturing boys and girls. Activities within physical education and recreational programs should be selected and organized in such a way that these pupils are grouped with others of similar skills and aptitudes. They should never be placed at a complete disadvantage to highly skilled players, which would result in embarrassment and a consequent dislike for these types of physical activities now and in the future. These students should be encouraged to participate in sport, dance, and exercise activities that are within their range of performance capability and in which they can demonstrate progress and skill development over time. The adult leader should provide continual positive emotional support and personal encouragement.

CHAPTER FIVE

This section on human growth and development would not be complete without selected comments on the aging process, which obviously occurs from the moment of birth to the time of death. Since primary emphasis elsewhere in this chapter has been placed on infants, children, and adolescent youth because this text is intended primarily for teachers and coaches of youngsters in those age brackets, this section refers to adults. The ultimate goal should be to provide viable physical education, sport, dance, and exercise programs for citizens of all ages, under professional leadership, and modified to each individual's needs, interests, abilities, and health limitations.

Definition of Aging. Aging is defined by Edington and Edgerton[12] as "the gradual loss of the organism's ability to respond to the environment — the loss accompanied by an increase in an incidence of disease and in the probability of death." Research on the aging process is conducted from various scientific, social, and philosophical perspectives. Selected generalizations of special interest to physical educators and athletic coaches follow.

A Possible Cause. Science has yet to determine exactly which physiological factors control aging. There are several theories that purport to explain the aging process. One fact of primary interest is that the muscle and nerve cells with which nature endows each individual do not reproduce when they die, whereas cells in the blood, skin, bone marrow, liver, and mucous linings in the intestinal tract are continuously being replaced with new cells. As a person ages, however, the replacement rate of these cells does not keep up with the rate of destruction. Thus, it is apparent that there is a decrement in function of many bodily processes as an adult ages.

Physiological Changes with Aging. According to Morehouse and Miller,[13] oxygen consumption during moderate physical activity does not change as one grows older. However, maximal oxygen uptake does gradually decrease with age during strenuous exercise. Other major physiological processes — such as those associated with the heart, the central nervous system, the lungs, and the kidneys, which function to maintain normal internal homeostasis of the human body — grow stronger from infancy through early childhood, are further strengthened in puberty and early adulthood, and then gradually decline from late adult life to the time of death.

Changes in Physical Capacity. In general, adults reach the peak of physical skill performances between the ages of 20 and 30 years, with gradual skill decrease of approximately 40 per cent over the next 40 years. The peak performance level for work is also attained at this time and thereafter declines about one per cent per year. With continual physical training, adults can participate in strenuous exercise or sports with little impairment of physical work capacity. However, it is dangerous for an adult in middle age to suddenly engage in a strenuous sport or exercise if he or she has been living a sedentary type of life up to that time. For optimum health, adults should maintain a regular program of appropriate exercises under the general direction of their family physician based on a yearly physical examination.

Exercise and Physiological Functions. Edington and Edgerton[14] report research findings concerning the relationships between exercise and physiological functions of adults at different ages:

> During near maximal exercise, maximum oxygen uptake of the aged (approximately 70 years of age) is reduced to 60% that of the

25-year-old; maximum heart rate is reduced 80% of the 25-year-old; maximum cardiac output is reduced; pulmonary ventilation is reduced; maximum respiratory frequency is reduced; and other energy support systems are impaired. Conditions in muscle and other peripheral tissues may be impaired to a great extent and may be the cause of the limitation of work capacity. It may be that the ability of the muscular system to extract oxygen is very low; therefore the exercising capability is limited.

In contrast to the above, during submaximal or low level work, there appears to be no difference in ability between the aged and the younger person to take up and use oxygen. However, a decreased efficiency of work has been demonstrated: for the same amount of work, the aged person requires additional oxygen.

Apparently, the nervous and muscular systems of the aged are subject to the greatest limitations in both submaximal and maximal types of exercises. On the other hand, it is possible to train older people to develop a higher degree of joint flexibility through motivated, controlled training programs.

It is clear that older persons can gain important health benefits from regimens of appropriate progressive exercises carried on continuously over time. However, it has not been scientifically demonstrated that such physical training programs directly increase the years of life expectancy.

EXERCISE PHYSIOLOGY

Definition

The term *physiology* refers to the study of the functions of human organic systems. Exercise physiology is a specialized branch of physiology concerned with the physiological effects of exercise stress on the human organism. Obviously, physical education teachers and coaches are fundamentally interested in the phenomena involved in exercise physiology and are guided by research concepts in this field to formulate their policies and their teaching and coaching practices.

Exercise physiology is also considered to be one of the academic areas of knowledge in physical education. Virtually every physical education major program includes the study of exercise physiology. Of course, physicians, medical researchers, physiologists, and other specialists have a fundamental concern for exercise physiology as well.

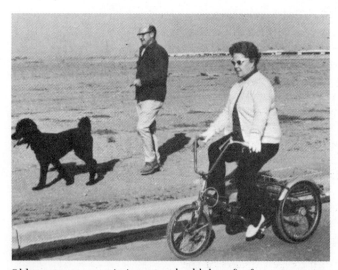

Older persons can gain important health benefits from appropriate exercise.

Tipton[15] states,

> My belief is that current and future exercise physiologists should concentrate their research efforts on better understanding the nature, mechanism and the consequences of homeostatic disruptions caused by movement and not on the resolution of man's problems. Since most, if not all, exercise physiologists are also educators, they should use classroom occasions, public forums or the media to indicate how exercise research findings can be employed to minimize and/or reduce health related problems.

He goes on to cite two concepts that are basic to the primary research goal of the exercise physiologist.

> The first is that most of the primary tissue types within the body (epithelial, connective, muscular, neural) are capable of adapting anatomically, physiologically, and biochemically to mechanical stimuli.... [Mechanical stimuli exert biological influences over these tissues.] The significance of the mechanical stimuli concept is that cellular and system modifications can be induced by acute and chronic periods of exercise. Thus, it is the responsibility of the exercise physiologist and other scientists to determine whether the changes noted are beneficial or deleterious for normal functioning.
>
> The second concept of importance to exercise physiologists is one of specificity.... [This term] is being used to mean that responses and adaptations of biological tissues to exercise must be interpreted and evaluated with regard to the *specific*:
>
> 1. Exercise conditions that prevailed when the movement was being performed (nature of exercise, type of contractions used, speed, duration, frequency, strenuousness, etc.).
> 2. Intrinsic characteristics of the individual who performed the movements (age, sex, health status, endocrine status, nutritional status, training status, level of motivation, fibre type profile, etc.).
> 3. Extrinsic conditions which prevailed when the movements were being performed (dry bulb temperature, wet bulb temperature, humidity, atmospheric pressure, wind velocity, time of day, locations, audience, etc.).[16]

Tipton goes on to say that the majority of exercise physiologists are interested in phenomena concerning the anatomical, physiological, and biochemical changes which occur within the cardio-respiratory, neuro-muscular, and metabolic systems.

Interdisciplinary Programs. A recent development in several American universities is interdisciplinary programs involving basic science departments in the universities. One reason for this alliance is to bring to bear greater resources upon instructional and research assignments of exercise physiologists because physical education departments generally do not have sufficient research facilities or a large trained staff. Also, there is a greater likelihood of receiving research grants from governmental agencies and private foundations through the departments in basic sciences and in medical schools than through physical education departments. Furthermore, the young physical education scholar will receive a practical and theoretical academic and laboratory experience of greater depth and breadth by using the broad resources of the university.

Dr. David H. Clarke[17] expands on Tipton's remarks and makes a special plea for the identification and development of what he calls "our own unique subject matter in exercise physiology."

Clarke reacts to the Tipton recommendation with a modified view by saying, "Clearly the way to go in my estimation is to develop a strong science-based curriculum and a vigorous and outstanding research program (in the physical education department), and if it is interdisciplinary as well, then there may indeed be a chance for additional support."

Exercise physiology is a rapidly expanding specialization within *Topics* physical education and its scope and content continue to magnify at a rapid rate. Examples of topics of major interest to exercise physiologists in physical education include the effect of exercise upon

— the cardiovascular system, including aerobic-anaerobic processes, temperature regulation, physical conditioning, physical fitness, gaseous exchange and transport, respiration, and circulation;
— the muscular system, including strength, endurance, flexibility, and warm-up and cool-down effects;
— the nervous system;
— the endocrine system;
— body composition and metabolism;

and the effects of the following on the body and exercise:

— physical work;
— nutrition;
— altitude;
— aging;
— ergogenic aids and drugs;
— physical handicaps and related problems;
— sex differences;
— new research and measurement developments.

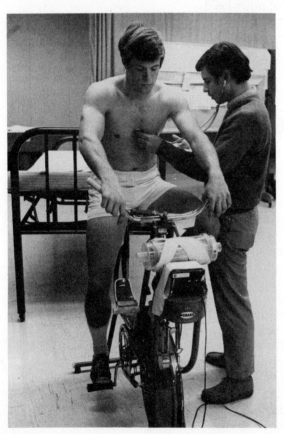

Exercise physiology is an expanding specialization within physical education.

CHAPTER FIVE

Nutrition. As the individual becomes more obese the number of adipose cells increases, as does the size of each cell. The individual who is obese as a baby will have a larger increase in the number of cells than the person who develops obesity several years later. Obesity frequently is the cause of degenerative disorders; however, sudden weight losses, such as by a wrestler, should not exceed 5 per cent of the normal body weight.

If an athlete regularly eats a normal diet that includes all of the essential vitamins, the ingestion of additional vitamin supplements will not improve physical performance involving strength and endurance.

Cardiovascular Function. As a result of regular exercise, the heart rate will become lower at all levels of submaximal effort. Also, the stroke volume becomes larger with each beat of the heart.

Interval Training. The interval training method is physiologically sound. More work can be performed in one practice session if practice is intermittent rather than continuous.

Warming-Up. Warm-up prior to "all out" muscular effort is generally recommended by physiologists. However, there is lack of agreement as to what constitutes appropriate warm-up for any particular individual engaged in a specific activity. Therefore, the best advice is for each athlete to engage in a warm-up routine with which he feels most comfortable psychologically.

Cooling Down. The purpose of cooling down gradually after intensive exercise is to deter blood pooling, which can cause severe muscle cramps and sometimes shock. It is now generally believed that vigorous exercise will not harm a normal heart.

Effect of Altitude. An athlete who participates in an event requiring

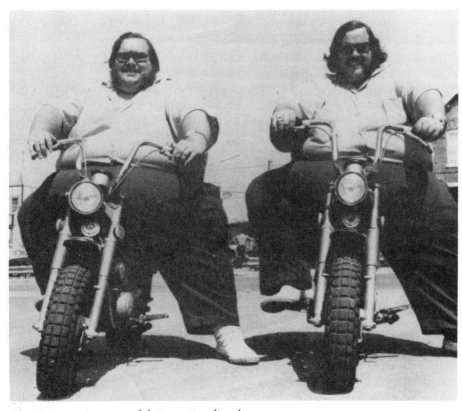

Obesity is a major cause of degenerative disorders.

continuous activity for more than two minutes in a high altitude area should train at that altitude for two to three weeks prior to the event. Apparently it is not advantageous to train at a higher altitude in an attempt to improve performance in an endurance event at a lower altitude.

Oxygen Administration. Laboratory tests have demonstrated that administering oxygen to an athlete immediately upon completion of a strenuous event has no significant effect upon normal cardiovascular recovery. The evidence concerning the administration of oxygen just prior to participation is contradictory.

Exercise and Cardiovascular Function. In 1977 Dr. Ralph S. Paffenbarger,[18] Professor of Epidemiology at the Stanford University School of Medicine, reported the results of a long-term study of 17,000 Harvard University male alumni. His basic finding was that men who participated regularly in strenuous sports such as tennis, mountain climbing, jogging, and swimming had fewer heart attacks than those who were less physically active. Strenuous physical exercise appears to result in a definite protective effect on the cardiovascular system. The physically active individuals engaged in strenuous activities three hours per week or more and expended 2,000 or more calories each week. Findings were similar among men ranging from ages 35 to 75.

Men who participated regularly in sports requiring only light exercise such as bowling, bicycle riding, golf, and boating received no more cardiovascular protection than men who did not engage in any sport activities.

Another interesting finding was that when Paffenbarger looked at other coronary risk factors among the men, including high blood pressure, cigarette smoking, over-weight, and family history of heart disease, he found that the protection offered by strenuous physical activity was largely independent of these considerations.[19]

The study also revealed that men who were very active in varsity sports in college received no more protection from heart attacks later on than other men if they did not continue participation on a regular basis in vigorous physical activity. Also, males who were not physically active in college, but who became so in later years, assumed a reduced risk of heart disease as they grew older.

Sex Differences. With regard to sex differences in athletic performances, perhaps it is in events requiring explosive power and muscular strength that the greatest difference in achievement occurs, as men

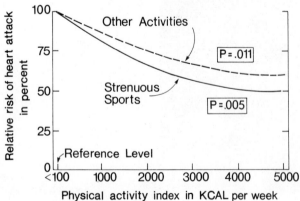

Relationship of physical activity to risk of heart attack.

CHAPTER FIVE

generally excel in these attributes. Also, women seem to be more adversely affected by high temperatures during athletic performance. Research results conflict concerning the phase of the menstrual cycle in which women athletes make peak performances.

Flexibility. In the development of increased flexibility both ballistic and static stretching exercises are effective. However, ballistic stretching is more likely to cause acute soreness in the muscles.

Drugs. Despite its apparent widespread use, there is no convincing scientific evidence that anabolic steroids significantly increase work capacity and physical strength of normal athletes.

Stress. Stress may be reduced by regular physical exercise. Also, regular exercise habits may contribute to satisfactorily coping with stress.

Research Equipment and Procedures

Exercise physiology researchers utilize a variety of sophisticated equipment and apparatus. Standard treatment of this subject can be found in several well-known texts. Examples follow.

The *bicycle ergometer* and the *treadmill* provide controlled exercise for the subject while the researcher computes energy expenditure and work output with a high degree of accuracy. Various types of work ergometers have been devised to measure work performance by the various muscle groups of the body.

The amount of energy expended and heat produced during work by a human subject can be measured by placing him in a closed chamber called a *calorimeter.* Or the subject can breathe into a *spirometer,* which measures the amount of oxygen used during the exercise. An athlete participating in a strenuous workout in swimming or running, or on the bicycle ergometer, can breathe expired air into a *Douglas bag* at the beginning and end of the workout. This air can be analyzed by a spirometer or by passing it through a *gas meter.* The difference between the pretest VO_2 value and the endtest value represents the oxygen utilized. Expired air can be collected during continuous exercise when the subject is on a stationary bicycle or on the treadmill. It can be analyzed by O_2 or CO_2 content.

Measures of body internal heat are taken by *thermometer* inserted into the mouth (oral) or the rectum (anal). A special thermometer using a thin needle can be inserted directly into the muscle tissue. The *Sling Psychrometer,* consisting of *wet* and *dry bulb thermometers,* is useful for determining environmental conditions of temperature and humidity, and can be used on the athletic field.

The vital capacity of the lungs is tested with a spirometer. The subject inhales the largest quantity of air of which he is capable. Then he forcefully expires it gradually, and for as long as he can, into the spirometer. The total amount of air expired can be ascertained, thus providing a measure of vital capacity.

The relationship between exercise intensity and blood circulation time can be measured by injecting a dye, *fluorescein,* into the blood so that the time it takes the blood to move from one area of the body to another during exercise can be recorded.

Chemical analyses of blood are made in the laboratory to determine the effects of exercise on pH levels, lactic acid, red blood corpuscles, erythrocyte sedimentation rate, white blood corpuscles, blood platelets, specific gravity of blood, blood sugar, phosphates, and cholesterol level.

The *sphygmomanometer,* an elastic cuff that is wrapped around the upper arm and inflated with air at various pressures, is used to measure blood pressure.

Variations in heart rates can be attained by directing the subjects to step up and down stairs or benches made for this purpose to a specified cadence. The pulse rate is taken before, after, and even during the exercising.

Special *calipers* have been designed to measure skin folds in different regions of the body to assess body composition. Also, calipers and measuring tapes are utilized to make accurate measurements of body segments.

Scales are used to measure gross weight. An under-water submersion apparatus has been developed so that the per cent of fat in the human body can be quite accurately measured.

Strength in various segments of the body is measured by *dynomometers* (leg, hand, back), a *manumometer* (grip strength), and a *tensiometer.*

Flexibility is measured by the *Leighton Flexometer* and by either a *manual goniometer* or an *electric goniometer.*

Radio telemetry has now been miniaturized so that it is contained in a very small package that can be strapped on the back of an active athlete. Electric signals can be relayed to monitoring equipment, thus recording the rate of respiration, heart beat and blood pressure during an actual sport performance by the athlete.

Computers can be connected with most of the equipment enumerated in the above paragraphs to record raw data. Data reduction, analysis, recording, reporting, and storage are other functions performed by the computer.

This brief summary of equipment and procedures customarily used in exercise physiology research demonstrates the necessity for sophisticated, unusually expensive equipment, facilities, supplies, and qualified personnel if quality basic and applied research studies are to be conducted. Today's exercise physiologist must have expensive, advanced graduate preparation in basic physiology as well as in exercise physiology and

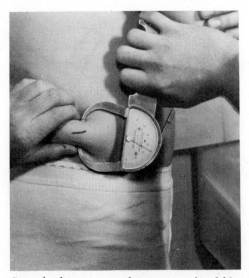

Special calipers are used to measure skin folds in different regions of the body.

CHAPTER FIVE

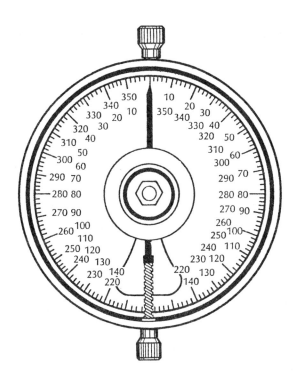

diverse laboratory experiences as prerequisites to a career in this physical education specialization.

Exercise physiologists are being employed by hospitals, medical centers, semi-public agencies such as YMCA's (Young Men's Christian Associations), sometimes in business and industry, as members of sport medicine units in colleges and universities, and in an ever-expanding array of alternative employment opportunities. It is a specialization with an exciting optimistic future for the interested candidate.

Future Research Directions

Recent discoveries in the physiology of muscular activity continue to provide a wealth of information. This knowledge guides the physical educator and coach in providing the types and amounts of physical activity that will be most appropriate for each individual. Exercise physiology serves as a basis for helping people plan sound, individual exercise programs and how to adapt them to varying personal needs throughout a lifetime.

Principles of physical education that guide our policies and practices should, to a large extent, be derived from present-day scientific knowledge. This discussion has touched only the fringes of knowledge in exercise physiology. However, it is hoped that enough has been said to stimulate the professional student to study intensively in this field. Coaches and physical educators should develop the ability to appropriately apply exercise physiology concepts to effective teaching, coaching, and administration in physical education and sport.

BIOMECHANICS OF HUMAN MOVEMENT

The athletic coach, the physical educator, and the physical education researcher have long been interested in what has been traditionally called kinesiology. The basis for study and application of research findings in kinesiology is the anatomy of the human organism and the application of laws of physics to its movements, particularly in the area of skilled movement.

In the early stage of teacher training the kinesiologist required the memorization of the actions of individual muscles and muscle groups and their mechanical relationships to the joints and body segments involved in a particular skilled movement. Hellebrandt,[20] referring to the early days in the development of kinesiology, reports that

> The movements comprising gymnastic maneuvers, and to a lesser degree sport skills, were described in anatomical terms, and lists were then compiled of the individual muscles which ought to contribute to the production of the joint positions assumed. This was a highly artificial kinesiology, based almost entirely on synthetic reasoning.

Eventually the emphasis changed from the anatomical basis of physical movements involved in skills to a biomechanical analysis of voluntary motor movements. The term kinesiology is being used less and less now, and is being superseded by the expression *biomechanics of human movement*. Of course, an understanding of basic human anatomy remains the foundation upon which the biomechanics approach rests.

Kinesiology. The word kinesiology traditionally has been defined as *Definitions* the scientific study of human movement. A detailed knowledge of human anatomy is basic. The application of laws of mechanics and physics to the movements and related actions of the human body, especially in areas of sport, dance, and designed exercise, is another essential component of this definition. Of course, the interrelationship with the central nervous system and sensory organs is implicit in this definition. One view is that there are two major types of kinesiology — anatomical and mechanical. It follows from this distinction that the term biomechanical eventually superseded the older phrase mechanical kinesiology.

Biomechanics. Northrip, Logan, and McKinney[21] state that

> Studying and analyzing humans in motion, sport object motion, and forces acting upon these animate and inanimate bodies is known as biomechanics.
>
> The term biomechanics has now gained general acceptance.

Miller and Nelson[22] indicate there are two major areas of research in *Two Areas of* biomechanics. The first they call the biological aspect, which is based on *Research* functional anatomy and studied primarily through electromyography. The second emphasis is on mechanical factors involved in human motion. These authors summarize the research parameters of biomechanics as follows:

> Research is conducted at three levels along the continuum: practical, fundamental, and theoretical. The first of these focuses upon the analysis of sport skills to provide a better understanding of the execution of those movements so that teachers and coaches can work more effectively. . . . Fundamental research deals with the study of simple movements and factors which influence them. Strength, limb length, mass and inertial properties, angular and linear velocity, and acceleration are examined. Results of this work form the basis for understanding the complexities of human motion and provide important insight into performance at the practical level. Theoretical research is relatively new to the field but will no doubt receive increasing emphasis in the future. It may involve the construction of a simplified mathematical model of a skill in a form which is suitable for computer analysis so that it can be simulated under several carefully controlled conditions. This leads to a thorough comprehension of the mechanics of the movement and has the potential for predicting more effective techniques.

Nelson[23] indicates that biomechanics is concerned with the objective measurement and evaluation of sport skills and that this special area of investigation is beginning to produce results which will have practical uses for teachers and coaches of sport, dance, and physical education. Biomechanics is now well established as one of the major disciplines of physical education. All teachers and coaches need to be well acquainted with selected, fundamental generalizations from biomechanics that have application to the effective teaching of correct performances of physical skills, as well as prompt identification of errors by performers, as a basis for future correction.

Mechanical Factors of Human Motion. One of the major advances in knowledge in this field has come about through the quantification of sport skills via analysis of slow motion pictures of performers in action. The analysis of sport techniques and an understanding of the biomechanics principles used by world class sports performers have been revealed through cinematographical analysis more clearly than by previous techniques.

Several principles of "correct" mechanics in performing standard sport skills which have long been held by a majority of coaches now are being overturned by the refined analysis provided through cinematography. Nelson points out it has long been taught that when projecting a missile in a sport event such as the discus, the optimal angle of 45° has been advocated to obtain maximum horizontal distance. Recent evidence indicates this advice is not sound in a majority of cases in various sports. Nelson[24] states that "distance in the shotput, for example, is dependent upon three factors: height of release, velocity, and the angle of take-off. Consequently, there is no single optimal angle which applies to all shotputters, and in no case would it be 45°."

Biological Factors. The increased use of electromyography has provided basic information that describes the electrical activity that activates muscle patterns. Thus, the physical educator now has a better understanding of the functions of various muscles as they move to fulfill a specific complex movement. Also, this research methodology has provided important basic knowledge about functional anatomy.

Another contribution of modern biomechanics research is to the improvement of mechanical characteristics of the equipment used by athletes. It is now possible to design sports equipment appropriately tailored to the specific strength and other bodily characteristics of an individual performer. Thus, sports skill instruction and performance become more efficient and effective.

Nelson[25] observes also that "The utilization of methods from modern biomechanics offers the motor learning expert possibilities for practical research which were formerly impossible. The integration of efforts of biomechanics specialists and motor learning specialists in sports skills research could provide the basis for a major improvement in the teaching of motor skills."

Finally, Nelson predicts that the use of computer simulation and mathematical modeling relative to complex sport movements are leading the way toward the discovery of the ultimate theoretical limits of human potential in the realm of sport.

Some biomechanics research specialists are combining their interests and talents with exercise physiologists.

A perusal of the standard textbooks on kinesiology and biomechanics *Biomechanics* of human movement, listed at the end of this chapter, will inform the *Topics* reader of the major topics of study, research, and application at the present time. For example, Northrip, Logan, and McKinney[26] give emphasis to the following topics in their comprehensive work:

1. Planes of the human body including anteroposterior, lateral, transverse, and diagonal
2. Anatomical land marks, or areas of special identification on the human body
3. Description of motions of the various joints
4. Linear motion, including velocity, acceleration, force, and mass
5. Pressure and friction
6. Energy and momentum, including work and power
7. Rotation
8. Angular measures and forces including torque
9. Gravity and inertia
10. Equilibrium, static and dynamic
11. Trajectories
12. Forces, including counter-forces and collision
13. Aerodynamics, including drag and lift
14. Hydrodynamics, including thrust (propulsive force) and buoyancy

With special emphasis on sport and physical education, biomechanics *Biomechanics* is making rapid strides in utilizing and adapting a wide range of newly *Research* developing electronic and mechanical measurement and research de- *Equipment and* vices. Miller and Nelson[27] provide a comprehensive listing and descrip- *Procedures* tion of the modern research equipment available to the biomechanics investigator. Examples follow:

1. Photoinstrumentation, including optical recording devices, motion picture cameras, videotape, still cameras, motion analyzers, digital computers, stroboscopic lights, three-dimensional photographs, photographs using mirrors, and stereo cameras
2. Electronic instrumentation, including timers (photoelectric cells, electronic counters), automatic performance analyzers, instrumentation systems, electrogoniometer, linear variable differentiated transformer (LVDT), force plate, accelerometer, signal conditioner, graphic recorder, magnetic tape recording
3. Digital computer techniques, including high-speed electronic digital computers, electronic programmable calculators, computer data processing, computer graphics, computer simulation
4. Photogrammetry
5. Radiation techniques, including gamma mass scanner
6. Mathematical models

Cinematography and Videotape. Cinematography is a basic mode of investigation in biomechanics research. High-speed motion picture cameras are available having the capability of shooting 10,000 frames per second. X-ray cameras and stroboscopic cameras add to the accuracy with which the researcher can follow the precise movements of the body and its components in complex skilled performances. Two or more cameras can be placed in different planes to record the movement on the same time line, which provides two- and three-dimensional analysis at the same instant. Various types of wooden and metal frames and grids with lines and squares marked off in specific units of distance can be placed behind the performer and recorded in the picture so that the researcher can measure accurately the distances, angles, and arcs any segment or specific area of the body moved over a specified time period. Specific parts of the body can be identified by markings on the body, such as the center of gravity, which then can be readily identified in the pictures so that an accurate tracing can be made, and mathematically analyzed, of the trajectory followed by that body part in the pictures over time. Accurate data from cinematographical analysis describe such phenomena of movement as force, power, velocity, and acceleration. These research findings lead the way to improved skill performances in sport, dance, and designed exercise.

With proper lighting conditions, cinematographical study can be conducted either indoors or out-of-doors. It can be used for minute analysis of skilled movements in controlled laboratory conditions either with respect to an isolated study of designated parts of the body or during complete, integrated performance of the total body. It can be used to analyze identifiable skilled movements in formal competitive sport situations or in demonstrations of sport, dance, and designed exercise. Film readers and analyzers and computers simplify the analyses and recording tasks of the investigator, although this job is a rigorous and time-consuming one at best. The researcher must work carefully with the measurements recorded and the analysis made of them to reconstruct the flow of the movements under study as related to the timed intervals, some of which may be 1,000th of a second or less in duration.

Cinematography is a valuable research asset to the biomechanics investigator and obviously is much more complex and difficult than indicated in this brief sketch. The equipment is expensive and the investigator requires much training and experience to become highly accurate and proficient. The standard biomechanics and kinesiology books and magazines, such as the *Research Quarterly,* report a wide variety of studies carried on by this type of research.

Descriptions of basic instrumentation, equipment, and research methodologies are also available in technical references and catalogs from companies manufacturing this equipment. Advanced formal training and considerable laboratory experience under supervision of professional researchers is prerequisite to entry into research of this nature. Gradually, more sophisticated analysis of human movement through cinematography is contributing to greater understanding of the potential for highly complex human movements and the exposition of the mechanical principles which undergird these performances.

VIDEOTAPE. Videotape can be considered as a special phase of cinematographical study and research. The investigator can make a series of analyses at any location on the tape at the rate of 60 half-scans per second, thus making it possible to study movement time and reaction time. A human performance can be observed while taking place through a monitor, and then can be "played back" for detailed analysis as a motion picture. Two cameras can be used simultaneously and played back on two split-screens, thus providing two-dimensional perspective. A timing device can be placed near the performer, such as a split-second clock scaled to .01 second so that movement can be analyzed in a time and sequence context.

The researcher can utilize the sound capability of the machine to make remarks while a performance is being filmed, such as identifying

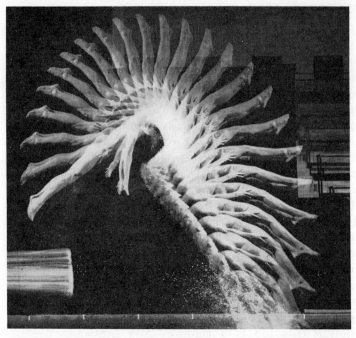

Cinematography has contributed extensively to greater understanding of complex human movements.

the performer, reciting information and data relevant to the performance as it is occurring, and recording any other necessary information occurring simultaneously with the action being visually recorded.

There are several administrative advantages in videotaping: The use of videodiscs reduces the possibility of inferior picture resolution and can provide a performance rate of 120 frames per second; a stroboscopic arrangement can eliminate the blurring effect during rapid movements; the original cost of the equipment is not as great as it is for other sophisticated biomechanics research apparatus (many schools and colleges already have the basic videotapes and recorders); the film can be used over and over again and there is no cost of development; and the subject can be transferred onto a 16mm film for permanent retention.

A Cinematographical Study of Running. An excellent example of the use of cinematographical research to assist in the improvement of execution of a specific sport skill is that of Nelson and Gregor[28] in studying the biomechanics of distance running. The authors stated the need for the accurate "quantification of the essential biomechanical components of running so that their relative importance can be ascertained." Five biomechanical components of running that could be accurately measured by cinematographic instrumentation were selected. They were stride length, stride rate, and three temporal components of stride time during periods when the foot was in contact with the ground and when it was not. Ten male runners from Pennsylvania State University were in this study for a period of five years. The runners were filmed at three speeds, sixteen fps (feet per second), twenty-two fps, and maximum speed. Nine of the ten runners demonstrated changes in their running styles, mainly with respect to a shortening of the stride length and a lessening of the stride time and an increase in stride rate. Every runner reduced his time of support.

The authors concluded,

> The results, however, have shown clearly that all runners studied did indeed demonstrate meaningful changes. These changes could not be attributed to direct intervention by the coach, since he made no direct attempt to alter their style of running.

This study is an excellent example of how fundamental cinematographic research can have important implications for the improvement of sport performance, in this instance, distance running.

Electromyography. Electromyography (EMG) employs a complicated electrical machine to record, analyze, and integrate recordings of the amplitude and duration of electrical impulses generated by muscles under contraction, or immediately prior to contraction. Electrodes are placed across the belly of the muscle under study, usually in the form of metal plates located on the skin over the area of investigation, or thin wire inserted into the muscles. Lead wires conduct electrical impulses from the muscle fibers as they are activated during a movement. A recording apparatus charts these electrical impulses by tracing irregular lines on fast-moving graph paper. These tracings can be studied to determine, with considerable accuracy, exactly when a muscle begins to "fire" (contract), when it ceases to move, and the varying amplitude of electrical impulses released. These impulses can be recorded electronically on electromagnetic tape and they can be viewed on an oscilloscope, from which photographs can be made as permanent records. Whenever an impulse from the central nervous system is conducted to a muscle, or muscle group, the thousands of motor units in the muscle are activated and an electrical potential is rapidly released, which is recorded on the tracings.

The study of the tracings, on a time scale, clearly depicts patterns of muscle actions and indicates when muscles contract and relax in a time relation with each other. It also informs the physiologist about the properties of muscle excitation. The exact role each muscle and muscle group plays as sets of muscles move limbs or other body segments through a range of motion can be accurately ascertained.

Physical educators, physical therapists, and sport medicine specialists are vigorously applying this type of biomechanics research to important phenomena occurring in sport and physical education in the United States and in many other countries. From these results, practical methods for the more effective teaching of voluntary, skilled movements, as well as instruction for corrective rehabilitation of pathologic and orthopedic problems, are evolving.

Electromyographical Research: The Landa Study. The Landa[29] study is an excellent example of the use of electromyography. The purpose of the study was to investigate the relationship of activity in selected shoulder muscles to the degree of body swing on the uneven parallel bars. A videotape picture was taken of the performance of each subject in order to determine the time duration and the distance range in the swing phase of each skill attempt.

A six-channel EM physiograph recorded the electromyographical data. Skin electrodes and a cable tensiometer were used to obtain the maximum strength of seven muscles involved in the gymnastic movement. The author presents detailed data and statistical analyses which accurately report her findings. The interested reader is referred to this article for complete information. Landa[30] reports the following conclusions and implications:

Based on the limitations of this experiment, muscle activity seems to increase with an increase in swing amplitude. The latissimus dorsi appears to contribute the greatest percentage of its maximal strength in all the skills performed.

Strength in the upper and middle back regions appears to be very important and crucial in controlling the swings. As a result, strengthening exercises for the muscles of this region should be an important part in the general conditioning exercises for the uneven parallel bars. For example, pull-ups and a weight training program to strengthen muscles such as the latissimus dorsi would be very beneficial for improved performances and control on the uneven parallel bars.

Although only four subjects were used in gathering data for this study, the results are useful in giving physical educators some direction to the activity of some muscles during the performance of certain gymnastic skills. To the author's knowledge, little or no work has been done to determine the extent to which muscles or muscle groups are active during the executions of gymnastic skills.

Computer Digitizer. Ariel[31] points out the ability of the computer digitizer complex to analyze total bodily motion by integrating slow motion cinematography, special equipment for tracing electromyographical data, and a high-speed computer. Ariel states,

> Appropriate programming results in a segmental breakdown of information of the whole motion including the total body center of gravity, segment velocities and accelerations, horizontal, vertical and resultant forces, moments of force, and a timing between the body segments. This analysis provides a quantitative measure of the motion and allows for perfection and optimization of human performance. Applications of biomechanical analyses permit an objective, quantitative assessment of performance replacing the uncertainty of trial and error, eliminating the element of doubt, and providing a realistic opportunity for improved performance.

This article provides several examples of a total analytical approach to sport skills analyses and is commended to the readers' attention.

Ramey[32] illustrates the use of digital computer simulation along with force place measurements and motion picture analyses to analyze body dynamics involved in the long jump. Basically, Ramey shows that, "given the proper angular momentum at take-off," the three major styles of long jumping are equally effective. He summarizes the benefits of this type of biomechanical analysis:

> When quantitative measures of the angular momentum are available and combined with simulations such as discussed in this paper, one can vary the parameters to either prescribe the angular momentum suited to the jumper's style or prescribe a style suited to the jumper's angular momentum. Further, the use of a dynamical simulation permits one to study the various motions used in a given style and to determine their influence on the overall execution of the jump.

Thus Ramey and other studies cited in this chapter not only indicate the theoretical capabilities of complex research techniques and instruments, but also demonstrate their practical applications to improve teaching and coaching methods, which in turn will result in improved skill performances.

Flexibility Assessment. Flexibility is the range of motion in a particular joint. Physical education teachers, coaches, and participants are vitally concerned about the phenomenon of flexibility, which refers to the range, degrees, and planes of movement possible in the various joint areas of the human body. This area of research in biomechanics is fundamental to improved methods of athletic training and conditioning as well as increasing sport, dance, and exercise performance skills.

Goniometer. The methodology for measuring joint flexibility depends primarily on three instruments. The double-armed goniometer resembles the well-known protractor. Two plastic or metal arms are hinged together so that a dial measuring degrees through a 180° radius indicates the degree of flexion in a joint when fully contracted and, at the other extreme, when the limb is fully extended. One arm of the goniometer is securely fastened to the limb just below the joint, and the other arm is fastened to the limb above the joint. When the joint moves the degree of flexibility registers on the dial. This manual method is easy to apply. However, it is not as accurate as is desirable. It is a gross method, subject to human error, and lacks high reliability.

Leighton Flexometer. Jack Leighton invented the well-known Leighton flexometer. Its operation is described in most biomechanics books and in the evaluation literature. It can be strapped onto most joint areas of the body. It consists of a complete rotary circle. There is a weighted point attached to the center of the dial. Both the dial and the pointer are free and independent of each other and both are affected and controlled by the force of gravity alone. The segment to which the flexometer is attached is placed in any desired stationary starting position of more than 20° deviation from horizontal. The zero point on the dial and the tip of the point float freely as the subject finds the position at which the zero point on the dial and the tip of the pointer coincide at rest. The dial is then locked into position. The limb is moved through the desired range of motion. At the end of that motion the needle is locked. Then the reading of the position of the needle indicates the number of degrees of the arc through which the motion has transpired. This instrument has proved to be highly reliable with coefficients well into the .90s. There are strict instructions about how to locate the flexometer on the various joints, how to direct the movements of the subject for accurate measurement, and how to read the results precisely. A period of training is necessary to use this instrument properly.

Electrogoniometers. Finally, Karpovich developed the electrogoniometer, called the "elgon." It provides for continuous measurement of movements of body segments through a range of motion so that patterns of movements can be analyzed minutely. A small potentiometer is attached at the center of the rotation of the joint. Two arms extend from it as with the goniometer. These arms are bound to the limbs involved on either side of the joint. As the joint moves, resistance is recorded electrically in terms of ohms, which can be analyzed to describe the movement of the joint quite precisely.

Coaches and teachers have always been concerned about the degrees of flexibility and stability in the various joints of the human body, particularly under exercise stress. Therefore, the phenomenon of flexibility will continue to attract major attention from researchers and instructors alike. Research data concerning various aspects of flexibility continue to be published by interested researchers and much of this information is being translated into desirable principles and practices of training, performing, and instructing.

In an intriguing article Nelson[33] describes how recent research by means of biomechanics research studies has overturned certain myths long held and practiced by American coaches, and he also reveals re-

Selected Research Findings

search data that will help coaches teach their athletes more efficient sport movements. Two examples of these myths are described.

Duration of Force Myth. The first long-held myth is that when an athlete takes off from the ground to perform a movement in the air, the movements that involve a change in velocity can be improved by lengthening the time during which the force is applied. Recent biomechanics research has demonstrated the opposite, namely, that take-off movements in such events as ski jumping, high jumping, water jumping in the steeple-chase, and the long jump should involve slightly less, rather than greater, time of application of a relatively high force value and a short application time.

Angle of Projection Myth. Another mechanical principle myth relates to the optimum angle of projecting implements, or the athletes themselves, into space in the performance of certain sport events. It has long been held almost unanimously by coaches that the optimal angle for a maximum projection into space is 45° from horizontal. However, recent studies show that the optimum angles in fact differ in various sports. In general, long jumpers leave the board at angles somewhat more than 20°. Divers leave the diving board at about 80°, and high jumpers take off from the ground at about 85°. Implements such as baseballs, softballs, and javelins, should be propelled at various angles other than 45°.

Nelson[34] projects his views of the lines future research will take in biomechanics of sport. He says there will be a close integration of research study by motor learning specialists and biomechanics researchers to evolve correct scientific principles for the teaching and learning of motor skills. So far, these research specialists have worked in too much isolation from each other. Also, there will be much closer interrelationship between the specialists in biomechanics and motor learning and the coaches and athletic trainers, with respect to applying research inquiries and findings to the improvement of coaching and training methods. *Future Research Directions*

Investigations in the future will emphasize computer simulation and mathematical modeling of sport movements to uncover the theoretical principles which will result in better sport performances. In turn, athletes will be taught by knowledgeable coaches how to modify their performances to approximate the new movement parameters revealed by research. Nelson cites one example discovered by biomechanics researchers in the German Democratic Republic (GDR) who have discovered that it is more efficient for ski jumpers to hold the tips of the skis together in mid-air to form a V rather than to hold the skis parallel as has been done in the past.

Undoubtedly, there are many discoveries remaining to be revealed which will result in improved sport performances through biomechanical applied research.

Physical fitness is often regarded as the major objective of physical education. Because the foundational areas of exercise physiology, biomechanics, and motor learning comprise major components of the concept of physical fitness, this section suitably concludes this chapter on the biological foundations of physical education. **PHYSICAL FITNESS**

The physical fitness of the American public of all ages continues to be a major concern not only of physical educators, but also of family physicians, other medical and educational specialists, and state and national governments. Organizations such as the American Medical Association and the President's Council on Physical Fitness and Sports conduct intensive campaigns to promote better health and well-being for all citizens through physical fitness activities. The various communications media keep the country informed of recent developments through professional and popular books, magazine articles, research reports, television and radio programs, and advertising.

Many attempts have been made to define physical fitness and to identify and describe its specific factors. The authors accept the widely held view that physical fitness refers to the organic capacity of the individual to perform the normal tasks of daily living without undue tiredness or fatigue, having a reserve of strength and energy available to meet satisfactorily any emergency demand. *Definition*

Physical Fitness: An Individual Matter. One obvious implication of this definition is that physical fitness is indeed an individual matter. The question "physical fitness for what?" must be answered for all individuals in terms of their general health, mental outlook, occupation, avocational activities, interests, needs and capabilities, and other contributing factors in order to arrive at a definition of an optimal condition of physical fitness.

It is fallacious to hold that there is one "best level" of physical fitness which all persons should strive to achieve. The inherent difficulties involved in identifying and then evaluating the status of the pertinent factors to be considered in setting a physical fitness goal for any individual constitute a formidable challenge to the physical education profession.

Total Fitness. Majority opinion holds that physical fitness should be

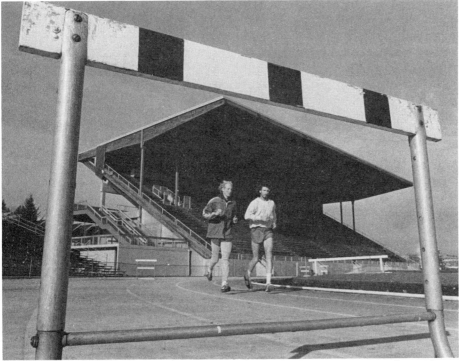

The physical educator has a primary interest in physical fitness as an essential ingredient of total fitness.

BIOLOGICAL FOUNDATIONS

considered as one aspect of total fitness, which has several components, intellectual, emotional and social, as well as physiological. Improvement in total fitness leads to more effective living. The physical educator has a primary interest in physical fitness as an essential ingredient of total fitness, as well as a general interest in the other components of total fitness that can be influenced favorably by a sound physical education program.

Clarke and Clarke,[35] after thorough analysis of the factors listed above, succinctly state that the basic elements of physical fitness are organic soundness, strength, freedom from disease, and nutritional adequacy. The professional student should formulate his own definition from a thorough consideration of all factors involved in this topic.

THE PRESENT
STATUS OF
PHYSICAL FITNESS

Background

Origins.   The physical fitness movement in the United States probably was first stimulated by Dr. William Anderson of the Adelphi Academy in 1885. Dr. Anderson was an instructor of Swedish medical gymnastics who invited 49 leaders of American youth to attend a conference held for the purpose of considering a scientific approach to the development of physical fitness. As a result of discussion at this conference, and because of inspiring addresses by Dr. Edwin Hitchcock of Amherst and Dr. Dudley Sargent of Harvard, the conferees organized the American Association for the Advancement of Physical Education. This organization was later to become our present-day American Alliance for Health, Physical Education, Recreation and Dance (AAHPERD).

Dr. Anderson and his colleagues returned to their universities with the task of describing "the ideal man" and with the objective of developing a program of physical education through which all people in the universities would study and work scientifically toward achieving this ideal.

Soon Dr. Sargent and his colleagues realized that merely making static measurements of body segments and proportions, and collecting strength test scores was not inclusive enough of a person's potential for physical fitness development. Sargent and his coworkers enlarged their study to include the measurement of efficiency, or the ability of the human body to perform physical skills while in motion. Identification was made of basic motor abilities that seemed to be common to the many forms of gymnastics and athletic events of that era. The result was a change of emphasis and interest toward a general athletic ability basis for physical fitness and a decline in the medical gymnastics approach.

The "Natural Program."   In the following decades, American physical education came to emphasize the so-called natural program, composed of a wide variety of sports, dances, and designed exercises, which in turn are composed of the fundamental skills and movements natural to humankind, such as running, balancing, jumping, leaping, throwing, hanging, climbing, catching, and dodging. This general philosophy is the basis for most physical education programs in American schools and colleges today.

World War II and the 1950s.   During World War II, with millions of young men serving in the Armed Forces, a renewed emphasis on physical fitness occurred both in the Armed Forces and in the schools and universities of the country. Although athletics and sports were retained in the schools and Armed Forces, there generally was a return to more formal

CHAPTER FIVE

gymnastic and exercise programs specifically for physical conditioning purposes.

Gradually, after World War II, the typical peacetime lack of interest in physical fitness returned to many school programs. Several states and many school districts relaxed, or eliminated, their physical education requirements, thus resulting in the report in the late 1950s that about one-half of the boys and girls in American high schools were not enrolled in any form of physical education. At the same time, many existing school programs moved so far in the direction of play, games, and sports that very little vigorous fitness activity was available. Studies that ascertained the extent to which students were engaged in vigorous activities indicated that many students in physical education classes were not active beyond the mild exercise and exertion required in walking for longer than two or three minutes in an entire physical education class period. In general, physical fitness became a lost objective in most school programs of physical education.

In 1955, for the first time in the national history, physical fitness in peacetime became a national concern of top federal government officials, including the President of the United States.

THE PRESIDENT'S COUNCIL

When the controversial Kraus-Hirschland[36]* research study was brought to the attention of President Eisenhower, the President was shocked at the unfavorable "minimum fitness level" test scores made by American children as compared with a sample of youth from selected European countries.

By executive order dated July 16, 1956, he established the President's Council on Youth Fitness and the President's Citizens Advisory Committee on the Fitness of American Youth. The purpose of these two groups was to promote physical fitness for all United States citizens through existing fitness programs and the launching of additional programs.

"The Soft American." President John F. Kennedy provided the strongest support the physical fitness movement had ever known in peacetime from a president of the United States. President Kennedy took an action that was unique in the field of physical education when, as President-elect, he wrote an article published under his own name in the December 26, 1960, issue of *Sports Illustrated* entitled "The Soft American," in which he cogently stated his deep concern for the fitness of the American citizenry and suggested steps for improving this deficiency. President Kennedy's unprecedented personal support for physical fitness gave the program national impetus. He continued to support the physical fitness movement during his tenure as President through speeches, television statements, references made at national conferences, and instructions to his staff to implement the program within their respective areas of jurisdiction.

The President's Council on Physical Fitness and Sports, since its inception, has provided outstanding national professional leadership in the development of appropriate physical fitness programs for the youth

Programs and Publications

---

*Many physical education authorities doubt the validity of the Kraus-Weber test for determining minimum fitness levels of youth. The flexibility item in the test as a determinant factor of fitness level is particularly subject to challenge. Students are referred to a study published in the *Research Quarterly* of October 1955, written by Marjorie Phillips and others, entitled "Analysis of Results on the Kraus-Weber Test of Minimum Muscular Fitness for Children."

and adults of this country. In 1962, the Council published an influential booklet, *Physical Fitness Elements in Recreation — Suggestions for Community Programs.*[37] This publication indicates how community recreation agencies can work to promote the physical fitness of all citizens, young and old alike, through expanded recreational programs.

In January 1963, the name of the Council was changed to the President's Council on Physical Fitness to emphasize its concern for the physical fitness of all Americans, not just of the youth. In 1967, the name was changed again to the President's Council on Physical Fitness and Sports, its current title.

In 1967, the Council published a booklet entitled *Youth Physical Fitness — Suggested Elements of a School Centered Program,*[38] which had a profound influence on strengthening physical fitness programs in schools across the country.

In 1967, the Council not only was renamed but also was moved into the Department of Health, Education, and Welfare. In October, 1970, C. Carson Conrad, the former director of the Bureau of Health, Physical Education, and Recreation, California State Department of Education, was appointed Executive Director of the Council. Capt. James A. Lovell (U.S.N. Ret.), the famous astronaut, was appointed Director of the Council and consultant on fitness to the President of the United States. Capt. Lovell and Mr. Conrad still hold their positions as of the date of the publication of this book.

In 1971, the Council appointed Professor H. Harrison Clarke, internationally renowned physical education scholar and researcher at the University of Oregon, to serve as part-time Consultant for Research and as Editor for the Council publication, *The Physical Fitness Research Digest.*

The Council works closely with a 100-member Advisory Committee on Fitness and Sport. Also, the presidents of well-known corporations and other business establishments have organized a Business and Industry Advisory Committee that works closely with the Council.

In 1969, the Council began to formally recognize selected junior and senior high schools across the country as Demonstration Center Schools because of their exemplary physical fitness programs.

Presidental Physical Fitness Award. Likewise, the Council has concentrated on encouraging strong physical fitness programs in the schools and colleges of the country. In order to motivate students' interest in physical fitness, the Council sponsors a Presidential Physical Fitness Award Program. Students who score at the 85th percentile or higher on each item on the Council's physical fitness test are eligible for this Award. In 1975–76, 406,448 students received the Award. The number of students qualifying for the Award increases each year, which shows a continuing interest in physical fitness, both by the instructors in the schools around the country and the students in the programs.

National Summer Youth Program. In 1970, the Council, in cooperation with the National Collegiate Athletic Association, began an extensive National Summer Youth Program, which involves participation of approximately 100 schools and universities and 35,000 boys and girls aged 10 to 18 years. The Department of Health, Education, and Welfare initially funded this Summer Recreation Program and continues to do so.

National Presidential Sports Award. In 1972, the Council established a National Presidential Sports Award for any man or woman 18 years of age or older. This award may be achieved in any one of 31 athletic events based on participation of at least 50 hours, in 50 or more different time periods, for at least 4 months.

For the past several years, the Council has sponsored regional fitness clinics throughout the nation and has provided a majority of the staff participating in these programs. Also, special symposiums have been held, such as the Medical Symposium on Exercise and the Heart.

Other Recent Publications. In April, 1972, the Council initiated a service which provides the 500 largest newspapers in the United States with material to use in a weekly physical fitness column. The Council has also been very active in producing its own informative publications and instructional films. The *Newsletter* was begun in November 1963 and is published several times yearly. The *Physical Fitness Research Digest* was started June 1971 and is published quarterly. Other valuable and timely pamphlets are published periodically and receive nationwide dissemination. Two pamphlets were published in 1976 — *The President's Council on Physical Fitness* and *Sports and Good Health is Good Business*. In addition to Council publications, educational films are produced with various fitness themes for use by schools, service clubs, and any other interested groups.

A Physical Fitness/Sports Medicine Research Service was organized in 1976 under the direction of the President's Council on Physical Fitness and Sports. It is composed of representatives of the American Medical Association, the American College of Sports Medicine, the National Library of Medicine, and the United States Olympic Committee, along with the Council. The Service publishes a physical fitness–sports digest quarterly.

In March, 1977, the President's Council on Physical Fitness and Sports *Newsletter* quoted Dr. Theodore Cooper, Assistant Secretary for Health for the Department of Health, Education, and Welfare, who said, "The incidence of fatal heart disease has decreased about 14% among Americans." Dr. Cooper said three factors contributed to the improved heart health: better dietary habits, less smoking, and more exercise. He noted that the most significant change was in exercise habits. He also commented about the change in physicians' attitudes toward exercise. He said that more doctors were prescribing regular vigorous exercise for their patients.

American Association of Physical Fitness Directors in Business and Industry. This Association was formed in 1974, and is affiliated with the President's Council. Its major purpose is to support and assist in the development of physical fitness programs in businesses and industry throughout the United States.

The AAHPERD Youth Fitness Test. The American Alliance for Health, Physical Education, Recreation and Dance* has filled a major leadership role in physical fitness in America throughout its long history. In 1959, Dr. Paul Hunsicker conducted a national study for the then AAHPER that established norms for the *Youth Fitness Test Manual*, published in 1961. In subsequent years the AAHPER Test has been administered to millions of pupils throughout the country.

AAHPERD
PHYSICAL FITNESS
PROGRAMS

---

*Formerly the American Association for Health, Physical Education and Recreation (AAHPER).

In recent years, the Alliance has expanded its activities in the area of physical fitness. It has established close working relationships with the President's Council, the American Medical Association, the American College of Sports Medicine, and other organizations having concern for the health and fitness of the citizens of the United States.

In order to ascertain the progress school pupils were making in physical fitness performance, Hunsicker and Reiff conducted another national study for AAHPER, which compared the results of fitness testing in 1958 with a national sample of test scores in 1965. In general, the physical fitness levels of this sample of American public school children were significantly improved over the 1958 national scores.

In 1975, the AAHPER Youth Fitness Test was revised for the second time under the chairmanship of Dr. Paul A. Hunsicker, in joint sponsorship with the President's Council on Physical Fitness and Sports. The softball distance throw was eliminated, the bent-knee situps for one minute were substituted for the unlimited straight-knee situps; the 600-yard run-walk was retained; and two optional runs were added, one-mile or a 9-minute run for ages 10 to 12 years, and a one and one half mile or a 12-minute run for ages 13 and over. This addition to the AAHPER Test has been adopted officially by the President's Council as part of its promotional and evaluation processes. More than 1 million boys and girls across the United States have earned the Presidential Physical Fitness Award sponsored by the Council by performing at the 85th percentile on all of the tests.

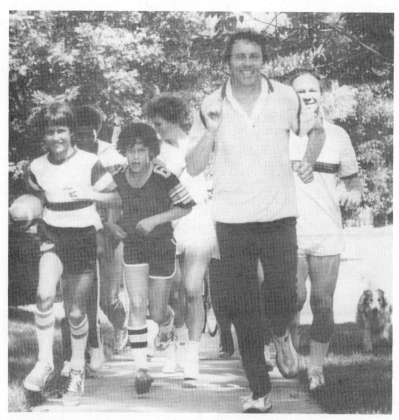

AAHPERD continues to maintain its influential leadership in promoting increased fitness among youth and adults.

CHAPTER FIVE

National Physical Fitness Award Program. In cooperation with the Joseph P. Kennedy, Jr. Foundation, the AAHPERD has developed a National Physical Fitness Award Program for the Mentally Retarded.

AAHPERD continues to maintain its influential leadership in promoting increased fitness among the young and adults of this country. This professional organization is serving the cause of fitness with distinction.

Today, physical fitness is generally accepted as one of the major objectives of any school or college physical education program. Many authorities would rank it as the primary objective.

A Shared Responsibility. Physical educators should not claim that physical fitness is their responsibility alone. The attainment by a student of an optimal level of physical fitness is not only a question of sufficient vigorous exercise. Fitness depends upon many other factors as well, such as freedom from disease, well-balanced nutrition, correction of remedial defects, a state of positive mental and emotional health, and other elements that are the concern of the family, school physician, the school nurse, counselors, administrators, and teachers, as well as parents. Thus, the physical fitness objective is shared with other school units, rather than being unique to the physical education department. It is recommended that the physical educator concentrate on improving the three main components of physical fitness, namely, circulatory efficiency, muscular strength, and muscular endurance.

There is considerable evidence that physical education programs, when properly conducted, can significantly improve the physical fitness status of the participants. The lack of proper physical education in public schools results in lower physical fitness levels for both boys and girls. Thus, as young men and women, they embark on university study or accept occupational roles in the adult world with a definite and potentially dangerous handicap, namely, a lack of normal physical fitness.

A fundamental contribution of physical fitness to the health of any individual is succinctly summarized by Clarke[39] as a result of an extensive analysis of research findings by various investigators, including his own studies. Clarke states, "it may be contended that a person's *general learning potential for a given level of intelligence* is increased or decreased in accordance with his degree of physical fitness."

A wide variety of physical fitness tests are now available to schools and colleges. Most states have prepared and officially adopted a physical fitness test or have accepted the President's Council Test in the publication *Youth Physical Fitness*. The American Alliance for Health, Physical Education, Recreation and Dance[40] likewise has a physical fitness test that is widely used in schools throughout the United States and in many foreign countries.

Schools, school districts, colleges, universities, and some states devise their own physical fitness tests and construct local norms pertaining to their own pupils — a procedure that the authors encourage. It is not sufficient to compare an individual pupil's results with national or state norms only. It may be even more important to know how a person is progressing in relation to his or her past performances, classmates, schoolmates, and the community.

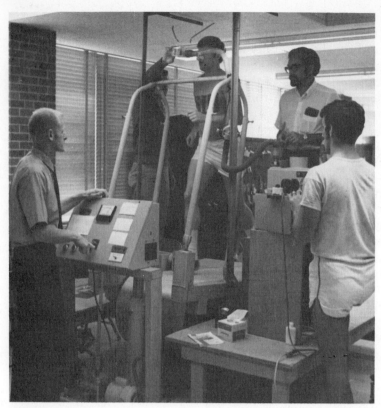
A physical fitness laboratory.

Physical Fitness Laboratory. A relatively new development in some schools throughout the country, as a way to increase interest in physical fitness testing, is the implementation of a Physical Fitness Laboratory. These labs are equipped with standard exercise physiology testing equipment so as to evaluate the effect of stimulating exercise upon pupils. Physical education teachers are returning to graduate school to study exercise physiology and laboratory techniques in order to administer and conduct instructional programs in these laboratories. Students serve as subjects and also as laboratory technicians. This program can be closely integrated with the science department and laboratory credit can be arranged for science classes. Students can learn important physiological concepts from interesting and challenging laboratory studies. They can learn selected, fundamental principles that underlie skilled physical performances. They can gain experience with some of the modes of inquiry of the biological sciences, which possibly could lead to the development of an interest in a career in this field. The potentialities of these laboratories are limited only by the imaginative, creative talents of the teachers and administrators in charge. This innovation seems to hold high promise to make physical education an even more varied, challenging, and interesting learning experience.

Finally, physical fitness testing and exercise programs are of personal interest to many young people and adults outside of the school environment. Personal physicians, medical clinics, community health agencies, community service organizations such as YMCAs and other groups are sponsoring physical education and physical fitness programs for very young children up through older adults.

Commercially, so-called health studios, private and semi-private sport and recreation clubs, racquet clubs, tennis clubs, swimming clubs, and other specialized sport and health organizations are rapidly proliferating in response to the ever-increasing interest and demand of the public for programs and services related to health, fitness, and recreational enjoyment and competence.

Armed Forces. The Armed Forces have increased their emphasis on physical fitness programs and evaluation in peacetime. The Marine Corps, the Department of the Navy, the Coast Guard Academy, and the United States Naval Academy have developed physical fitness tests and require practice and periodical test administration by all troops under their command.

Fitness for Older Americans. On November 28, 1975, the President signed into law the Older Americans Act. It includes a statement on fitness for older Americans that encourages services to assist old people to develop and maintain physical and mental health with programs in regular physical fitness activities and a variety of forms of exercise. The Administration on Aging provided a grant to the National Association for Human Development to sponsor projects concerning fitness for the aging. This project is being carried on in cooperation with the President's Council on Physical Fitness and Sports.

National Athletic Health Institute. This institute was established in Inglewood, California, in 1975. It is a non-profit organization for research and education in sport medicine, recreation, and health.

Vita Parcours. This organization is rapidly spreading in popularity throughout the United States. "Vita" means life and "Parcours" means course or track. A course can be set up around an existing quarter-mile track or can be laid out in any area where there is running room and areas

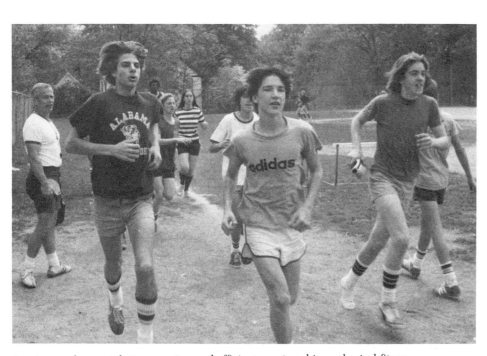

Jogging can be a quick, inexpensive, and efficient way to achieve physical fitness.

alongside for any length desired. The participant jogs along the selected path and stops to perform designated exercises at exercise stations located alongside the running trail. Directions for carrying out the exercises correctly are located on a weatherproof bulletin board at each exercise station. Also, a description of health benefits to be derived is included.

The National Library of Medicine originated in 1975 as a "physical fitness/sports medicine information service." It contains the most comprehensive list of printed materials concerning physical fitness and sport of any known agency in the United States.

The National Jogging Association, a non-profit organization, was founded in 1968. Its purpose is to promote the least expensive, quickest, and most efficient way to achieve physical fitness for most persons — by jogging.

Many other individuals and institutions throughout the United States have developed and revised physical fitness tests and programs.

The previous sections of this chapter emphasize the importance of the physical fitness objective in proper focus and balance with the other valuable objectives of physical education, recreation. and health education programs. The physical education curriculum should not be based primarily on physical fitness testing programs. Overemphasis on this objective might jeopardize gains made in the achievement of other equally valuable objectives discussed in other chapters.

Finally, emphasis on the physical fitness objective should not erode the fundamental educational aim of physical education and its major contributions to pupil learning and development by presenting only a limited program of physical training.

CONCLUSION

Darwin's theory states that living organisms must adapt to their changing environment or become extinct. The cooperation principle explains natural selection by asserting that organisms are most likely to survive and develop in relation to their ability to work together among themselves and with their physical environment to facilitate their chances for survival. Humans are unique among animals because they have developed a culture.

Physical educators and coaches should be knowledgeable about major concepts concerning the growth and development of babies, young children, adolescents, and young adults. There is considerable evidence that normal children need vigorous, daily physical activity for a period of four to six hours if optimal growth and development are to occur. Older persons can gain important health benefits from regimens of appropriate progressive exercises carried on continuously over time.

The term *physiology* refers to the study of the functions of the organic systems of an individual. *Exercise physiology* is a specialized branch of physiology that is concerned with the physiological effects of exercise stress on the human organism.

Evidence confirms the need of normal children for vigorous, daily physical activity for a period of four to six hours if optimal growth and development are to occur.

SUMMARY

CHAPTER FIVE

Coaches and physical educators should develop the ability to effectively apply exercise physiology concepts to teaching, coaching, and administration in physical education and sport.

Physical fitness refers to the organic capacity of the individual to perform the normal tasks of daily living without undue tiredness or fatigue having a reserve of strength and energy available to meet satisfactorily any emerging demand suddenly arising.

It is recommended that the physical educator concentrate on improving the three main components of physical fitness, namely, circulatory efficiency, muscular strength, and muscular endurance.

The physical education curriculum should not be based primarily on physical fitness testing programs. Overemphasis on this objective might jeopardize gains made in the achievement of other equally valuable objectives.

Northrip, Logan, and McKinney define *biomechanics* as the study and analysis of humans in motion, sport object motion, and forces acting upon these animate and inanimate bodies.

Cinematography is a valuable research asset to the biomechanics investigator. Videotape can be considered as a special phase of cinematographical study and research.

FOOTNOTES

[1] William E. McElroy, Carl P. Swanson, and Robert I. Macey, *Biology and Man.* Englewood Cliffs, N.J.: Prentice-Hall, Inc., 1975, pp. 334, 335.

[2] Claude A. Villee, Warren F. Walker, and Robert E. Barnes, *General Biology* (4th ed.). Philadephia: W. B. Saunders Company, 1973, pp. 843, 844.

[3] William E. McElroy, Carl P. Swanson, and Robert I. Macey, op. cit., p. 358.

[4] Ibid., p. 54.

[5] Ibid., p. 4.

[6] Harry Munsinger, *Fundamentals of Child Development* (2nd ed.). New York: Holt, Rinehart and Winston, 1975, p. 11.

[7] Ibid., p. 84.

[8] Ibid., p. 83.

[9] Ibid., p. 27.

[10] Ibid., pp. 413, 414.

[11] Ernest R. Hilgard, Richard C. Atkinson, and Rita L. Atkinson, *Introduction to Psychology*, (6th ed.). New York: Harcourt, Brace and Jovanovich, 1975, p. 93.

[12] D. W. Edington and V. R. Edgerton, *The Biology of Physical Activity.* Boston: Houghton-Mifflin Company, 1976, p. 335.

[13] Laurence E. Morehouse and Augustus T. Miller, *Physiology of Exercise* (7th ed). St. Louis: The C. V. Mosby Company, 1976.

[14] D. W. Edington and V. R. Edgerton, op. cit., p. 340.

[15] Charles M. Tipton, "Exercise Physiology: Today and Tomorrow," Academy Papers No. 10, *Beyond Research — Solution to Human Problems.* Louisville, Ky: The American Academy of Physical Education, 1976, pp. 70, 71.

[16] Ibid., p. 72.

[17] David H. Clarke, "Reaction to Tipton's Paper: Exercise Physiology — Today and Tomorrow," The Academy Papers, No. 10, *Beyond Research — Solution to Human Problems.* Louisville, Ky: American Academy of Physical Education, 1976, pp. 75, 80.

[18] Ralph S. Paffenbarger, Alvin L. Wing, and Robert T. Hyde, "Physical Activity as an Index of Heart Attack Risk in College Alumni," *American Journal of Epidemiology*, 108:161–175, 1978.

[19] Ibid., p. 5.

[20] F. A. Hellebrandt, "Living Anatomy, *Quest,* I:44 (December, 1963).

[21] John W. Northrip, Gene A. Logan, and Wayne C. McKinney. *Introduction to Biomechanic*

Analysis of Sport. Dubuque, Iowa: Wm. C. Brown and Company, 1974, p. 3.

[22]Doris I. Miller and Richard C. Nelson, *Biomechanics of Sport: A Research Approach.* Philadelphia: Lea & Febiger, 1973, pp. 3, 4.

[23]Richard C. Nelson, "Contribution of Biomechanics to Improve Human Performance," The Academy Papers No. 10, *Beyond Research — Solution to Human Problems*. Louisville, Ky: American Academy of Physical Education, 1976, pp. 6–15.

[24]Ibid., p. 9.

[25]Ibid., p. 10.

[26]John W. Northrip, Gene A. Logan, and Wayne C. McKinney, op. cit.

[27]Doris I. Miller and Richard C. Nelson, op. cit.

[28]Richard C. Nelson and Robert J. Gregor, "Biomechanics of Distance Running: A Longitudinal Study," *Research Quarterly*, 43:417–428 (October, 1976).

[29]Jean Landa, "Shoulder Muscle Activity during Selected Skills on the Uneven Parallel Bars," *Research Quarterly*, 45:120–127 (May, 1974).

[30]Ibid.

[31]Gideon Ariel, "Method for Biomechanical Analysis of Human Performance," *Research Quarterly*, 45:72–79 (March, 1974).

[32]M. R. Ramey, "Significance of Angular Momentum in Long Jumping," *Research Quarterly*, 44:488–497 (December, 1973).

[33]Richard C. Nelson, op. cit., pp. 6–15.

[34]Ibid.

[35]H. Harrison Clarke and David H. Clarke, *Application of Measurement to Health and Physical Education* (5th cd.). Englewood Cliffs, N.J.: Prentice-Hall, Inc., 1976.

[36]Hans Kraus and Ruth P. Hirschland, "Muscular Fitness and Health," *Journal of American Association of Health, Physical Education, and Recreation*, 24:17–19 (December, 1953).

[37]*Physical Fitness Elements in Recreation—Suggestions for Community Programs.* Washington, D.C.: President's Council on Youth Fitness, U.S. Government Printing Office, 1962.

[38]*Youth Physical Fitness—Suggested Elements of a School Centered Program*. Washington, D.C.: President's Council on Physical Fitness and Sports, U.S. Government Printing Office (rev. ed.), 1973.

[39]H. Harrison Clarke, *Application of Measurement to Health and Physical Education* (4th ed.). Englewood Cliffs, N.J.: Prentice-Hall, Inc., 1967, p. 51.

[40]American Alliance for Health, Physical Education, and Recreation, *AAHPER Youth Fitness Test Manual* (2nd ed.). Washington, D.C.: AAHPERD, 1975.

SELECTED REFERENCES

Albinson, J. G., and Andrew G. M. (Eds.), *Child in Sport and Physical Activity*. International Series on Sport Sciences, Vol. 3. Baltimore, MD: University Park Press, 1976.

Arnheim, Daniel D. *Athletic Training—A Study and Laboratory Guide*. St. Louis, MO: C. V. Mosby Company, 1978.

Barham, Jerry, *Mechanical Kinesiology*. St. Louis, MO: C. V. Mosby Company, 1978.

Broer, Marion R., and Zernicke, Ronald F., *Efficiency of Human Movement* (4th Ed.). Philadelphia: W. B. Saunders Company, 1979.

Clarke, David H., *Exercise Physiology*. Englewood Cliffs, N.J.: Prentice-Hall, Inc., 1975.

Cooper, John M., and Glassow, Ruth B., *Kinesiology* (4th Ed.). St. Louis, MO: C. V. Mosby Co., 1976.

DeGaray, Alfonso, L., Levine, Carter, and Linsay, John E. (Eds.), *Genetic and Anthropological Studies of Olympic Athletes*. New York: Academic Press, 1974.

"Drugs and the Coach," (rev.) Washington, D.C.: American Alliance for Health, Physical Education and Recreation, 1977.

Fox, Edward L., *Sports Physiology*. Philadelphia: W. B. Saunders Company, 1979.

Hay, James G., *The Biomechanics of Sports Techniques* (2nd Ed.). Englewood Cliffs, N.J.: Prentice-Hall, Inc., 1978.

Howe, Michael, *Learning in Infants and Young Children*. Stanford, CA: Stanford University Press, 1976.

Jensen, Clayne R., and Garth, Fisher A., *Scientific Basis of Athletic Conditioning* (2nd Ed.). Philadelphia: Lea & Febiger, 1978.

Katch, Frank I., and McArdle, William D., *Physiological Conditioning for Women — An Equal Load*. Boston: Houghton-Mifflin Co., 1976.

Klafs, Carl E., and Arnheim, Daniel D., *Modern Principles of Athletic Training: The Science of Sports Injury Prevention and Management*. St. Louis, MO: C. V. Mosby, Co., 1977.

Lamb, David R., *Physiology of Exercise: Response and Adaptations*. New York: Macmillan, Company, 1978.

Leyson, Glynn A., *Programmed Functional Anatomy*. St. Louis, MO: C. V. Mosby Co., 1974.

Logan, Gene, and McKinney, Wayne C., *Anatomic Kinesiology* (2nd Ed.). Dubuque, IA: Wm. C. Brown Company Publishers, 1977.

MacIntyre, Christine and Wessel, Janet, *Body Contouring and Conditioning through Movement* (2nd Ed.). Boston: Allyn & Bacon, Inc., 1977.

Malina, Robert and Johnston, F. E., *Human Physical Growth and Development*. Philadelphia: Lea & Febiger, 1975.

Mathews, Donald K., and Fox, Edward L., *The Physiological Basis of Physical Education and Athletics* (2nd Ed.). Philadelphia: W. B. Saunders Company, 1976.

Nelson, Richard C., and Morehouse, Chauncey A., *Biomechanics IV*. Baltimore, MD: University Park Press, 1974.

Rasch, Philip J., and Burke, Roger K., *Kinesiology and Applied Anatomy: The Science of Human Movement* (6th Ed.). Philadelphia: Lea & Febiger, 1978.

Ryan, Allan J., and Allman, Fred L., Jr. (Eds.), *Sports Medicine*. New York: Academic Press, 1974.

Stone, William J., and Kroll, William A., *Sports Conditioning and Weight Training: Programs for Athletic Competition*. Rockleigh, N.J.: Allyn & Bacon, Inc., 1978.

Strauss, Richard H., *Sports Medicine and Physiology*. Philadelphia: W. B. Saunders, Company, 1979.

Wilmore, Jack H., *Athletic Training and Physical Fitness: Physiological Principles and Practices of the Conditioning Process*. Rockleigh, N.J.: Allyn & Bacon, Inc., 1978.

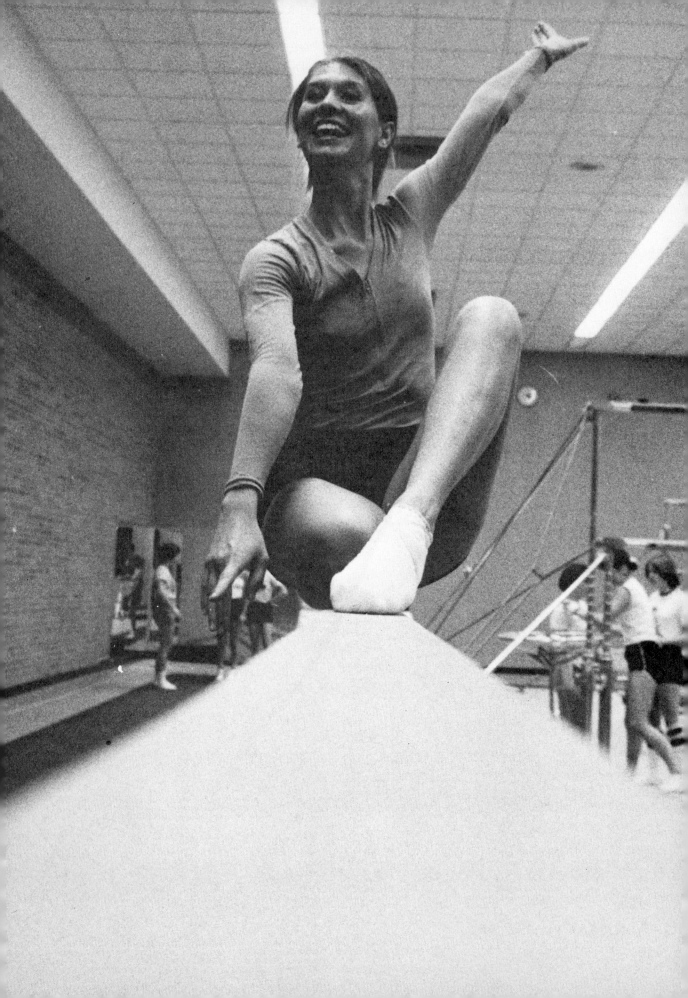

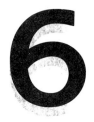

PSYCHOLOGICAL ———— ———— FOUNDATIONS

Introduction. Psychology is one of the academic disciplines of the behavioral sciences. Its main focus is the behavior of human beings, although some psychologists also study the behaviors of animals. Among the wide-ranging topics of interest for psychologists are

— the organic processes that control the activities of humans and other animals;
— the growth and developmental patterns of the young of a species;
— the way in which humans perceive their internal and external environments through their sensory systems;
— the way in which humans learn, think, and solve problems;
— motivation and emotional responses;
— personality development and individual differences;
— the ways in which humans cope with stress, conflict, and frustration;
—and, finally, the study of how individuals relate to each other in groups, a discipline known as social psychology.

The physical educator is also interested in all of the above phases of psychology. The psychological foundations of sport and physical education now occupy a primary role in the preparation of major students and the inservice education of teachers and coaches in the field.

Motor learning is of special interest and emphasis in physical education and sport. How humans can most effectively learn complex motor skills now occupies central emphasis in the study of physical education and sport.

Because the term *behavior* is fundamental to psychology, it should be noted that it refers to overt activities engaged in by persons, or other organisms, which are observable by another person or by appropriate recording instrumentation.

Psychology contributes to the educational background of the teacher and coach by (1) developing competence to accurately assess and classify student knowledge and abilities as a basis for planning and evaluating instruction; (2) providing information about internal and external influences and conditions which elicit and control human behaviors, so that optimal learning opportunities will be planned and provided to best accomplish educational objectives; and (3) offering insights into methods of research for further investigations of human behaviors related to sport, dance, and exercise.

Learning, particularly motor learning, and thinking are areas of special interest to physical education research specialists.

NEUROLOGY

The Central Nervous System

Voluntary and reflexive human movements are controlled and directed by the central and peripheral nervous systems. For most effective instruction the physical education teacher and the athletic coach should study these basic control mechanisms and how they function as communication channels. Physiology, anatomy, physiological psychology, and kinesiology contribute to an understanding of these complicated and minute neural components and systems.

The central nervous system (CNS) is composed of a spinal cord, the brain, and the brain stem which are located in the skull and the vertebrae. The cerebro-spinal fluid and the ligamentous connections in the spine assist in protecting the spinal cord from injury.

The Neuron. The neuron is the basic functional unit of the nervous system. Neurons receive and transmit nerve impulses. Thus, one of their major functions is to transmit impulses or messages from one bodily part to another through electro-chemical processes.

Interneurons are located within the central nervous system. Afferent neurons are outside of the central nervous system and carry nerve im-

A typical motor neuron.

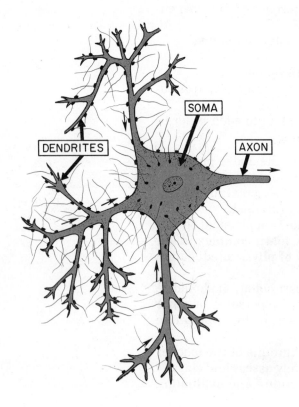

DENDRITES

SOMA

AXON

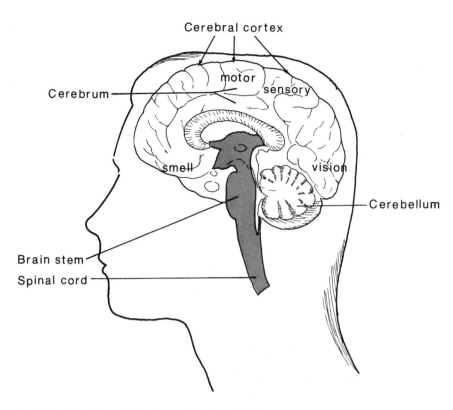

Sagittal section through the human head and brain.

pulses from the sensory receptors to the spinal cord or brain. Efferent neurons conduct messages from the central nervous system outward to the muscles and glands.

The central nervous system has two central purposes: (1) to carry information from the external environment and from the body to the brain for storage and integration with previous knowledge; and (2) to relay information from the brain to glands and muscles that produce movements and bodily adaptations to cope with environmental inputs.

Cerebrum. The cerebrum constitutes the largest portion of the brain (upper portion) and is composed of millions of cell bodies (gray matter). It is divided into right and left hemispheres, which are symmetrical. In general, the bodily functions on the left side are controlled by the right hemisphere, while functions on the right side are under the direction of the left hemisphere. Human thought and consciousness are controlled in the cerebrum.

Cerebral Cortex. The cerebral cortex is the outer layer of the cerebrum. Curiously enough, it contains approximately nine billion neurons. All sensory systems of the human body relay messages to the cortex, each to a specific region. A major portion of the motor control of muscles and glands is located in specific regions of the cortex. The cortex exerts the highest level of motor control.

The *motor cortex* is the area of integration and control of motor messages. The premotor area lies anterior to, or in front of, the primary area. Together, the motor cortex and the premotor area coordinate the outgoing messages which have originated in other parts of the CNS to initiate highly complex skilled movements.

The *prefrontal* area of the cortex is responsible for crucial regulatory directions to the muscles so that accurate movements will be made in

PSYCHOLOGICAL FOUNDATIONS 193

response to the environmental evaluation made by the precortex. This area may also be important in the control of judgment, ambition, consciousness, abstract thought, and speculation about the future.

The *somatosensory cortex* is the portion of the cerebral cortex that receives sensory stimuli from cutaneous and proprioceptor afferent nerves (nerves in the skin and muscles). This area controls the basic sensations of touch, pressure, heat, and cold. It also detects changes in spatial relationships of the body and its segments relative to joint movements and touch sensations. This area controls reflex movements resulting from visual stimulation and from auditory stimulation. It controls the tonic contraction of muscles.

Cerebellum. The cerebellum, or "little brain," is composed of two hemispheres, each of which has a cortex and a complicated network of internal nerve fiber connections. It is believed that the cerebellum is mainly responsible for coordinating skeletal movements. It also coordinates movements that originate in other sectors of the CNS. However, it cannot initiate movements. It is involved in the reflex control of bodily balance or equilibrium, as detected by the inner ear. Apparently it coordinates postural movements and locomotor activities. As the body moves in space, the cerebellum monitors the constantly changing positions and provides a continuous flow of rapid feedback information concerning the direction and amplitude of these movements. Whenever a segment of the body starts to deviate from an intended movement goal the cerebellum sends out a corrective signal and the body attempts to adjust its movements to its original intentions. The cerebellum also anticipates what positions the body and limbs will be in within a few seconds and thus alerts the body to sudden danger in time to take corrective action to avoid injury. Finally, the cerebellum is highly instrumental in the control of bodily equilibrium and coordinates information from the vestibular (balance and hearing) system, the proprioceptor system, and the visual system.

The Brain Stem. The brain stem connects the cerebellum and cerebral cortex, which send out motor fibers, and the spinal cord, which ascends into the brain stem. It also plays an important role in controlling hand, neck, and eye reflex movements. It is associated with the coordination and involuntary aspects of posture and other automatic movements and appears to assist with the control of head and upper body movements. It regulates certain vital processes such as artery flow, blood pressure, and respiration. Finally, the brain stem influences the control of sleeping and waking and contributes to attention and to the activation of the individual.

The Spinal Cord. The spinal cord also contributes to the control of muscular movements. It is primarily a transmission pathway. All sensory messages from bodily organs and receptors are transmitted to the brain and all motor commands are sent from the brain to the muscles and glands via the spinal cord. It also is fundamental to reflex function; it is the center for reflexes that have been innately developed and that are continuously active as modifiers of human movement. An example is the well-known "knee jerk." There are many other types of reflex movements controlled at the level of the spinal cord.

The peripheral nervous system consists of the spinal and cranial nerves. The peripheral system controls bodily functions not directly concerned with skeletal movements, such as the heart, blood vessels, glandu-

The Peripheral Nervous System

CHAPTER SIX

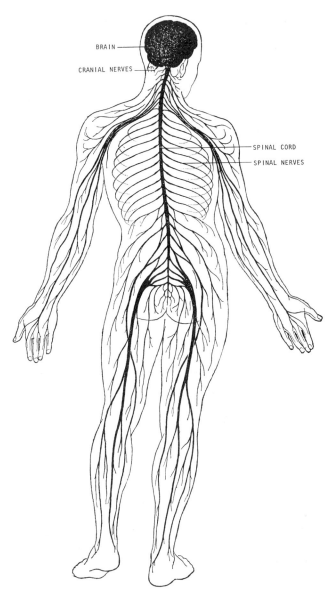

BRAIN

CRANIAL NERVES

SPINAL CORD

SPINAL NERVES

The peripheral nervous system.

lar secretions, and smooth muscles. There are 31 pairs of spinal nerves that enter the spinal column at various levels. They all receive sensory messages from various bodily parts, transmit these messages to the spinal cord, and return the message to the muscles in the area of the original stimulus. There are twelve pairs of cranial nerves, which carry sensory information to the brain from the regions of the mouth, nose, ears, and eyes. Likewise, motor fibers control the movements of the throat, tongue, face, mouth, and eyes, and also control the smooth muscles and glandular functions in the viscera.

From the moment of birth the infant learns about the external world through the sensory systems. Experiences (sight, sound, smell, pressure, balance, etc.) are transmitted to the central nervous system in the form of **PERCEPTION**

PSYCHOLOGICAL FOUNDATIONS

sensation. These sensations are received at various levels in the central nervous system and are stored for later recall by a process of classification that converts them into *perceptions.* Perceptions give meaning to individual instances of incoming sensate data. A process of mediation occurs that converts specific sensory inputs into meaningful perceptions. Perceptions, in turn, are organized into *concepts.* Concepts range from highly concrete to broadly abstract ones. The individual continually uses stored perceptions and concepts as data for generating responses to stimuli constantly received from the internal and external environments.

Perception is "man's awareness of sensory stimuli, his attention to them, and the meaning he attaches to them." It is frequently noted that, although two individuals may observe the same measurable reality, they perceive it differently. The individual's perception is discriminatory, depending upon past experience, state of attention, emotion, and other sensory stimuli. Movement is one medium through which perception can be extended. The teacher can help the student to broaden perceptions through making available experiences that are appropriately challenging and interesting.

Perceptual abilities are developed with experience. Movement is very important in enabling the individual to develop a wide repertoire of perceptual abilities. On the other hand, voluntary human movements necessarily involve some degree of perceptual awareness and information provided by the sensory systems. The more accurate the perceptions, the more likely the individual is to evoke successful, coordinated motor behaviors. A rapid feedback system serves as message carrier that keeps information continuously flowing between the source of the perception and the motor nerve center; thus, there is a constant relationship between the incoming perceptual information and the outgoing messages that guide voluntary motor acts. The central nervous system utilizes this feedback information to correct errors in movement in order to assist the person to perform more accurately a specific motor task.

Sensory Systems.   All of the sensory systems contribute to perceptual and conceptual development. These systems continually monitor our internal and external environments and relay messages to the central nervous system to keep us informed of all that is transpiring around us as well as within all of our bodily systems.

The Sensory Systems and Their Functions

auditory	hearing
visual	seeing
olfactory	smelling
gustatory	tasting
tactile	touching
kinesthetic	spatial awareness, bodily position, muscle stretch
vestibular (inner ear)	balance

The terms perception and kinesthesis are defined in different ways by various authorities; because of this inconsistency, it is at times confusing to read about these concepts. Sage[1] helps to distinguish between the two, pointing out the kinesthetic functions of *proprioceptors,* which are complex sensory receptors located in muscles, tendons, joints, and in the labyrinth of the inner ear.

Visual versus Tactual-Manipulative Behaviors. Researchers in Russia have demonstrated a direct relationship between visual behaviors and tactual-manipulative behaviors as children develop their perceptual abilities. One such notion is called *motor copy theory.* This theory contends that in carefully examining an object manually, a child is simultaneously accruing a visual image, or motor copy, of the object. Apparently, the child is comparing the impressions he or she receives about the object both from tactile manipulation and by visual features, such as size, form, and texture. In other words, the child is creating a more precise impression or knowledge or "copy" of the object. Research clearly indicates the importance of active motor exploration as the child develops perceptual abilities in a continually more refined manner. There is an obvious relationship between tactual manipulation and other types of sensory input into the central nervous system. Children should be encouraged to engage in active tactual manipulation as well as visual and other sensory manipulation in learning about new objects. As the child grows older it is probable that motor behaviors become somewhat less important than visual attention in the development of perceptual refinements of objects in the environment.

Perception takes place when the sensations received by the various sense organs of the body are processed by the central nervous system. Each incoming "raw" sensation from the various sensory organs is promptly processed and given a meaning. These meanings are referred to as *perceptions.* Perceptions provide a basis for comparison and decision making, used in coordination with future incoming sensations and the meaning the individual attaches to them.

Perceptual-Motor Learning

The important point here is that nonverbal sensations are continually being received in the central nervous system, and transformed into perceptions, as a result of our movement experiences. Likewise, perceptions are being formed from input provided by all of the other sensory systems. The brain integrates all of these perceptions into *concepts,* which are stored and thus are available for later retrieval as we cope with our internal and external environments.

Perception and Movement. The physical educator is particularly concerned with visual and kinesthetic perceptions. Unless one is blindfolded, or is blind, the sense of vision continually provides input into the central nervous system during the performance of a sport skill. Likewise, the athlete is continually receiving incoming messages from the proprioceptors, the sensory nerve endings located in the muscles, tendons, and joint surfaces of the human organism. Sensory stimuli from the inner ear also are essential to give direction to dynamic and static balance and to maintain equilibrium during movements involving changing bodily positions. These sensory messages are received from the inner ear, namely from the three semicircular canals and from the utricle, all of which continually assist the human organism in maintaining an upright, balanced position against the stress of imbalance, the force of external objects, and other factors seeking to upset our equilibrium, particularly during fast moving sport activities. Sense, or appreciation, of position on the part of the muscular system, particularly during movement, is termed *proprioception.*

Perception and the Physical Educator. All skilled learning is *perceptual-motor learning.* Indeed, it seems redundant to use the term "perceptual" in this designation of the skilled learning of human movements; however, this terminology is frequently employed in physical education textbooks. The physical education major should study intensively the subject of perception and concept development in relation to human movement experiences and the learning of skilled motor performances.

The complex area of perceptual-motor learning is of special significance to the physical educator. It is an area of psychology essential to the professional education of teachers of elementary school-age infants and young children in particular. Of course, all physical educators are directly concerned with the perceptual-motor learning of the individuals with whom they work, whatever the stage of life of these persons.

It is well established that skilled physical performances are highly dependent upon a variety of internal perceptual mechanisms. As Sage[2] says,

> The concept of perceptual-motor behavior, then, refers to the extracting of more and more refined information to produce greater control over one's overt motor behavior.

It is evident that motor behaviors are dependent upon the richness of perceptual bases which have developed in each individual. It is also believed that voluntary movements which are available for instant use by any individual are highly dependent upon an early life rich in a variety of perceptual experiences. It has been demonstrated that perceptual abilities at a very early age can be improved and expanded by concentrated movement education programs. Also, perceptual-motor programs are used to assess pupils with learning disabilities in their formative years. Some theories suggest that by enriching the repertoire of experiences of a child with a learning disability through an exposure to a wide variety of perceptual-motor skills and activities, specific learning disabilities will be remedied, at least to some extent. Today, the evidence is contradictory concerning the efficacy of perceptual-motor skills programs producing significant improvement in intellectual and language skills.

Learning Disabilities. In recent years specialists in early childhood education, psychologists, ophthalmologists and other interested physicians, as well as physical educators and elementary classroom teachers, have become intensely interested in the study of perceptual-motor development. They are particularly concerned with learning disabilities which appear to be related to serious perceptual deficiencies in the early years of many children. Recent research offers some hope, supporting the theoretical construct that a fundamental motor development program in the first six years of life is basic to long-range normal perceptual and conceptual growth and development. It is postulated that a child who has suffered a paucity of motor experiences in the early years will not develop perceptual abilities in the normal sequence or quantity, and thus will be handicapped in undertaking academic and intellectual learning tasks assigned in daily school work, such as reading, arithmetic, composition, and other basic abstract subjects.

Perceptual-Motor
Education
Programs

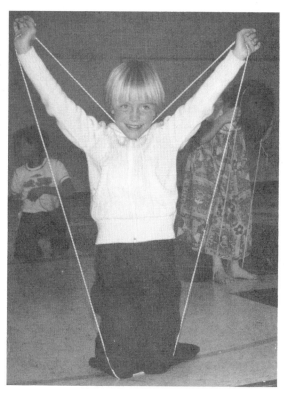

Many physical educators and elementary classroom teachers believe that current physical education programs are, in reality, perceptual-motor programs.

Teachers, consultants, physicians, and psychologists have developed and implemented a variety of perceptual-motor training programs in the hope of improving general intellectual development as well as specific skills in reading, spelling, and handwriting.

Screening Tests.　An assortment of perceptual-motor screening tests are available and are proliferating each year. These tests purport to indicate behavioral deficiencies with respect to perceptual-motor development. They concentrate on skills such as directionality, laterality, depth-perception, balance, spatial discrimination, time-awareness, locomotor movements, and manipulative skills. It is hypothesized that, through intensive perceptual-motor training programs involving the above physical behaviors and exercises, children's perceptual-motor behaviors will be in the normal range for this stage of development, and that as a consequence their intellectual abilities will likewise conform to the norm for their age group. These hypotheses have not been conclusively verified by research to date, but there is suggestive evidence to support them.

Physical Education Programs as Perceptual-Motor Programs.　Finally, many physical educators and elementary classroom teachers are of the belief that current physical education programs are, in reality, perceptual-motor programs.

The above discussion is reflected in the following summary by Gallahue.[3]

> There are two primary aspects of cognitive development that may be dealt with effectively through the movement education portion of the child's day. The first of these aspects is the various perceptual-

motor concepts involving the development of body awareness, spatial awareness, directional awareness, and establishment of an effective time-space orientation. The second aspect of cognitive development involves the development and reinforcement of increased understandings and appreciations of fundamental academic concepts involving science, mathematics, language arts, and social studies through the medium of movement. The bulk of available evidence indicates that both types of cognitive concepts, whether perceptual-motor or academic in nature, may be enhanced through active involvement in carefully selected and directed movement activities. It should be noted, however, that there is little support for the notion that increased movement abilities will have a correspondingly positive affect on the native intelligence of children. The use of movement as a method of enhancing cognitive development is *not* a panacea. Only through the combined and coordinated efforts of parents, classroom teachers, and the physical education teacher will truly positive inroads be made into the child's development of cognitive abilities.

Kinesthesis

Kinesthesis refers to the perceptual experiences resulting from the transmission of information from receptors in the muscles, tendons, joints, and vestibular apparatus.

Sage[4] defines kinesthesis as

> the discrimination of the positions and movements of body parts based on information other than visual, auditory, or verbal. The immediate stimuli arise from changes in length and from tension, compression, and shear [*sic*] forces arising from the effects of gravity, from relative movement of body parts, and from muscular contraction. It includes the discrimination of the position of body parts [and] the discrimination of movement and amplitude of movements of body parts, both passively and actively produced.

Thus, all voluntary motor performances are basically *perceptual-motor* acts.

Kinesthesia is the sense of position perceived through movements of the joints. Receptors, called *Golgi tendon apparatus,* are located in the tendons near their muscular origin and also are in the connective tissue of muscles. Whenever the connective tissue or tendons are stretched, the resultant pressure acts on nerve endings and causes messages to be relayed to the central nervous system. Pacinian corpuscles are spread throughout the fascia of the muscles and are especially concentrated beneath the tendon insertions to the joints. They are embedded deeply in skin layers. When muscles stretch or contract, the nerve endings are stimulated and messages are relayed to the central nervous system. Also under the skin lie touch and pressure receptors that also are important to skilled movements. They aid in the identification of the location of limbs, and the position of the body while moving. Some of these neural impulses set off by touch or pressure will result in reflexive movements; others will be transmitted to the cerebellum for integration into complex voluntary movements.

The *vestibular apparatus* in the inner ear is another sensory system that has a central role in the control of skilled motor movements. The semicircular canals of the inner ear act reflexively to help the body maintain its balance at all times. The utricle is reflexively sensitive to the varying head positions in relation to the forces of gravity and enables the individual to maintain an upright, balanced position, and to prevent falling. Thus, movements in all planes of space are sensed continuously and this information is steadily relayed to the central nervous system.

Vision is obviously another very important source of sensory information although it is not essential to human existence. For those fortunate to have partial or full sight, crucial information is relayed to the central nervous system, adding to the sensory stimuli that enable the CNS to initiate and control voluntary, purposeful physical movements.

Kinesthetic information seldom is acted on by the CNS in isolation. Rather, it is combined with information provided almost instantaneously from other sensory systems. In experiments where kinesthesis and other sensory modalities were manipulated for combined and partial efficiency of human movement skills, it was found that reduction in proprioception alone resulted in greater decrement of physical skill performance than when any one other sensory system was reduced or eliminated. Whether or not kinesthesis can be improved with practice is debatable. Kinesthesis can be deleteriously affected by heavy fatigue and excessive muscular tension. Various forms of motivational stimuli do not seem to improve kinesthetic perception.

SENSORY-MOTOR DEVELOPMENT

Piaget believes early sensory-motor experiences have lasting effects on later intellect. He thinks infants start with a few innate reflexes and construct sensory-motor functions and sophisticated cognitive operations from these simple beginnings. He also argues that simple sensory inputs and responses are combined to allow the use of symbols.[5]

Piaget's Six Stages of Sensory-Motor Development. Jean Piaget, a world-famous child psychologist, theorizes that sensory-motor development in children occurs through six stages. There is no rigid age prescribed for each of these stages; however, each child moves through these stages in the same progression.

Stage 1–Birth to one month: Reflex actions. Simple, primitive reflexes change gradually through growth and experimentation with environment. All later intellectual development is based on these early behaviors.

Stage 2–One to four months: Primary circular reactions. The baby acquires simple habits based on gradual modification of reflexes through experimenting with environment. Elementary sensory-motor coordinations develop.

Stage 3–Four to eight months: Secondary circular reactions. In this stage the child engages in more voluntary activities rather than reacting to external stimuli. The child becomes able to develop motor representations of external events although in a crude way. The child's behavior is controlled by the results that are produced. Greater awareness of external events enables the child to engage in sensory-motor acts specifically directed toward external objects. For the first time the child is now engaged in the intentional act of attaining a goal. This instrumental behavior is evidence of the use of intelligence. The child is now ready to adapt to novel situations rather than simply repeating learned responses.

Stage 4–Eight to twelve months: Sensory-motor coordination. During this stage the child is able to establish new goals and to discover many methods for reaching these goals through motor activities. The discovery of new movement patterns leads to the ability to carry out intentions. Eventually the child is able to anticipate circumstances and thus moves from mere trial and error into tentative combinations of movement until success is attained.

Stage 5–Twelve to eighteen months: Tertiary circular reactions. Now the child can deal with objects in the environment by using new variations of movements according to the specific situation. No longer a random explorer, the child develops new behaviors through active experimentation and soon comes to realize the permanence of objects in the environment.

Stage 6–Eighteen months to two years: Mental operations. This stage creates a basis for creative thinking. The child begins to use mental operations, conceiving new relationships in the environment and novel ways to solve movement problems, and no longer relying solely on trial and error. Sometimes the infant literally grasps the solution to a movement problem very quickly. This phenomenon is called *insight*.

Piaget also postulates that the child engages in six particular types of learning *interaction* with the environment during the early stages of development enumerated above. These special areas are: (1) play, (2) conception of space, (3) conception of time, (4) imitation, (5) causality, and (6) object concept. Space does not permit description of these areas. The interested reader is referred to Piaget publications.

Sheppard and Willoughby[6] give an excellent summary of Piaget's theory of cognitive development:

> At the core of Piaget's theory is the assumption that all cognitive growth results from the child acting upon the environment. The infant learns about the world by acting upon it. Later in childhood, these overt actions go underground and become internalized in the form of thought. But, according to Piaget, such thoughts have their beginnings in the actual physical, manipulative contact with the environment. In this regard, Piaget shares a common view with Bruner that the infant's first way of representing the environment is *active*. Because Piaget views the acquisition of all knowledge — whether in infancy, childhood or adulthood — as an active, ongoing process, his must be considered an *interactionist theory*. An interactionist theory sees the child engaged in continual interplay with the environment — as acting upon, transforming, and modifying the world, and in turn, being transformed and modified by the consequences of his own actions. It is this dynamic interaction between individual and environment which Piaget views as the essential, adaptive basis of all intelligent behavior.

According to Mussen,[7]

> Piaget believes that several factors influence the child's growth through his stages of intellectual development. They include (1) exercise and activity with objects, (2) detection of the salient aspects of experiences, and (3) logicomathematical experiences which result in the discovery of abstract properties of objects that do not belong to the objects themselves.
>
> Piaget's theory implies that a normally endowed child who could not use his arms or legs would have great difficulty growing intellectually, for Piaget assigns an important role to the infant's motor actions. These actions subsequently become internalized as operations.

As we have seen in previous chapters, the term "physical education" ORGANISMIC UNITY is a misnomer. It implies that the human being can be subdivided into a physical and a mental entity; and some authorities also would add a separate spiritual dimension. There is, however, considerable scientific evidence indicating that each act we perform—be it thinking, feeling, or moving — is a total human organismic experience, involving the *whole person* and not confined to some specific part of the body, such as the brain or the heart or a special muscle group.

Current findings from biology, anatomy, physiology, psychology, genetics, and other physical and medical sciences combine to demonstrate the validity of the organic unity of the human organism. Each and every part and function of the human organism is in some way related to all of the other parts and functions. In other words, the human organism is highly integrated in vastly complex ways.

Earlier in this chapter we saw how important early childhood movement experiences are to the development of basic concepts that will provide the basic framework for the child's thought life in the future. Steinhaus' famous observation, "Your muscles see more than your eyes,"[8] expresses vividly the importance of the sensory systems of kinesthesis, proprioception, hearing, vision, and the other sensory systems of the body, all of which combine their input to the central nervous system to inform the individual and to contribute to the sum of perceptions, concepts, and generalizations.

These scientific facts provide strong arguments for all areas of education to scrutinize their methods and activities, to determine the extent to which a particular learning experience is desirable for any individual as an integrated human being, rather than whether or not it is desirable only for the development of mental abilities, physical coordination, or ethical and moral standards. We must understand that any form of education will have an effect, favorable or unfavorable, upon the total individual, regardless of how specifically it is aimed at one phase of the development of that individual. In view of these facts, physical education can no longer be looked upon as purely muscular training or physical fitness development. Every muscular movement sets up reactions within the organism which ultimately influence, in some measure, the total living organism.

In summary, modern scientific evidence validates the concept of the human body as a network of highly intricate and effective systems of intercommunication, control, and coordination that have their bases in the nervous system and in the glands of internal secretion; these systems produce a highly developed integration of the various functions of the human body. This concept reveals one of the most amazing and significant understandings about the life of each human being. The physical educator should become thoroughly knowledgeable about these scientific facts. With this knowledge, the physical educator can, and should, become a leading interpreter of the new knowledge about the total, integrated human being and the role of movement activities and other forms of nonverbal experience and learning in the overall growth, development, and education of the individual.

MOTOR BEHAVIOR AND LEARNING

MOTOR BEHAVIOR

Behavior, as applied to human beings, refers to all of the activities engaged in by men, women, and children of all ages. Behaviors are generally amenable to some type of human measurement or assessment. Some behaviors are external and can be observed; others take place within the body, and many of these can now be monitored by sophisticated research equipment.

Physical educators and coaches are particularly interested in motor behaviors, especially behaviors which occur while the individual is engaged in a sport, dance, or exercise. Teachers and coaches help individuals improve, or become more skillful, in specific aspects of motor behaviors in sport, dance, and exercise. They seek the most efficient methods of practice and performances leading to acquisition of higher and more complex skills. When changes in skilled performances appear to be consistently more accurate and persistent than previously, it may be inferred that skill *learning* has taken place.

Physical educators and teachers are not only interested in motor skill performances and learning per se, they are also concerned with concomitant behaviors that can influence motor skill performances and learning either negatively or positively. Examples are the various types of eating, drinking, resting, sleeping, relaxing, dietary, and other health-seeking behaviors that have known effects, one way or the other, on skilled performances in sport, dance, and exercise.

Sage[9] states that

> The study of motor behavior is specifically concerned with motor skill acquisition and performance. This subject consists of a body of knowledge, compiled in the use of the scientific method, about the psychological aspects of human motor behavior. Thus, it may be viewed as a subfield of psychology.

Sage and other authorities point out the necessity for coaches and physical educators to have a thorough knowledge of motor behavior and recent research as guides to effective teaching and coaching. Psychological phenomena, such as incentives, motivation, stress, motor learning, perceptual processes, and relaxation, are essential elements to high level skill performances in sport and dance. Instructors must understand them thoroughly in order to instruct the pupils effectively and to apply these concepts in action on the playing field or in the dance studio. Psychological variables such as the ones listed above are under at least partial control of coaches and teachers of pupils learning physical skills. It is self-evident that teachers and coaches must be highly knowledgeable about these concepts and adept at translating them into practice and performance in the movement repertoires of sport contestants and dancers.

Child psychologists broadly agree that infants and young children should have opportunities for interacting with their environment through unrestricted movement activities, within bounds of safety, if normal developmental processes are to unfold. A child's motor development is basic to early trials of talking and communicating and there is a motor base underlying language development for many years after childhood.

There is compelling evidence from child growth and development research that motor skills in children improve with age, at different rates for boys and for girls. These differences may be explained by the distinct muscular and physical endowments of the sexes as well as by differential social experiences in early youth.

In general, girls mature physically more rapidly than boys and thus their visual-motor coordination is more advanced at the same age level. This generalization is most apt when coordination and fine muscle control, rather than strength, are required in particular physical skill performances. Again, there may be important cultural influences operating to determine which activities are deemed suitable for girls to participate in or to avoid.

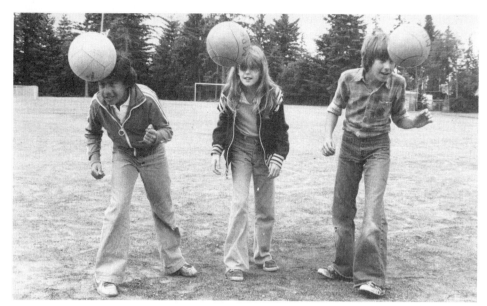
Gross motor skills.

Drowatsky[10] defines motor learning as "the adaptation process involving movement and muscular responses." The three components of muscular responses are postural, transport, and manipulative movements.

Motor patterns should be distinguished from motor skills. *Motor patterns* are broad, common elements used in the performance of various fundamental skills. A *motor skill* is a specific motor response developed to attain a desired result or outcome. Many authorities also distinguish between gross motor skills and fine motor skills. *Gross motor skills* involve several muscle groups of the body in such activities as running, swinging a baseball bat, jumping on the trampoline, and catching or hitting a moving ball. The active participation of the entire body is involved in gross motor skills. *Fine motor skills* involve the smaller muscles of the body where more minute precision is required, as in repairing a watch or playing a musical instrument. These skills are frequently employed in research exercises with such apparatus as pursuit rotors and finger mazes.

Cratty[11] defines motor learning as "that which includes the rather *permanent change* in motor performance brought about through practice and excludes changes due to maturation, drugs, or nutrients." Note the emphasis on stable change in behavior and the necessity for practice and repetition to bring about the change. Cratty defines similar terms such as movement behavior, motor performance, motor skill, motor fitness, motor educability, sensory-motor skill, and perceptual skill. The physical education major will learn these definitions and the basic concepts related to them in courses on motor learning. There is an abundance of current literature on the vast topic of motor learning and its elements.

According to Sage[12] motor learning occurs as an individual improves his motor skill in attempting to accomplish a particular set of goals with precision and accuracy. The learning process consists of a variety of motor and perceptual responses acquired through practice and repetition. Eventually, through the process of practice and repetition the learner develops a set of motor responses into an integrated and organized movement pattern.

PSYCHOLOGICAL FOUNDATIONS

The participants working under the direction of the physical educator usually are motivated by the desire to improve and to become more skillful in the specific motor performances in which they are engaging. Therefore, a definition of a skilled performer is a crucial concept for teachers and coaches to understand. Sage[13] succinctly describes the skilled performer:

> A skilled performer is characterized as one who can produce a fast output of high quality, and this is the criterion of skilled performance with which most assessment is concerned. Skilled performance is also characterized by an appearance of ease, of smoothness of movement, an anticipation of variations in the stimulus situation before they arrive, and an ability to cope with these and other disturbances without disrupting the performance — indeed, increasing skill involves a widening of the range of possible disturbances that can be coped with without disturbing the performance.

Open, Closed, Discrete, Serial, and Continuous Skills. In addition to citing the categories of gross and fine motor skills, recent literature also refers to open and closed skills, and to discrete, serial, and continuous skills.

An *open skill* is performed in an environment in which conditions are continually changing, thus requiring the performer to adapt constantly to novel stimuli during a performance. In effect, flexibility of movement responses performed very rapidly is required while engaged in an open skill.

Closed skills, on the other hand, require the performer to consistently repeat skilled movements as accurately as possible in an environment that changes little and does not have many stimuli which interfere with the concentration of the performer. The performer knows in advance exactly what movements are going to be required, and he or she can count on a stable environment throughout the performance.

In recent years the work of Poulton[14] stimulated interest in, as well as controversy over, the notion of open and closed skills. Sage[15] summarizes this system as follows:

> Closed skills are those which require a consistency of movement pattern and are performed under an unchanging environment. A gymnastic routine, a platform dive, a shot put or discus throw is an example of a closed task. On the other hand, "open" skills are externally paced in the sense that they must be done under varying environmental conditions each time they are executed, so they require a flexibility of movement response. . . . The handball player is never able to use exactly the same movement pattern for two shots. Proficiency in open skills requires a diversification and versatility of movements to meet the demands of the particular task.

Another category of sport and dance skills is based on a temporal dimension. *Discrete skills* have an obvious beginning and ending. One example would be the throwing of a technical foul shot in basketball. A *serial motor skill* consists of several discrete events occurring one after another in rapid succession and is employed in many sport events, such as the dribbling of the ball as the basketball player progresses up the floor. Finally, a *continuous skill* is repetitive and essentially the same movements are used over and over again. Various types of swimming strokes and the pace at which a runner attempts to move according to the length of a sprint or an endurance event are examples.

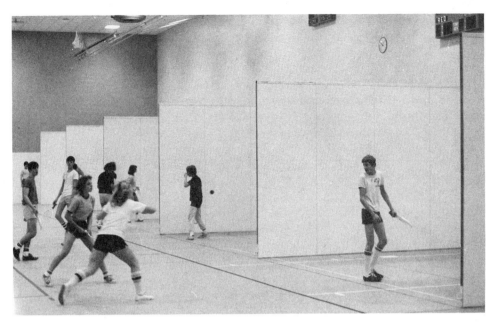

An example of "open skills."

Practice refers to the repeated efforts on the part of the individual to engage in the activity of interest for the purpose of increasing the degree of skill and its retention over time. Self-practice is commonly employed and, as the term indicates, refers to repetitions of sport movements and the evaluation of their accuracy and speed without the help of another individual. It is possible to improve in sport skills through self-practice, particularly if the individual has studied recently recommended fundamental movements and their integration into the sport pattern. The participant must have a mental picture of the correct movements and of the movement sequences involved from the start of the skill until its completion. Obviously, while using autoinstruction the participant lacks the benefit of verbal feedback from a knowledgeable observer; however, it is possible to make a videotape of one's practice performance for later review.

In schools and colleges most practices are planned, conducted, and evaluated by a coach or teacher charged with this responsibility. In general, practice is essential for improvement in the learning of physical skills. Examples of important principles relating to practice follow. The interested student should study recent motor learning books for complete details.

Principles of Practice:

1. *Motivation:* The learner must be motivated to improve the skill; thus, practice must be purposeful.
2. *Model:* The learner must have an example or mental picture of how the skill should be performed prior to making the practice attempt.
3. *Meaningful feedback:* After each practice attempt the movements made should be compared with the model movements.

Of course, in a class or team with several members present, the teacher cannot provide individual feedback after each practice attempt.

On the other hand, certain activities provide a degree of feedback automatically owing to the nature of the required skills, as for example, when shooting a basketball, the ball either goes through the hoop or it does not, a result that is apparent to the shooter.

Massed versus Distributed Practice. Massed versus distributed practice is a topic of continuous debate. As the terms suggest, *massed practice* involves concentrated instruction and repetition of certain skills within a short period of time. *Distributed practice* utilizes a less intense schedule, providing instruction and repetition alternately with time periods of no practice. Distributed and massed practices appear to have approximately equal value up through some optimal length of time of practice. Beyond that point, distributed practice appears to be more beneficial. It seems likely that distributed practice is more beneficial for the learning of motor skills which emphasize accuracy.

Sage[16] provides a summary of principles gleaned from recent research:

1. Distributed practice produces superior performance.
2. There is very little difference in learning between distributed and massed schedules, but distributed schedules have a slight advantage.
3. Distributed practice is preferable when the energy demands of the task are high, the task is complex, the length of the task performance is great, the task is not meaningful, and motivation of the learner is low.
4. Massed practice is preferable when the skill level of the learner is high and when peak performance on a well-learned skill is needed.
5. Massed practice may be preferable when the skill is highly meaningful, when motivation is high, and when there is considerable transfer from previously learned tasks to the new task.

Simply put, feedback refers to the information the individual receives either during or upon completion of the performance of a motor act. Information concerns the behavior itself and the consequences of that behavior as well. As a result of this feedback, the performer decides whether or not to revise various movements on the next attempt or whether or not the performance is satisfactory.

Feedback

Intrinsic and Augmented Feedback. Feedback is commonly referred to as knowledge of results. Different authors have developed models naming several types of feedback.[17] Basically, feedback can be labeled as either intrinsic or augmented. *Intrinsic feedback* is available to a performer during his performance or almost immediately thereafter, such as in serving a volleyball or swinging at a baseball and striking out. In some cases, the behavior does not provide clear feedback to the participant. In this case, the teacher will provide *augmented feedback* through a verbal explanation of what occurred during the movement or through slow motion pictures or instant television replay, which can be used to demonstrate the errors made by the athlete. There are many subtopics within the general concept of feedback. Physical education teachers and coaches should be aware of the most recent research findings. Some examples follow.

Research Findings on Feedback. It is frequently suggested that *knowledge of performance* (KP) is emphasized in the teaching of closed skills, while *knowledge of results* (KR) is more valuable for learning open skills.

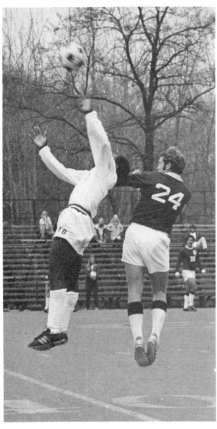

The athlete must be taught to "feel" body position through proprioceptive feedback during performance of the total skill process.

The more clear and accurate the feedback is, the more value it will have for the athlete. There is a limit to each case, however, and it is possible for the instructor to overload the participant with too much feedback. Likewise, there may be an optimal level of precision beyond which the learner cannot comprehend and utilize the information in subsequent movements.

Feedback should be as *specific* as possible and communicated in language that is understood by the pupil. Feedback should be given as *promptly* as possible, as it becomes less effective with delay in time.

The student should be taught to depend upon the intrinsic cues that are most fundamental to making the proper movement. For a participant practicing a closed skill, the feedback should assist the learner toward being able to perform the movement patterns in a repetitious manner as identically as possible. In other words, consistency of response is a key teaching technique. The athlete must be taught to "feel" body positions and the locations of the body and its segments in space through proprioceptive feedback as he or she is engaged in the total skill process.

In summary, feedback appears to have three major functions: information, motivation, and reinforcement. Nixon and Locke[18] summarize recent research findings on feedback by noting that "the motivational and corrective influences of feedback ensure that it will be the strongest and most important variable controlling motor performance."

This subject is discussed in more detail under the section Sport Psychology later in this chapter. However, selected comments are appropriate here concerning this essential psychological concept related to teaching and learning in school physical education classes and in informal non-school physical education and sport settings.

In order to learn effectively in a physical education class a student must be motivated to desire to make progress toward the goals the teacher has established for the pupils in the class. A *motive* is an inner urge to accomplish a goal or to attain a satisfactory emotional state in a specific environmental situation. The teacher attempts to *motivate* all pupils to make progress toward the program objectives, general and specific. Many factors can be manipulated by the teacher in an attempt to motivate each pupil in a positive direction. Selected motivational principles follow.

Clarify Individual Objectives. The general objectives of the physical education curriculum and the specific goals of each instructional unit must be made clear to all pupils. Students must understand how they will benefit from the participation, practice, and evaluative processes they will be involved in throughout the unit. Teachers must communicate to students verbally and nonverbally at various levels of comprehension necessary to clearly inform each student of the objectives and goals to be attained. Students should be given opportunity to discuss the goals and objectives with the teacher and with each other. Some teachers have pupils write down a set of behavioral objectives to be achieved by the end of the unit. This list can be modified during the course of the unit as the students actually practice, participate, and evaluate their progress toward their personal goals, with teacher guidance.

Adapt to Individual Ability. The learning activities in the curriculum must be within the potential abilities of each class member to gradually accomplish through successful performances and learning throughout the unit. The instruction, and opportunities for practice and participation, must be individualized so that each pupil gradually improves in skill performances, knowledge, and understanding, and in attitudes associated with each learning activity. Students should be grouped with other pupils of similar ability range. Pupils with poor skills in a complex sport will be embarrassed and, in many cases, "turned off" if more expert players clearly outperform them.

Supply Positive Reinforcement. Teachers and student aides should offer helpful hints concerning major constant errors the student is making. Positive reinforcement should be provided for proper execution of a skilled movement, or even for a practice attempt which is an improvement over previous attempts.

Increase Opportunity for Practice. Teachers should provide as many practice trials as can possibly be arranged for each member of the class in practice sessions. If nine pupils have to stand in line while one student at a time makes one attempt to walk across the balance beam, boredom and lack of attention will soon set in. Most important, little or no learning can possibly occur under such sparse practice conditions. One of the major deficiencies of many public school physical education classes is the lack of provision of equipment, facilities, and supplies necessary for each pupil to engage in many practice repetitions of important sport, dance, or exercise skills.

Fair but Rigorous Evaluation. Formal grading systems should be constructed which accurately inform students as to their progress toward realistic individual goals. Grades should not be used as a punitive measure or to embarrass a pupil who is poorly skilled in comparison with other students. The rationale underlying grading systems in physical education needs to be carefully analyzed (see the chapter on evaluation).

Schools and colleges should provide academic credit and should employ the same system of grading student accomplishment in physical education as for any other subject matter area in the school curriculum. If physical education is not as rigorously evaluated, the students will soon presume that this subject field is not as important as the other subjects.

Required Physical Education Classes. Physical education course credit should be required as a qualification for graduation from elementary school, junior high school, and senior high school, along with the other basic subjects. The same academic standards for course completion should apply to physical education as to the other required subjects in the school curriculum. As with academic credit mentioned above, students will not be as motivated in physical education if school and district policies infer, or explicitly state, that this subject is less important, is non-academic, or is not basic to a well rounded public school education.

Teacher education courses and field experiences devote heavy emphasis to student motivation principles and to effective teacher behaviors. Many textbooks discuss this vital topic in detail.

Motivation in Informal Settings. In informal settings such as playgrounds, community swimming pools, tennis courts, golf courses, and parks, as well as programs and facilities provided by semiprivate and private organizations, motivation is again a basic concept. One big advantage regarding the motivation of individuals who attend these programs is quite obvious. In most cases the participants have voluntarily decided to come to the sponsoring agency and to engage in the available program either on a free basis or subject to an attendance fee or a membership stipend. Some are coerced by parents, friends, or peer group pressures to engage in physical education activities in nonschool settings. However,

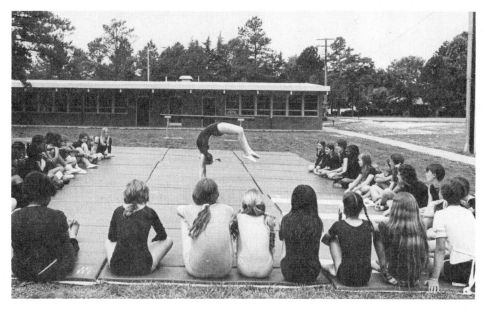

Large participant groups should be avoided.

in general, one can expect them to be more self-motivated and enthusiastic than pupils in required school programs. If properly instructed and personally well treated, participants find these experiences to be highly motivating and self-satisfying. Unfortunately, in some cases, the instructional personnel are not as professionally qualified as they should be and some of them may be violating well known teaching and learning principles. Also, sometimes there is a tendency to make a participant group too large in terms of the number of instructional personnel or the facilities and equipment to be employed, which can soon cause motivational problems among the clientele.

In summary, internal motivation, personal satisfaction with one's performances, and overall enjoyment of the group situation in which the person is participating will ultimately determine the pleasure, fun, degree of learning, and overall personal benefit gained from this type of sport or dance experience.

Retention refers to the length of time learned information can be retained and recalled for future use. It also can refer to continued ability in an improved skill in sport, dance, and other forms of activity involving skilled performances. This concept is obviously of fundamental importance to teachers and coaches and to curriculum planners. If there were little or no long-term retention of the motor skills learned in physical education classes there is little likelihood the program would occupy an important role in the total school and college curricula as it does today. *Retention*

The opposite of retention is forgetting, or the psychological term *extinction*. Singer[19] indicates that retention of physical skills will be increased if they are *overlearned*. Overlearning refers to the amount of practice provided in the performance of a specific movement after it has been learned according to some preestablished criterion. Fortunately, motor skills are usually retained for a long time because we really do not learn a large number of them. Also, several of them are unique, are practiced for a great length of time, and thus involve many repetitions, such as learning to ride a bicycle, to bowl, to swim, and so on. Singer summarizes factors contributing to the retention of physical skills:

1. Material should be well organized for the benefit of the learner, so there will be ease in internally organizing it for storage and retrieval.
2. Material should be meaningful as perceived by the learner.
3. Material should be well learned (overpracticed).
4. Competing activities should be minimized, from time of practice to time of retention.
5. Time lag from practice to retention should not be too long, or else some related task experience should occur in the interval.
6. Material should be presented in such a way as to be compatible with the information-processing abilities of the learner considering transition from short-term memory to long-term memory.
7. Retention tests should encourage the opportunity for the person to reorient.
8. The use of covert rehearsal or observation of others performing the task in the rest interval can be beneficial.

One of the basic assumptions of a school curriculum is that the skills, competencies, understandings, attitudes, and appreciations learned in the various subject-matter fields will "carry over" or *transfer* to similar *Transfer* situations in nonschool environments. It is obvious that one of the major purposes of teaching motor skills in physical education and sport programs is the use of those skills in similar situations and in a variety of other life situations, in school and out. Therefore, physical education teachers and coaches should be thoroughly familiar with basic principles of transfer of motor skill learning and should teach for such transfer in their classes and in their athletic practices. Examples of principles of transfer of motor learning which appear to have a research basis are listed in the following paragraphs.

Types of Transfer.   There are three general types of transfer of learning. The first type is called *positive transfer,* wherein the motor skills learned in one situation can be applied with success in a new, similar situation. A second type is *negative transfer,* where the original motor skills are not directly usable in a different situation. Also there are occasions when there is neutral or *zero transfer,* during which time previous learning appears to have no effect on the performance or learning in a new situation. Some authors postulate a *net transfer* in a complex motor skill situation wherein both positive and negative transfer components are present.

Conditions Affecting Transfer.   Singer[20] discusses important conditions which affect the transfer of training in the performance and learning of motor skills. The most important principle may be that the more similar the tasks the greater the positive transfer probably will be. The time spent in learning the original motor skills usually is directly related to the degree of transfer to be expected. Motivation is another essential element in transferring a skill from one situation to another. There is some experimental evidence that the types of training used may be positively related to transfer results. The degree to which the students understand the motor learning tasks to be performed and can develop mental understandings of principles which can be applied in the transfer of one task to another may be an important factor in developing positive transfer. The ability of the instructor to bring out such insight and understanding is crucial.

Coaches and physical educators are constantly seeking effective instructional methods for the teaching and learning of sport activities which require the development of speed or quickness as well as accuracy, such as hitting a backhand tennis shot. Reviewing available research studies on this topic in physical education, Nixon and Locke[21] summarize:

> Nowhere in the literature is research in more perfect and happy agreement. Instructions for either speed or accuracy produce the intended effects. Tasks that demand equal emphasis profit from equal emphasis throughout the learning process. Certainly the natural proclivity of the teacher to stress accuracy in early trials is contraindicated. In general, physical skills should be practiced at the speed which will be employed during an actual contest. To practice at a slower or faster speed is to increase the possibilities of negative transfer.

Bilateral Transfer

The phenomenon of bilateral transfer has always interested physical education teachers and coaches. The question is, when a player learns to throw a baseball right-handed, to what extent is his skill in throwing the ball left-handed facilitated in the absence of left-handed practice? In other words, how much positive transfer has occurred between limbs?

Electromyography studies have demonstrated the transfer of electrical pulses from one part of the body to another in the performance of the same physical skill. Several studies in sport support the notion of the bilateral transfer of specific skills, not only between arms but also transfer from hand to hand, and from hand to foot.

Research Results on Transfer of Learning. Sage[22] refers to the large body of research studies that have been made on many aspects of transfer of learning phenomena. His summary of principles from these studies follows:

1. Transfer of learning is greatest when two tasks are highly similar.
2. When a second task requires the learner to make different, incomparable responses to identical or similar stimuli which appeared in the original task, initial negative transfer will likely result.
3. When a second task is quite dissimilar to the original task, little or no transfer usually results.
4. When successive tasks of the same type are given, the tasks will tend to be learned more and more quickly.
5. Positive transfer increases with increasing initial mastery of the original task.
6. Practice with one limb usually results in positive transfer to all the other limbs.
7. The research on task difficulty and transfer is contradictory; optimal conditions must be established for each task.
8. An understanding of the general nature and basic principles which are important to task performance produces positive transfer.
9. When two tasks involve similar movement patterns, they should not be learned at the same time, for a maximum positive transfer.
10. Practice of nonspecific "coordination" or "quickening" tasks will not produce positive transfer for specific sport skills.

Complex Skills

Another consideration is whether or not the learner should practice a modified, easier version of a total complex physical skill, gradually increasing the complexity during the practice period until he or she is finally practicing the actual skill to be used in a game situation. Limited research in sports seems to indicate that complex skills should be practiced and taught using the same level of complexity and difficulty that will be encountered in the actual game situation. In other words, a skill should not be modified in practice to a more simple version, nor should it be made more complex than it will occur in a game situation. An example would be practice-putting on a putting green with holes which are larger or smaller in diameter than the regulation holes on the golf course.

Whole-Part Practice. *Whole-part practice* is a major controversy in the sport skills research literature. The main difficulty is to come to a common agreement about the terms "whole" and "part" in any discussion on this topic; in fact, there is a third type of skill learning called *progressive part* learning. Space prohibits a detailed explanation of this complex problem. Drowatzky[23] summarizes this issue with tentative conclusions from available research with which the authors of this text agree:

Studies have indicated that there is no superiority for either method in all situations. The part method appears to be best suited for more complex skills, and the whole method is best for less complex skills. In any event, both the part and whole methods must involve skills that are meaningful; the part instructions should use skills that are easily separated from the whole, such as the lay-up in basketball. The part method might be used to advantage in overcoming the problems of fatigue or boredom if the whole would involve long practice sessions. It may also give more rapid feedback and reinforcement.

214

On the other hand, the whole method appears to be best used when the material is so meaningful that it hangs together well and when the students have enough intelligence to learn quickly. In fact, the whole method appears to be better in most learning situations; the notable exception is team games. Probably the best recommendation is for the teacher to find a flexible plan of instruction that begins with materials organized in larger units but moves to smaller units of instruction when students experience difficulty in learning. If the part method is used, the instructor must plan for the parts to be combined into a whole rather than expecting the integration to occur through incidental learning.

The model by Nixon and Locke[24] divides "critical events in motor learning" into seven stages as well as preactive decisions and postactive events and combines recent research findings in a variety of phases of motor learning. This model (see p. 216) should assist the teacher or coach in organizing recent knowledge and principles for teaching and coaching gleaned from available research literature.

Conclusion

Nixon and Locke[25] conclude:

> Research does not tell the physical education teacher how to teach motor skills — no matter how attentively he listens. The research we now have contains: (1) some suggestions that the teacher may pursue with confidence, as in the case of demonstrations through film and augmented knowledge of performance for closed skills; (2) some suggestions for experimental alterations to traditional practice, as in the cases of programmed learning and the use of distraction; (3) some strong suggestions about what is not effective, as in the case of progressive part practice, extended verbal analysis for beginners, and task simplification; (4) some information, as yet so incomplete and subject to qualification that it can mean little more than "it all depends," as in the case of mental practice and distribution of practice; (5) some great voids where the teacher's operations must now depend on tradition, chance, intuition, and native wit, as in the case of teacher observation and the guidance of student response to feedback; and (6) some suggestions for the improvement of pedagogy through the development and use of empirically based models, as in the few studies that utilize the power of learning theory or the control over treatment provided by systematic descriptions of teaching.

Definition. There is division of opinion about the use of the terms sport psychology and motor behavior. Some authorities prefer the use of the latter term because the present state of knowledge about human motor behavioral performances in physical education is so sparse that teachers and coaches must make the application of principles and generalizations from studies conducted in nonsport situations in the majority of cases. There is a growing body of knowledge about principles of psychology developed from research studies conducted in physical education environments.

SPORT PSYCHOLOGY

Sport psychology is defined by Lawther[26]: "Sport psychology is an area which attempts to apply psychological facts and principles to learning, performance, and associated human behavior in the whole field of sports."

Loy[27] indicates that formal interest in sport psychology started more than 75 years ago with publications emphasizing theoretical and empirical studies by scholars from various disciplines, both nationally and internationally, interested in the psychological phenomena associated

SCOPE

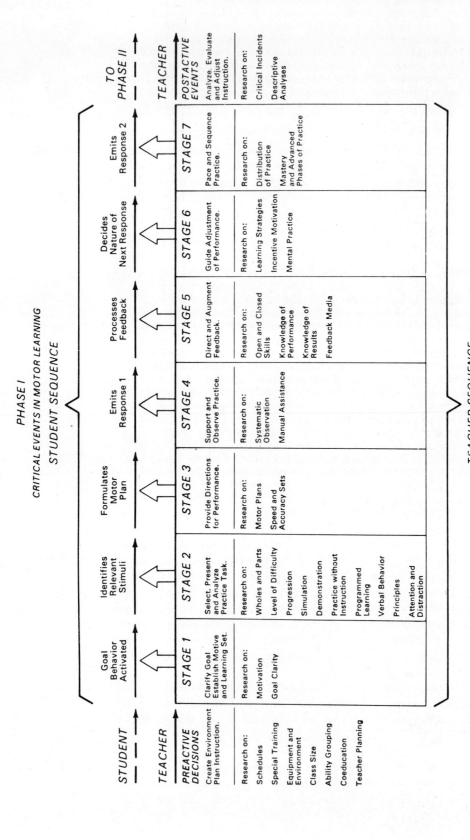

Model for Critical Events in Motor Learning.

CHAPTER SIX

with sports. Examples of topics which have undergone research scrutiny over the years are: social facilitation, the psychology of coaching, the psychology of the athlete, the personality of the athlete, sport skills learning, the roles of sports and games in culture, the educational values of sport, psychological dimensions of women's participation in sports, social psychology, self-concept, body image, and fundamental physiological concepts.

Cratty[28] indicates that the topics generally studied in sport psychology are subsumed under the major headings of psychological and social dimensions in coaching, psychological demands in athletics, teaching skills and conducting practices, personality and sport, activation, aggression and anxiety, and social dimensions in sport.

Contemporary Readings in Sport Psychology, edited by William P. Morgan,[29] offers a wealth of interesting topics concerning sport psychology and physical education; included among them are comparative and physiological psychology, engineering psychology, learning theory, measurement, mental health, motivation, motor learning, perception, personality dynamics, psychophysiology, and social psychology. Morgan observes in his preface,

> Because of the embryonic nature of sport psychology, it is difficult to predict just what course the growth of this field will ultimately take. Indeed, perusal of the program of the Second International Congress suggests that workers in this area are presently concerned with many different specialized facets of psychology. Therefore, it seems appropriate to regard sport psychology as being multidimensional.

In a more recent book Tutko and Tosi[30] have narrowed the focus of their work to the application of principles from psychology to success in athletic competition. These authors are straightforward in stating that "this book offers a coordinated system of techniques used by successful athletes for turning stress energy into better sports performance."

The major topics included in this book are

— how to handle stress in sport performances;
— the types of pressures which exist and how to cope with them;
— how psychological pressures are intrinsically related to physical performances;
— how one's emotions can be controlled for optimal performance in sport;
— how to identify and cope with seven psychological traits during a sport performance — desire, assertiveness, sensitivity, tension, confidence, personal accountability, and self-discipline;
— "peaks" and "slumps";
— relationships between the instructor or coach and the athlete;
— winning, what it is and what it isn't.

The authors conclude by relating the lessons learned in sport practice and participation to other areas of living, or what they call "life psyching."

Sport psychology as a subdiscipline of physical education has expanded rapidly in recent years. Many young people are electing to enter this specialization and are preparing themselves accordingly in doctoral programs. The scope of this field has never been accurately delineated nor has its content been adequately described. There is a rapid proliferation of research emanating from young scholars, and one is struck by the wide range of subjects being studied. Examples follow.

Cross-Cultural Studies in Motor Development. Some physical educators with special training in anthropology are studying cross-cultural child rearing practices and motor development of selected samples of young children in various countries. Apparently, motor development in infants and young children progresses at differing rates of time in various cultures according to the specific types of upbringing by the parents. As yet, little work has been done at higher age levels and cross-cultural comparisons are lacking.

Studies in Competition. Competition is an area studied by several investigators. One common finding is that both individual attitude and the sex of the athlete account to some extent for differences in competitive attitudes and strategies in young athletes. Rapid changes in attitudes toward sport competition are accompanying changes in social expectations and legal requirements.

Female Athletes. There has been considerable research activity concerning female athletes. Many studies have investigated the psychosocial aspects of the female athletes' experiences in sport. Athletes, as well as other females who excel, have been found to express self-descriptions that are considered psychologically androgynous. That is, these women identify characteristics in themselves that our culture ascribes to members of both sexes; for example, female athletes describe themselves as nurturant (a characteristic associated by our culture with femininity) as well as achievement oriented (a characteristic associated with masculinity). In addition, it has been found that female athletes who describe themselves as androgynous display greater self-esteem in comparison to subjects who express self-descriptions characterized as stereotypically feminine. There is evidence in the literature to support the observation that characteristics associated with masculinity correlate well with self-esteem.

Social Facilitation. A topic of several studies, *social facilitation* is described as the enhancement of athletic performance by the mere presence of other people. In general, these studies indicate that the presence of other persons serves as a source of motivation and tends to enhance the performance of athletes in tasks that are well learned, though it may hinder or lower performance in early task learnings.

COACTION. Closely related to social facilitation is the possible influence of *coaction*, or the effect of group involvement in the same activity. It has been suggested that the beneficial influence of *coacting groups* is distinct from, for example, the effect of an audience. Findings to date, however, have been largely contradictory and offer few, if any, practical conclusions.

GROUP COHESION. Along the same lines, several investigators are interested in the roles of leadership by various members of teams and the extent to which *group cohesion* relates to the percentage of wins the team achieves. In general, teams having members who interact well and often with each other, and thus develop high social cohesion, are more successful in achieving victories.

A subject closely related to these just discussed is the human need for *affiliation*, which is discussed later in this chapter.

The Role of the Coach. Some investigators are studying the role played by the coach in providing emotional support for athletes and the effect of this support on winning. Preliminary evidence suggests that coaches of very successful teams emphasize personal attention and individual emotional support. Players of lesser ability fare best with coaches who assist them in directing attention to the skills of the game, to the ultimate goal of playing their best, and in making every attempt to win. Obviously, there is a subtle distinction between styles and purposes of coaches working with athletes of varying skill abilities.

Another phenomenon which is of interest is the extent to which long and varied experience by the coaches, both as former athletes and as coaches, contributes directly to the success of their athletes. It has generally been assumed that there is a direct relationship between coaches' experience in participating and coaching, and the success of their teams. Apparently there is little or no research to uphold this contention.

Achievement Motivation. Other investigators are interested in achievement motivation, which is identified as the extent to which any sport performance is related to both the immediate and future expectations of success and failure (winning and losing).

The term *motivation* is generally defined as a desire by the individual to behave in such a way as to satisfy a need or to engage in goal-seeking behavior. The term motivation derives from the word "motive" which refers to any condition of the human organism which has an effect upon its readiness to begin or continue a sequence of behaviors desired by that individual. Thus, motivation consists of a series of motives sometimes called needs or drives. The conditions provoking motivation may originate either from within the organism or from the outside environment.

Goals are related to motivation. Persons are motivated to strive for specific goals. Also, the individual may desire to avoid a situation that has a negative end. The participant attempts to meet biological needs and social needs through goal-directed behavior, and the success of these actions will be mediated by the strength of the motivation to reduce the needs.

Incentives are material or symbolic objects or conditions to which a person is attracted or from which a person withdraws. Athletes on school teams are given the opportunity to earn letters, medals, and trophies for outstanding performances in their sports. The possibility of public recognition through the media, sport banquets, and in other ways also serves as an incentive in sport.

Pep talks are frequently used in sport as verbal encouragement by the teacher or coach. Little research has been done upon the effect of "pep talks" by coaches to their athletes prior to a game or at half-time; therefore, the matter is still subject to individual opinion and experience. It seems plausible that each situation is "iffy." In general, teachers and coaches should not expect an emphasis on verbal encouragement to produce maximum skilled performance.

In some cases, coaches combine verbal incentives with material incentives. It may be that incentives vary in effectiveness with different individuals and in differing sport environments. There may be no general procedure currently valid that all coaches should follow with all athletes. If one had to speculate, perhaps it would be prudent to believe that verbal exhortation has little or no positive effect on sport performance. As yet we have no scientific evidence concerning this controversy.

COMPETITION AS AN INCENTIVE. On the other hand, competition has been found to be a powerful incentive and, of course, coaches frequently make the most possible use of it. However, not in all cases does competition improve performance. Some studies have indicated that intense competition may produce such a high state of arousal that the athlete is not capable of performing at an optimal level. Also, if the team members firmly believe they do not have much of a chance to win a particular game it may not be an effective incentive to emphasize the competitive function and the importance of winning in that particular contest. It does seem that when individuals or teams are approximately equal in their abilities, competition frequently elicits top level performances by many of the athletes. Sage[31] reports a series of principles and conclusions concerning motivational techniques including the following: Threats by coaches can have powerful influences, either positive or negative, on athletes. However, some athletes may react by overly depending on the coach, while others will resent such treatment.

INTERNAL MOTIVATION. Perhaps the most agreed upon principle is that the best motivation is the internal incentive to desire to perform as well as possible. This incentive, in general, will produce higher skilled performances than will external incentives such as prizes, sweaters, and public adulation. Many athletes can be motivated not only to identify and strive to achieve their goals, but also to be a part of accomplishing team goals.

Coaches should encourage team members to set goals because of the involvement of two very strong social needs, namely self-esteem and social approval. Being asked to help set goals gives the individual a sense of identity and good feeling.

ASPIRATION. Aspiration is another element of motivation that is very important for some. It is seen in athletes who estimate what their performance will be during the next contest or possibly in the future; they set performance goals players believe to be within their capability of achievement. Research has shown what may seem to be the obvious, namely, that individuals who are successful according to some outside criterion tend to increase their levels of aspiration for higher levels of excellence. Likewise, when the athletes do not perform at the expected level, their aspiration level may decrease. Social group and parental aspiration levels also influence aspiration levels of children.[32]

ANXIETY AND STRESS. Anxiety and stress in motor performances is another area of interest for researchers as well as for coaches. One major topic is the extent to which athletes should develop a state of arousal prior to a contest and while actually participating.

Studies have been done on the effects of stress on performance in competitive sports. Three experimental variables can be introduced into these studies: physiological measurements, performance measurements during execution of specific skills, and phenomenological measurements or self-reports from the athletes as to the degree of tension they felt. The evidence of these early studies is so ambiguous as to lead to no worthwhile tentative conclusions at this time. However, the topic is of considerable interest and as the research methodology improves perhaps the results will become apparent in the years ahead.

Spectators. In the past, physical education literature generally has stated the view that spectators at formal, competitive athletic contests may benefit from the release of tensions and feelings of aggression as a result of enjoying the game. This explanation has been known as the *catharsis* theory. In recent years young scholars in physical education, and in allied disciplines, have begun to question this notion. They contend that exciting games involving considerable aggressive activity on the part of the players may well increase the feeling of aggression on the

Sport: Catharsis or Instigator?

part of the spectators. Overt behaviors by spectators, such as running onto the field, tearing down football goal posts, running away with the bases from the baseball diamond, attempting to struggle with players leaving the athletic field, and similar activities would seem to support this latter interpretation. The apparent explanation is that some people do become emotionally activated during certain types of athletic contests and thus tend to become more aggressive in their behaviors during and after the game. Therefore, it is recommended that schools and colleges undertake spectator appreciation education to ensure an environment of self-control among spectators.

Participants. A similar controversy arises concerning the athletes in sports contests. There are conflicting assertions made by coaches, psychologists, and other interested observers; some contend that the catharsis theory operates with respect to the contestants, while others believe that certain sports may train the participants to be more aggressive and that this behavior will carry over into other areas of their personal lives. There is no valid research to resolve this debate with a high degree of confidence. Again, it seems obvious that teachers, coaches, and administrators should make every effort to demand acceptable social behaviors from athletes during contests, where they must abide by legal rules and by the decisions of the game officials. Likewise, it is hoped that there will be transfer of desirable personal feelings and attitudes toward fair play, emotional control, and appropriate controlled aggression as sanctioned by the society at large.

PERSONALITY

There is a widespread interest in the extent to which successful athletes have personalities that differ in major respects from those who are nonathletes. Investigations have been conducted of athletes in a variety of sports, at different levels of schooling, and in different categories of competition, all the way from local to national and including international contests. Singer[33] summarizes this research by stating that "the champion athlete obviously possesses superior skills and personal characteristics when compared to the average athlete. Why else is he superior? However, attempts at determining personality traits or profiles unique to the champion have resulted in disagreement in research findings."

Likewise, the question of the extent to which participation in athletics contributes to marked permanent personality change has been argued and discussed frequently in physical education and sport literature in recent years. The postulated changes in personality that occur can be either positive or negative. If sport experience directly affects personality change, are there differences in the influence of different sports, or in different levels of sport competition? What is the influence of a host of other factors that are present in any sport scene which could contribute to personality change? It is indeed a complex research question. Individual studies have recorded results in both directions, some showing a positive development of personality, while other studies report a deterioration in personality related to a sport experience. Again, Singer[34] provides a realistic summary of the present state of research on the question:

> Common sense suggests that the athlete decides to experience a given activity and then becomes competent due, at least in part, to the personality he brings to the situation. Sport and fulfillment must be somewhat compatible with an individual's personality. . . . Because so many environment situations affect us, it is dangerous to attribute specific characteristic changes to sport involvement alone. Not until

more precise measuring instruments are developed, studies planned, and variables controlled, can we posit any definitive statements.

Alderman,[35] in a comprehensive review of research concerning the personality of athletes, supports the generalization that studies fail to verify a causal relationship between experiences in sports and changes in personality traits. He also points out that the personality tests used include personality traits that may be very little influenced by participation in sports.

Alderman also agrees with Singer that research today does not demonstrate that specific personality types are related to high performance in particular sports.

Morgan[36] summarizes important research on what he calls the *consequences of participation* in sports. He also points out that sport activity influences psychological *states* and *traits* in different ways. He says that "*states* such as anxiety or depression can be influenced almost immediately by a variety of stimuli such as pharmacologic agents, electroconvulsive shock, exercise, hypnosis, meditation, biofeedback, and progressive muscular relaxation, whereas *traits*, such as extroversion-introversion, neuroticism-stability, augmentation-reduction, or field dependence-independence, are relatively immune to these same stimuli."

The following are selected generalizations from the research literature in sports psychology concerning participant consequences as reported by Morgan.

1. Persons who participate in sports report that they "feel better."
2. Vigorous exercise does reduce the degree of anxiety in men and women suffering from anxiety neurosis.
3. Morgan quotes Rarick[37] as follows: "Based on the evidence to date, one could not with confidence conclude that competitive sports constitute an emotional danger to the young participant." It should be noted that Rarick is one of the most prominent physical education researchers in the area of growth and development of young children and has a special interest in sports and physical fitness at this age level.
4. A comprehensive review of research literature in the area of the acute effects of sports participation on young people leads to the conclusion that the evidence is equivocal.

Concerning what he calls "chronic considerations," Morgan[38] goes on to report

1. Individual young persons who elect to participate in highly organized competitive sports are likely to possess particular psychological characteristics which differ from those held by non-participants. This difference exists from a very early age.
2. Morgan summarizes considerable research as follow: "It seems reasonable to propose that (a) athletes differ psychologically from non-athletes and (b) these differences exist from the outset; that is, sport does not provoke the observed differences. In this context, it also seems likely that many young boys and girls who do not possess the necessary psychological prerequisites for intense athletic competition are probably eliminated from sport very early."
3. "Acute and chronic physical activity of a vigorous nature offers a unique and effective method for reducing tension (state anxiety) and depression. In this respect vigorous physical activity can be

PSYCHOLOGICAL CONSEQUENCES OF SPORT PARTICIPATION

CHAPTER SIX

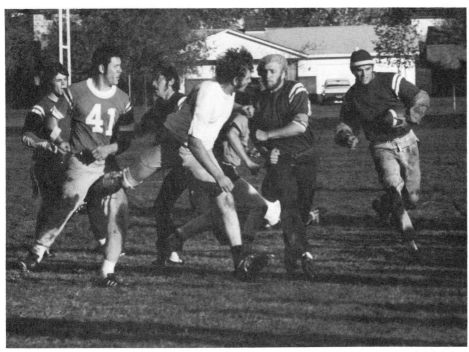

Physical activity of a vigorous nature offers a unique and effective method for reducing tension.

regarded as one practical and parsimonious 'coping strategy' in man's creative adaptation to the stress characteristics of our time." Involvement in sport does not appear to provoke consequences (good or bad) which do not occur with physical activity *per se.*

Over the years, psychologists have established that every human being has a strong need for interaction with others having similar interests, aspirations, attitudes, and ideals. This need is known as *affiliation,* and it constitutes one of the major psychological foundations of sport. Of affiliation in sport, Alderman[39] writes:

AFFILIATION

> The love and affection people have for each other, and the feelings of belonging to an important group, tend to be emphasized when the group faces a common external threat. Nowhere can this be seen as well as in the strong camaraderie and friendship developed in competitive sports teams. When one trains, practices, sacrifices, and dedicates oneself, day in and day out, alongside close friends who are doing the same thing, a strong bond is forged. This becomes a significant motivational drive in the behavior and performance of these people. In order to gain insight into athletic behavior, then, it is obviously necessary to take into account the strong affiliative tendency operating in sport and physical activity.

Many sport participants at all age levels would empirically concur with the above contention. The entire social context is surely one of the most powerful motivations attracting millions of Americans to participate in and to "spectate" at innumerable sport activities.

The central nervous system (CNS) is composed of a spinal cord, the brain, and the brain stem which are located in the skull and the vertebrae. The peripheral nervous system consists of the spinal and cranial nerves.

SUMMARY

Kinesthesis refers to the perceptual experiences the individual has as a result of the transmission of information from receptors in the muscles, tendons, joints, and vestibular apparatus.

Physical educators and teachers are not only interested in motor skill performances and learning per se, they are also concerned with concomitant behaviors which can influence motor skill performances and learning either negatively or positively.

Feedback appears to have three major functions: information, motivation, and reinforcement. Nixon and Locke summarize recent research findings on feedback by noting that the motivational and corrective influences of feedback ensure that it will be the strongest and most important variable controlling motor performance.

Lawther defines *sport psychology* as an area which attempts to apply psychological facts and principles to learning, performance, and associated human behavior in the whole field of sports.

Perhaps the most agreed upon principle concerning motivational techniques is that the best motivation is the internal desire to perform as well as possible.

Research into the psychological effects of sport participation and viewing has for the most part proved inconclusive. There is, however, much evidence substantiating *affiliation*, the human need for interaction with others in striving for a common goal, as in sports competition.

FOOTNOTES

[1]George H. Sage, *Introduction to Motor Behavior: A Neuropsychological Approach* (2nd ed.) Reading, MA: Addison-Wesley Publishing Co., 1977, p. 88.

[2]Ibid, p. 229.

[3]David L. Gallahue, *Motor Development and Movement Experiences for Young Children.* New York: John Wiley & Sons, Inc., 1976, pp. 10, 11.

[4]George H. Sage, op. cit. p., 296.

[5]Harry Munsinger, *Fundamentals of Child Development* (2nd ed.). New York: Holt, Rinehart and Winston, 1975, p. 103.

[6]William C. Sheppard and Robert H. Willoughby, *Child Behavior — Learning and Development.* Chicago: Rand McNally College Publishing Co., 1975, p. 492.

[7]Paul H. Mussen, John J. Conger, and Jerome Kagan, *Child Development and Personality* (4th ed.). New York: Harper & Row, Publishers, 1974, p. 314.

[8]Arthur H. Steinhaus, "Your Muscles See More Than Your Eyes," JOHPERD, 37:38–40, (September 1966), p. 39.

[9]George H. Sage, op. cit., p. 1.

[10]John N. Drowatzky, *Motor Learning–Principles and Practices.* Minneapolis, MN: Burgess Publishing Company, 1975, p. 2.

[11]Bryant J. Cratty, *Movement Behavior and Motor Learning* (3rd ed.). Philadelphia: Lea & Febiger, 1973, pp. 10, 11.

[12]George H. Sage, op. cit., p. 336.

[13]Ibid., p. 337.

[14]E. C. Poulton, "On Prediction in Skilled Movement," *Psychological Bulletin,* 54:467–478, 1974.

[15]George H. Sage, op cit., pp. 338, 339.

[16]Ibid., pp. 400, 401.

[17]Ibid., p. 414; John N. Drowatzky, op. cit., pp. 88, 89. Robert N. Singer, *Motor Learning and Human Performance* (2nd ed.). New York: Macmillan Company, 1975, p. 430.

[18]John E. Nixon and Lawrence F. Locke, "Research on Teaching Physical Education," in Robert M. W. Travers (Editor), *Second Handbook of Research on Teaching,* AERA. Chicago: Rand McNally & Company, 1973, p. 1222.

[19]Robert N. Singer, op. cit., pp. 465, 471.

[20]Ibid., p. 445.

[21]John E. Nixon and Lawrence F. Locke, op. cit., p. 1222.

[22]George H. Sage. op cit., p. 454.

[23]John N. Drowatzky, op. cit., pp. 215, 216.

[24]John E. Nixon and Lawrence F. Locke, op. cit., p. 1213.

[25]Ibid., pp. 1227, 1228.

[26]John D. Lawther, *Sport Psychology.* Englewood Cliffs, N. J.: Prentice-Hall, Inc., 1972, p. 7.

[27]John W. Loy, "A Brief History of the North American Society for the Psychology of Sport and

Physical Activity." Proceedings of the North American Society for the Psychology of Sport and Physical Activity, 1973, pp. 2–10.

[28]Bryant J. Cratty, *Psychology and Contemporary Sport: Guidelines for Coaches and Athletes.* Englewood Cliffs, N.J.: Prentice-Hall, Inc., 1973.

[29]William P. Morgan (Editor), *Contemporary Readings in Sport Psychology.* Springfield, Ill: Charles C Thomas, Publisher, 1970, p. xi.

[30]Thomas Tutko and Umberto Tosi, *Sport Psyching – Playing your Best Game All of the Time.* Los Angeles: J. P. Tarcher, Inc., 1976, p. 1.

[31]George H. Sage, op. cit., pp. 528–530.

[32]Ibid., p. 530.

[33]Robert N. Singer, op. cit., p. 95.

[34]Ibid., pp. 97, 98.

[35]R. B. Alderman, *Psychological Behavior in Sport.* Philadelphia: W. B. Saunders Co., 1974, p. 151.

[36]William P. Morgan (Editor), op cit., p. 16.

[37]G. Lawrence Rarick, "Competitive Sports in Childhood and Early Adolescence," in G. Lawrence Rarick (Editor), *Physical Activity: Human Growth and Development.* New York: Academic Press, 1973, p. 375.

[38]William P. Morgan (Editor), op. cit., pp. 23–25, 27.

[39]R. B. Alderman op. cit., p. 259.

SELECTED REFERENCES

Christina, Robert W., and Landers, Daniel M. (Eds.), *Psychology of Motor Behavior and Sport – 1976, Vol. I.* "Motor Behavior" — Proceedings of the North American Society for the Psychology of Sport and Physical Activity Annual Conference, May 1976. Champaign, IL: Human Kinetics Publishers, 1977.

Christina, Robert W., and Landers, Daniel M. (Eds.), *Psychology of Motor Behavior and Sport — 1976, Vol. II.* "Sport Psychology and Motor Development" — Proceedings of the North American Society for the Psychology of Sport and Physical Activity Annual Conference, May 1976. Champaign, IL: Human Kinetics Publishers, 1977.

Cronbach, Lee J., *Educational Psychology* (3rd Ed.). New York: Harcourt, Brace, Jovanovich, 1977.

Dacy, John W., *New Ways to Learn: The Psychology of Education.* Stamford, CT: Greylock Publishers, 1976.

Evans, Ellis D. (Ed.), *Contemporary Influences in Early Childhood Education* (2nd Ed.). New York: Holt, Rinehart and Winston, 1975.

Fisher, Craig (Ed.), *Psychology of Sport — Issues and Insights.* Palo Alto, CA: Mayfield Publishing Company, 1976.

Gentile, A. M., "A Working Model of Skill Acquisition with Application to Teaching," *Quest,* Monograph XVIII:3–23 (January 1972).

Harper, William A., Miller, Donna Mae, Park, Roberta J., and Davis, Elwood C., *The Philosophic Process in Physical Education* (3rd Ed.). Philadelphia: Lea & Febiger, 1977.

Hilgard, Ernest R., Atkinson, Richard C., & Atkinson, Rita L., *Introduction to Psychology* (6th Ed.). New York: Harcourt, Brace, Jovanovich, 1975.

Hulse, Stewart H., Deese, James, and Egeth, H., *The Psychology of Learning* (4th Ed.). New York: McGraw-Hill, 1975.

Hunt, David E., and Sullivan, Edmund V., *Between Psychology and Education.* Hinsdale, IL: Dryden Press, 1974.

Klausmeier, Herbert J., Ghatala, Eliabeth S., and Frayer, Dorothy A., *Conceptual Learning and Development: A Cognitive View.* New York: Academic Press, 1974.

Lieberman, Josefa N., *Playfulness: Its Relationship to Imagination and Creativity.* New York: Academic Press, 1977.

Lindsay, Peter H., and Norman, Donald A., *Human Information Processing: An Introduction to Psychology* (2nd Ed.). New York: Academic Press, 1977.

Martens, Rainier, Burwitz, Les, and Zuckerman, Joshua, "Modeling Effects on Motor Performance," *The Research Quarterly,* 47:277–291 (May 1976).

Morgan, William P., "Psychological Consequences of Vigorous Physical Activity and Sports," *Beyond Research — Solutions to Human Problems, Academy Papers, No. 10.* Louisville, KY: American Academy of Physical Education, 1976.

Sahakian, William S., *Learning: Systems, Models, and Theories.* Chicago: Rand McNally Publishing Co., 1976.

Sheppard, William C., and Willoughby, Robert H., "Motor Behavior: The Child's Emerging Repertoire," *Child Behavior—Learning and Development.* Chicago: Rand McNally College Publishing Co., 1975.

Thoresen, Carl E. (Ed.), *Behavior Modification in Education.* Seventy-second Yearbook of the National Society for the Study of Education, Part I. Chicago: University of Chicago Press, 1973.

Travers, Robert M. W., *Essentials of Learning* (4th Ed.). New York: Macmillan, 1977.

Wade, Michael G., and Martens, Rainier (Eds.), *Psychology of Motor Behavior and Sport.* Proceedings of the North American Society for the Psychology of Sport and Physical Activity. Urbana, IL: Human Kinetics Publishers, 1974.

West, Charles K., and Foster, Stephen F., *The Psychology of Human Learning and Instruction in Education.* Belmont, CA: Wadsworth Publishing Co., Inc., 1976.

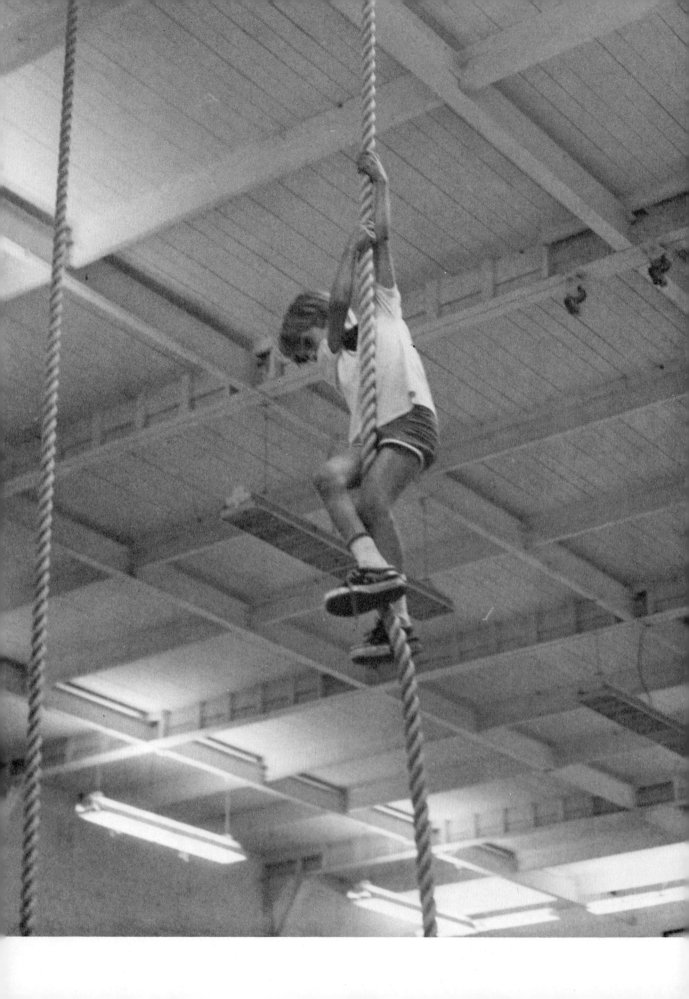

PHYSICAL EDUCATION —— ——— CURRICULA

Voluntary movement is a significant human function; it serves many roles in human life. Motor development is of crucial importance in the growth and learning of the preschool child. Physical recreation is important to elementary school children and secondary school youth in their out-of-school hours. Physical activity plays a vital role in the lives of all adults during the productive career years and into retirement living. Professional physical educators are concerned with the importance of their discipline to all of these contexts. School programs of physical education, however, must be thought of as primarily educational.

Introducton

Formal education helps the individual to develop the capacity to function successfully in the environment, to contribute to the improvement of that environment, and to realize his or her full personal, human potential. Because the time available for schooling is comparatively brief, there exists the problem of which types of contributions the school should concentrate upon. To what extent is physical education an essential element of a contemporary liberal education?

People need physical education to help them live well in today's world. We need efficient body mechanics, especially optimum body alignment for long periods of sitting or standing or specific physical work tasks. We need skills of conscious neuromuscular relaxation to renew enthusiasm and maintain productivity through long periods of stress. We need perceptual-motor training to help us produce appropriate motor responses to the variety of stimuli we are constantly bombarded with. We need direct survival skills of water safety and personal self-defense. We need satisfying physical recreation experiences to find personal joy in movement and to share fully in group living in our society.

Not only do we need physical education to live in today's world, we need a physical education to cope with tomorrow's world. Tomorrow's world will certainly require us to adapt movement patterns to conditions of weightlessness, to develop new movement skills for tasks yet undefined, and to condition ourselves for unfamiliar forms of stress. We will need men and women with the knowledges, skills, and physical training, not just to enjoy underwater sport, but to work and maintain themselves

227

for long periods of time far below the ocean surfaces. Human beings will need to learn to adjust to temperature extremes and variability. We will need many experts competent to investigate different factors of human performance.

We need physical education relevant to today's living and tomorrow's coping. But, more important, physical education is needed in this computer space age to emphasize our humanity. Humanness is retained only as one is a fully integrated person. Education that emphasizes the wholeness of the individual — as expressed through movement as an avenue of self-actualization, movement as a form of participation in wholesome group activity, movement as a means of communication among persons, movement as one aspect of our common humanity — is sorely needed in this contemporary world.

Originally, the function of the school in America was to teach children to read, write, and figure. The other phases of education were assumed to be taken care of through the media of the home, church, and community life. But as the social order became increasingly complex, and as the pattern of home and community life underwent many changes, the school assumed wider responsibilities.

During the past 20 to 30 years, the school has come more and more to be regarded as a place where students gain experience in better living and learn to become more effective citizens in a democratic country. These objectives developed as the public school's responsibilities grew to include more than the traditional task of teaching of the "three R's." Recently, in celebration of the nation's bicentennial and rededication to its traditional values, there has been an important ongoing reevaluation of the purposes and function of public schools in America. Many individuals and groups advocate a return to the "fundamentals," a deemphasis on social adjustment and citizenship as major aims of the schools, and a primary emphasis on learning the basic concepts and modes of inquiry of the academic disciplines.

There is a real danger that current curricular emphases and the rapid, widespread use of instructional technology will lead to the "dehumanization" of the individual. This potential danger has been recognized and discussed publicly and in professional literature by perceptive scholars of curriculum and by authorities in the fields of mental health, sociology, and social psychology. Phenix, Maslow, Benne, Pilder,[1] and others urge a redress in the balance of curriculum directions, and they predict that we will see a return to a "humanized" curriculum in the years ahead.

Physical Education and Personalized Learning. The education essential to each person includes learning how human movement functions in personal experience and in the achievement of common human goals. Physical education has long been viewed as the series of school programs concerned with the development and utilization of the individual's movement potential. Currently, physical educators, attempting to realize the full potential of this area of human experience, are seeking to extend concepts of physical education to the needs of learners of all ages in both school and non-institutional contexts. Physical education is increasingly viewed as personalized, self-directed learning, using selected movement learning media to achieve individual human goals. Physical education provides instruction and selected experiences in human movements that help the individual to learn more about his or her self as a fully integrated

CHANGING CONCEPTS OF SCHOOLING

person and to increase the meaning and significance of life within the surrounding social milieu.

As it is increasingly recognized that education is a continuing life activity, more professional educators are referring to institutionalized aspects of education as *schooling*, thus distinguishing the organized, relatively formal phases of education that are the primary responsibility of teachers from the limitless range of experiences that may properly be considered education. The focus of this chapter is upon schooling as contrasted with education and upon the place of school programs of physical education in total school programs.

SOCIAL RESPONSIBILITY

Although many educators plead for narrowing the scope of school responsibility and many legislators and taxpayers seek limited and specific definitions of school accountability, it is a fact that the American general public, launching into the third century of the nation's existence, insists upon school involvement in broad social programs and curricular attention to the more critical social problems of our times. People are demanding that school personnel find ways of assisting with the resolution of urban ills, ecological crises, and the continuing problems of those children and youth disadvantaged by our social system and its institutions.

Changing Conditions and New Demands

Changes in Lifestyle. Under the changing conditions of the present and the predictable future, we tend toward a vastly different type of life from that of the past. While it is true that our advancement in civilization has brought a multitude of advantages to the human race, it has also produced many conditions of living that are fundamentally detrimental.

The Urban-Suburban Situation. A large percentage of the people are crowded together in cities or in suburbs of tract and row houses which afford them little incentive or opportunity to lead the type of life that is normal for human beings. In the cities, lack of open space inhibits the normal, free play life of children and adults alike. One of the greatest dangers in fast-developing suburban areas is that cities, school districts, recreation districts, and counties will fail to acquire sufficient outdoor space for educational and recreational use while such areas are available, prior to becoming subdivisions or business zones.

Reduction in Physical Activity. Everywhere, mechanical means of transportation tend to make walking a lost art. Housework, chores, and errands rarely involve any considerable amount of vigorous activity. The motion picture, radio, stereo, and television offer sedentary forms of entertainment and recreation, providing vicarious emotional experiences as substitutes for the active enjoyment and genuine emotional experiences of the more natural pursuits of hunting, fishing, play, games, and the like. Machines have replaced thousands of workers who previously performed routine tasks with human muscle power. The development of automation in industry has reduced the amount of physical energy supplied by human beings.

The Modern Labor Paradox: More Leisure, More Stress. In industry, the trend toward a shorter work week, longer periods of paid vacation time, earlier retirement, larger retirement benefits, and similar changing conditions is providing millions of Americans with previously unheard-of amounts of leisure time. Still, many persons, particularly those in executive and leadership positions, are working long, strenuous hours under pressure and strain. Leaders in the professions and in business may work seventy or more hours per week, and at a fast pace. Others, who work a forty-hour week or less, seek a second job. Such individuals actually may work 60 to 80 hours per week at two jobs. In many cases, this extended strenuous effort results in deleterious physical and mental fatigue.

Changing Family Lifestyles. The labor market is changing rapidly and drastically. More women are working; more of them are becoming long-term members of the work force. The professions and other occupations are no longer limited to single career women and women working to support dependents in single-parent households; the number of two-income families is growing rapidly. Particularly in middle-class families, Americans are choosing family lifestyles which depend upon two incomes; full-time work outside the home for both husband and wife throughout the productive work years is built into long-range planning.

Unemployment and Job Insecurity. Problems in the area of career entry by high school graduates remain serious; and the frustrations caused by lack of career progression and need for re-education for mid-career adults, particularly women, demand solution. The complexity of our present-day social and economic order and the lack of predictability of particular job status and opportunity develop much insecurity and undesirable emotional tension, for which there are insufficient acceptable outlets.

An inflationary economy has created serious unemployment problems, greater numbers of persons living at poverty levels, higher crime rates with disturbing increases in violent crimes, and particularly heavy financial pressures on middle-class families and retired persons. All of this has bred a climate of retrenchment, conservatism, and tax revolt. The strains in the national economy have made it increasingly difficult to implement needed social programs in equal employment opportunity, affirmative action, national health care, welfare assistance, and services to the disadvantaged.

Disadvantages of a Mobile Society. A large portion of the American public is on the move. Individuals and family units move to new areas for various reasons. Many of them make multiple moves over a period of several years, creating for schools the problem of maintaining a program of continuity for the child who transfers from one school to another, in different cities and frequently in different states. This easy mobility in turn tends to foster less stable friendships and neighborhood life. Deprived of a stable "home base," many people become lonely and depressed. Dehumanization has been identified as a more and more common social problem by sociologists who have studied these present-day patterns of working and living conditions.

Spending Cut-backs: A Challenge for Educators

The United States has entered its third century as a republic, with a spirit of confidence in its heritage and optimism for its future. At the same time, the American public is asking for less spending at all governmental levels, while maintaining the expectation that the public schools will continue to play a key role in the resolution of our most significant social problems and in enhancing the quality of individual living and of our common life.

This climate poses an almost impossible challenge for educators, school and university authorities, and boards of education. Federal legislation demands certain reforms in the schools. Girls and women are to

CHAPTER SEVEN

receive equal opportunities and equal benefits; but additional funding is not available even to make up the inflationary deficits in presently operating boys' and men's programs. Minority children and youth need supplementary educational assistance and high-cost individualized special studies programs at a time when it is exceedingly difficult to generate additional revenue. The handicapped are to be mainstreamed and provided genuinely equal educational opportunity; yet this goal can be accomplished only through extensive remodeling of educational facilities and significant added expenditures for specialized personnel and technical services. New outlays of public funds are needed to introduce and expand educational programs to counter important social problems such as smoking, alcohol and drug abuse, teenage pregnancy, care of the aged, and death education. Neither educational nor political leaders have yet found answers to these real and continuing problems. It is especially difficult to project solutions in the face of organized demands for tax relief such as the successful 1978 campaign to support California's Proposition 13.

Competency-based education is controversial, yet increasingly accepted, as we approach the 1980s. Public concern for low academic achievement has led to strong demands for educational accountability. Phrases and terms frequently seen and heard in both professional journals and the popular media include functional literacy, "back to basics," "right to read," behavioral objectives, performance goals, competency-based learning, minimum standards, exit examinations, competency-based teacher education, and accountability.

MINIMUM COMPETENCY STANDARDS

Accountability. The term *accountability* first appeared in the *Education Index* in June, 1970. The entry reflects changing concepts of the responsibility of the school to its constituents and the accountability of school agents to external authorities. Proponents of behavioral accountability are urging that the effectiveness of schools be judged by results achieved, measured in terms of student accomplishments. In many instances, not only effectiveness, but also efficiency, in the form of relating dollars spent to student accomplishment, is required. A program of behavioral accountability provides for a systematic attempt to specify objectives in measurable terms, the control of educational outputs to coincide with these objectives, and an external program evaluation of the extent of achievement of objectives.[2] The techniques used include program evaluation and review technique (PERT), program planning and budgeting system (PPBS), management by objectives (MBO), and management information systems (MIS).

The notion that high school graduates should be expected to demonstrate by actual performance that they have acquired knowledges and skills that can be used in real life situations appeals to parents and the general public as eminently reasonable. The competency movement is a response to the demand for social accountability. Public opinion has supported the idea that education could become more effective and more efficient by modeling itself after business and industry; competency-based education appears to be highly compatible with the computer technology and systems approaches which have facilitated giant steps in the development of the American industrial complex.

Competency Legislation. Between 1975 and 1978, 33 states passed mandates requiring minimum competency standards for elementary and secondary students; all other states now have legislation pending or studies under way.[3] Competency testing for teachers is also growing. Mandates for performance-based pre-service training programs have been legislated in seventeen states; Georgia and Florida now require competency testing for recertification. Sandefur and Westbrook[4] conducted a survey of 816 American Association of Colleges for Teacher Education (AACTE) institutions during the summer of 1977. Fifty-eight per cent of the 686 institutions responding were involved in CBTE (Competency-Based Teacher Education) programs. Programs had not declined since a similar survey in 1975; in many instances they had been expanded.

The adoption of a policy on minimum competency testing requires answering certain difficult questions, seven of which are identified by Brickell[5] as follows:

The Issues Involved in Competency Standards

What competencies?
How to measure?
When to measure?
One minimum or many?
How high the minimum?
Minimums for students or for schools?
What to do with the incompetent?

Many other issues are involved in this controversial movement. It is being led by noneducators who may lack insight into special problems created by certain programs. Many educators have criticized the lack of a sound theoretical base for this approach and have pointed to the lack of evidence that educational outcomes will improve in any significant way. Many programs have been authorized by mandates with little or no financial support although the costs of test development and security are certain to be heavy and results unsatisfactory if expensive remediation activities do not follow. Many programs are based on the unwarranted assumption that the school skills tested will transfer automatically to on-the-job or life skills. Numerous groups and individuals have expressed concern that the minimum competency movement violates the traditionally-valued principle of a locally controlled American education system.

Wise[6] offers helpful insight into the contradictions and controversy created by the competency standards movement:

> It is ironic that at the very moment when state and federal legislators are seeking rationalistic approaches to school management, many educational researchers are intensifying their criticism of the feasibility of such approaches. . . .
> The two major problems of American schools are inequality in education and low academic achievement. Generally, problems associated with equality in education . . . are political problems. . . . The proper distribution of opportunities and resources is a goal that can be promoted through legislation and litigation. . . .
> Policy designed to solve the problem of low academic achievement is different from policy designed to solve the problem of unequal educational opportunity. The solution to the problem of low achievement is more technical than political. . . . Serious research on the problems of poor learning and poor teaching is required. . . . Reason and evidence provide little, if any, justification for the belief that minimum competency testing will help poor students to learn or poor teachers to teach.

While performance-based education and competency-based teacher education may indeed have genuine potential for upgrading public education, it is apparent that much research is needed and that programs of minimum competency testing should be adopted only after careful study, with caution and commitment to responsible review.

Looking Ahead. It is anticipated that the current pressures on schools for behavioral accountability will continue in the 1980s. Responsible educators accept the desirability of shifting the focus from teaching to learning. The real challenge of the next decade, however, is to find a balance between protection of the public interest and the maintenance of an educational environment conducive to creative teaching and the continuous growth and development of learners as self-actualizing individuals.

Another special challenge that physical educators will face is demonstrating to educational policy-makers and the general public that physical education is one of the basic essentials in school programs. Knowledges, skills, and attitudes relating to movement education, lifelong fitness, and motor performance are basic curriculum content that must be maintained through periods of economic stress and educational reform efforts. Any acceptable series of minimum competencies will include essential physical education learning outcomes; standardized criterion-referenced tests for high school graduation must certainly require the demonstration of a satisfactory level of performance in selected physical education activities.

HUMANISTIC EDUCATION

Most educational philosophers, authors, journalists, and critics endorse greater humanism in education. While thinking persons are challenging the schools to take increased responsibility for the resolution of major practical social problems, they are concurrently urging a clearer, more sensitive focus on the individual. While taxpayers, boards of education, legislators, and social critics are seeking greater accountability in competency-based education, they are also demanding humanistic schools that "work to free people so that they may make wise choices, utilize and choose from the options that are open to them, and become all that they potentially might become."[7]

Differing Perspectives

Humanistic education has been described and defined in many ways. Orlosky and Smith[8] have provided a useful analysis of present views, classifying three forms of humanism that are influencing current thinking about the curriculum. *Psychosocial humanism* emphasizes the self as an achievement rather than a given, that is, the realization of self as a supreme condition of well-being. *Classical* or *traditional humanism* is usually expressed as a study of the humanities in contrast to vocational studies. *Scientific humanism* asserts that the well-being of humankind is served by extending our knowledge and using it to improve social, moral, and material life.

Bridges[9] summarizes the three predominant perspectives in humanistic education as follows:

> *Classroom milieu.* Here the emphasis falls on giving the learner the freedom to learn what he needs to know, and to do that in his own way. This concern leads to a focus on "unstructured" situations: open classrooms, flexible time schedules, free choice of subject. The teacher's role in this learning pattern is that of a facilitator or resource person. . . .

Humanistic education emphasizes freedom to learn.

The learner as a person. Here the main concern is for ways in which the traditional cognitive approach to learning . . . can be reintegrated with the other ways in which a person apprehends his situation. These ways include his feelings about what he learns, his intuitive reactions to it, the ways in which it fits into his purposes in life. . . . Here we find terms like "affective," or "psychological" or "confluent" education. . . .

The subject matter. As the needs of the total person are taken into account, it becomes clear that the traditional subject matters are simply bodies of information with varying degrees of significance for the person's situation. . . .

Recognizing that humanistic education has been "more honored than practiced," the Association for Supervision and Curriculum Development has published a timely monograph summarizing humanistic goals and objectives and offering guidelines for their assessment. This report of the ASCD Working Group on Humanistic Education suggests the following definition of humanistic education and a series of seven major goals through which it may be more explicitly approached:[10]

Putting Humanism into Practice

Humanistic Education is a commitment to education and practice in which all facets of the teaching-learning process give major emphasis to the freedom, value, worth, dignity, and integrity of persons.

Humanistic Education:
1. Accepts the learner's needs and purposes and develops experiences and programs around the unique potentials of the learner.
2. Facilitates self-actualization and strives to develop in all persons a sense of personal adequacy.
3. Fosters acquisition of basic skills necessary for living in a multicultured society, including academic, personal, interpersonal, communicative, and economic proficiency.

CHAPTER SEVEN

4. Personalizes education decisions and practices. To this end it includes students in the processes of their own education via democratic involvement in all levels of implementation.

5. Recognizes the primacy of human feelings and utilizes personal values and perceptions as integral factors in educational processes.

6. Develops a learning climate which nurtures growth through learning environments perceived by all involved as challenging, understanding, supportive, exciting, and free from threat.

7. Develops in learners genuine concern and respect for the worth of others and skill in conflict resolution.

A task force of the ASCD Working Group on Humanistic Education devised a checklist[11] of 100 rank-ordered items for assessing the humanistic orientation of a local school or classroom. Items relating to such areas as teacher-student interactions, student activities, student-student interactions, materials and facilities, and other persons in school can be used to determine the degree to which the goals quoted above are being implemented by school systems, schools, teachers, and students.

The Foshay Grid.   Foshay proposes an approach to curriculum design and evaluation that systematically categorizes the operational goals of teaching according to psychological categories of development. He identifies the four elements of the operational goals of teaching as fluency, manipulation, confidence/value, and persistence, and points out that these are important teaching concerns that are independent of the particular subject matter. On the basis of research in developmental psychology, the six elements of the human condition are stated as intellectual, emotional, social, aesthetic, spiritual, and physical. Foshay arranges these elements on a grid and focuses on the intersections of the two dimensions — What does it mean to be human? What does it mean to teach? — to raise questions which lead to the development of a curriculum for the humane school that we are seeking. Twenty-four cells constitute the grid; consequently twenty-four questions must be confronted by educators. Foshay concludes:[12]

> The great preponderance of our current curriculum design and evaluation efforts deal with only two of the cells. . . . We have projected a monstrous version of the human condition by our failure to examine seriously twenty-two out of the twenty-four elements that belong in comprehensive curriculum design and evaluation. . . .

In summary, we support the need for more emphasis on humanistic education. We believe that humanistic education strives toward individual self-actualization and transcendence and that the desired goal for every learner is to become all that he or she is capable of becoming. Humanistic education is concerned with two modes of knowledge. It seeks what Bronowski[13] describes as "the single identity of man" through scientific knowledge and self-knowledge. Scientific knowledge uses empirical tests to provide us with a thinking language. The self-knowledge that underlies the arts provides "a second language in which a man converses with himself." Scientific knowledge is single-valued, while the knowledge of the arts is many-valued. The two modes of knowledge complement each other to create an ethic that unites respect for what is done with respect for what we are.

Humanistic education seeks individual identity through the development of those qualities and abilities which are characteristically human. Humanistic education focuses on the interests and ideals of people in contrast to technological efficiency or the maintenance of a social status system. Humanistic education places the integrity of persons above the structure of knowledge or the quality control of material objects. Humanistic education helps each learner to find personal meaning in the confluence of cognitive, affective, and motor experience.

Changing Questions about the Future. Another force which modifies our concepts of schooling is the development of the field of futures research. Futuristics is becoming an increasingly respected professional specialization. Educators traditionally have not taken futures research very seriously; but the field of futures research is changing and moving in new directions, and educational planners now recognize its potential significance in curriculum development. Futurists first became visible in a period of economic growth as a group of forecasters who were responding to questions posed primarily by business and industry relating to markets, sales, and larger production outputs. The questions of the past were mainly *know-how*; today the questions are more often *know-why* and they are attracting the concern of the general public as well as government, industry, and organizations.[14] For example, we can no longer be satisfied with forecasting ways of producing and consuming energy and enlarging the economy; we must ask whether we should consume energy at the present rate and, if not, what rate of energy consumption should be planned. Futures research is now addressing itself to the formulation of the right questions.

Futures research and planning has become vital to our very survival. The World Future Society celebrated its tenth anniversary in 1976 with over 20,000 members. It publishes two society periodicals and a dozen section newsletters, and provides excellent book and conference services. Its Special Studies Division has sections in business, communications, education, food, government, habitats, health, human values, international affairs, lifestyles, population, energy and natural resources, technology, and work and careers. A growing number of distinguished scholars have committed themselves to this area of study and the body of literature in the field is substantial. All of these factors have gained futuristics acknowledgment in the intellectual community and have made futures research important in the thinking of educational planners.

Two Outlooks. Two major perspectives of the future characterize current theorizing. Most persons agree that we are living in a period of social transition. And both the prophets of hope and the prophets of doom have their followings. From one perspective the future is viewed with despair. Impending world disaster is predicted through atomic holocaust, overproduction of energy, biochemical destruction, environmental pollution, overpopulation, or some combination of these potential crises. On the other hand, those who view the future with optimism believe it will be better than the past. They look toward a world with adequate sources of energy, food, and mineral resources, and the technical ability to meet the needs of the world's next generation. They insist that the real problems are political and institutional, not scarce resources. The curriculum planner with a futuristic orientation calls upon the futures researcher to pose appropriate questions and to provide information which can help us to structure desirable modifications in both school organization and curriculum for future decades.

What should be the response of the school to currently available knowledge about the future? Fifty years ago Harold Rugg had a profound influence on educational thought with his view that the social sciences curriculum should be based on what the "frontier thinkers" believe the persistent problems and issues of the future will be. Recently, Harold Shane summarized the conclusions of a panel of 50 distinguished world citizens and educators, supplemented by a panel of 96 high school students, in "America's Educational Futures 1976–2001" as follows:[15]

> Emergent educational development, 1976–2001, presumably would help young learners acquire a knowledge of the realities of the present, an awareness of alternative solutions, an understanding of consequences that might accompany these options, development of insights as to wise choices, and help U. S. youth to develop the skills and to acquire the information that are prerequisite to the implementation of examined ideas, policies, and programs. In short, five terms to remember in developing new curricula are: realities, alternatives, consequences, choices, and implementation!

Shane[16] has discussed his own recommendations for educational response to the futurists in a direct and challenging style. *The Educational Significance of the Future* is recommended to the reader. Shane proposes a "seamless curriculum" in which the child's first direct contacts with the educational community would begin somewhere near the second birthday and advancement would proceed without interruption through overlapping segments of the school continuum through secondary education. A "paracurriculum" of out-of-school experiences would be provided, for some as early as age 13, throughout retirement years, guaranteeing lifelong exit and reentry privileges. Credentialing university programs would continue; in addition, a communiversity program would greatly expand continuing postsecondary education. Staff deployment would emphasize flexible teaching partnerships.

In anticipating new content and curricular emphases based on futuristics data, Shane identifies the following: clarification of new values, reversal of our culture's misplaced confidence in materialism, the dangers and problems of the naive use of technology, adequate response to the threat of damage to the biosphere, sensitivity to the dangers in unrestricted breeding, assistance for learners in coping with the potential power of mass media in shaping opinions and attitudes, and recognition of the need to view democracy as a social order which emphasizes greater equity but which also emphasizes that success is not necessarily defined by rising above one's father's status in life. Shane cites some of the controversial changes which the future may demand in curriculum content and instruction:

1. Presenting the concept of the "true-costing" of consumer goods. We do not repay the biosphere at present for what our consumer goods really cost. . . .
2. Interpreting to youth the growing need to reverse our "growth-is-good" doxology in favor of the need for "dynamic contraction. . . ."
3. Excellence versus growth. . . .
4. Developing a sense of fulfillment based on satisfaction rather than possession. . . .
5. Yet another challenge is to create, at least in part through schooling, a recycling society. . . .
6. We need to help the young to understand the potential richness of a service-oriented society. . . .
7. Refining the merits of simple communal living today to match the virtues of pioneer life in a younger America. . . .

8. Make more effective use of educational TV, packages, and school-and-home learning techniques. . . .

9. Recognizing that a measure of mutual coercion will be necessary for the general welfare if we are to bring off and to enforce the social and educational changes that the future demands. . . .

We must recognize that the future is not determined by the forecasts of the futurists, nor can the course of our destiny be shaped entirely by our minds. But this does not mean that people have no control over the directions in which they move into the future. Within our social milieu, and with a recognition of trends which futuristics can help us to know and understand, we do have choices to make. As individuals, and as a profession of educators, it would be foolish to fail to give serious attention to the recommendations of the futurists.

Many models have been developed by those seeking to improve the processes of schooling or to increase its effectiveness. Proposed models run the gamut from traditional grade-placement models, through cybernetic-systems models, to futuristic models and "alternative schools." Joyce has popularized the notion of a variety of educational models appropriate to a spectrum of educational missions. He proposes a pluralistic world of education composed of programs designed in accordance with differing models to further a large number of educational missions.[17]

MODELS FOR SCHOOL PROGRAMS

Conceptual Models. Many curriculum models of the 1960s and 70s have been designated *conceptual models* and have emphasized analyses of the bodies of knowledge of the various disciplines. Key concepts have been identified in mathematics, biology, physics, chemistry, social studies, health education, and in physical education; instructional units are then organized in terms of selected key concepts and subconcepts. Schools place great stress on acquiring knowledge of those concepts as the most efficient means for the human central nervous system to receive, collect, classify, store, retrieve, and utilize essential elements from a vast reservoir of rapidly increasing and changing human knowledge.

The Systems Analysis Approach. Systems analysis is currently being applied in educational management by many who believe that this technique can help to create outcomes which dedicated professionals have sought for years. Kaufman[18] defines the system approach as

a process by which needs are identified, problems selected, requirements for problem solution are identified, solutions are chosen from alternatives, methods and means are obtained and implemented, results are evaluated, and required revisions to all or part of the system are made so that the needs are eliminated.

System planning requires description of predictable learner-oriented results, clarification of inputs as well as outputs, and the use of such tools as mission analysis, function analysis, task analysis, and methods-means analysis. Those who support a system approach to schooling argue that precision and planning can be our best assurance that learners are not forced into arbitrary molds through ignorance or lack of adequate instructional tools. Whether or not a system approach is humanizing depends upon the people using it and whether they use its tools appropriately for making education individually responsive.

Models for Greater Relevancy. The youth rebellion of the 1960s forced education decision-makers to realize that schooling had in fact been largely irrelevant for many and had "miserably failed the individual student in his search for self-fulfillment."[19] More relevant programs are being developed through interdisciplinary approaches that attack key human problems through creative curriculum designs and innovative instructional arrangements; such programs are being introduced in many schools. Programs in early childhood education, parent and family life education, human sexuality, family economics, consumer education, race relations, drug abuse, and death education are examples. School programs in ecology and the control of pollution have reoriented many established offerings in the sciences and suggested new models for laboratory experience and outdoor education. Emerging concepts in continuing and adult education have provided new models for off-campus learning and school-community cooperation and stimulated educational change in equivalency certificates, creative leisure activities, apprentice training, public affairs education, "women's world," "schools without walls," and "education about education."

Career Education. The Federal government mounted a major effort in the 1970s to strengthen programs of career education in the nation's schools.[20] The fundamental concept of career education is that all educational experiences, curriculum, instruction, and counseling should be geared to preparation for economic independence and an appreciation for the dignity of work. It is designed to increase the relevance of school by focusing on the learner's career choice.

> The main thrust of career education is to prepare all students for a successful life of work by increasing their options for occupational choice, by eliminating barriers — real and imagined — to attaining job skills, and by enhancing learning achievement in all subject areas and at all levels of education.

Under the career education concept, the elementary school child explores the world of work through a wide spectrum of occupational "clusters"; in the middle grades the student explores those in which he or she is most interested. During the secondary school years, all students develop elementary job entry skills and have opportunities to enjoy actual work through cooperative arrangements with business, industry, and public institutions.

Remodeling for Title IX and Public Law 94-142

Many school programs are currently undergoing remodeling to conform to federal legislation relating to equality of opportunity for girls and women and for the handicapped. Title IX of the Education Amendments of 1972 requires that all instructional opportunities and participation in school-sponsored activities be equally available to students of both sexes. The impact of the HEW guidelines for implementing Title IX is noted in more balanced enrollments in courses traditionally encouraged for one sex only, mergers of physical education programs for male and female students, and major changes in the organization of activity programs, particularly efforts to expand opportunities for girls and women in organized sports and athletics. Such changes have necessarily led to numerous adjustments in school staffing arrangements and to many modifications in specific curricular content.

Public Law 94-142, directed toward protecting the rights of the handicapped, requires schools to ensure that the handicapped have access to all educational facilities and such technical and professional assistance as may be needed to provide full educational opportunity. In practical terms,

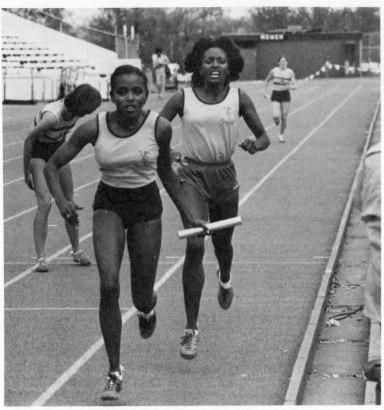

Title IX requires that all instructional opportunities and participation in school-sponsored activities be open to students of both sexes.

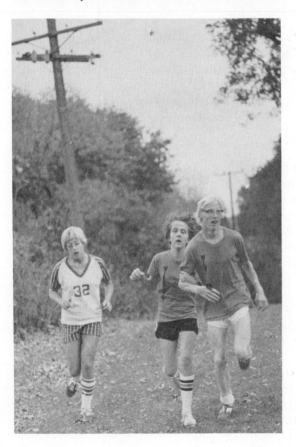

Previously served by special schools, the handicapped are now being "mainstreamed" into regular classes.

this legislation leads to a variety of models for "mainstreaming" for those students whose educational needs previously were served through special classes or special purpose schools or, in too many cases, were not equitably served.

Alternatives is a key word in contemporary writings about education. Some of the current models for alternative curricula and programs within today's schools have been identified in the preceding paragraphs. Other proposals and models have been offered as alternative schools. The concept of the private school that provides an option for the individual child or family not satisfied with the manner in which the public school meets individual needs is not new. But the interest in attending and supporting alternative schools has greatly increased recently in the context of concern for individual freedom and the preservation of cultural pluralism; of criticism of state and federal regulation of schools and of inflexible certification and curriculum requirements; and of disenchantment with local schools and the frustratingly slow pace of educational change. Today, some alternative schools are publicly supported within the system, offering these wider options to individual learners without the financial resources to attend private institutions. On the higher education level, the free university, the external degree, and new alternative programs through state university extension divisions are expressions of the alternative school concept.

Alternative Education

Curriculum modifications have characterized American schools since their beginnings. Actual study of the process of curriculum improvement is a relatively modern feature, however. Curriculum change is social change. Planned curriculum change is typically viewed as a problem-solving process directed toward changes in people, changes in the structure of the school as a social institution, and changes in human relationships within local groups.

CURRICULUM CHANGE

The question of procedures for curriculum change began to receive formal attention from social scientists about 1960.[21] In the 1960s and early 1970s many analyses for examining roles in educational innovation and strategies for effecting curriculum change were proposed, tried, and reported. These efforts do not appear to have had the results desired by the would-be innovators. Curriculum change is an exceedingly complex phenomenon and it is difficult to identify with confidence why this has been the case. Probably too much attention was given to the improvement of managerial practice in the educational enterprise at the expense of focus on better understanding of the interactive teaching-learning process. It is likely that too many of the models for innovation underemphasized the need for curriculum improvement to begin with the concerns of teachers. Possibly the major reason for limited success in introducing workable procedures for curricular change is that professional educators no longer have sufficient power to make and implement decisions basic to significant curriculum change.

Although the teacher plays a key role in curriculum change, teachers and administrators, and even school boards, actually have less direct control and unfettered power to make their own curriculum decisions than at any previous time. For over 25 years it has been considered desirable for students, parents, and citizens' advisory committees to offer recommendations; today these groups are playing an even more decisive role. Every teacher should recognize and learn to deal with these sources of pressure for curriculum change. It is an inescapable fact of life today that public school curricula are under continuous political influence not only at the local school board and city levels but also through county, state, and federal levels of government.

Doll[22] has identified four forces affecting curriculum change that have become especially prominent. Although he includes among these four "the needs and concerns of people in schools, within surrounding social and cultural milieus," and recognizes that this is the most satisfying and meaningful force with which educators deal, it is clearly acknowledged that the other three forces are strong. The drive for power, the appeal of the dollar, and growth in knowledge, with corresponding efforts at evaluating acquisition of knowledge, are also significant variables affecting the success of attempted curricular reforms.

In many instances power has shifted to groups other than teachers, administrators, and school board members. Doll identified

> scholars in the subject fields, conductors of summer inservice institutes, people who complain most loudly, those who have special programs to promote, the inner councils of teachers' unions and associations, self-appointed community leaders, paraprofessionals, and other climbers on career ladders, designers and reviewers of project proposals, bureaucrats at state and federal levels of government, and specialists at sitting-in, impeding, and taking over meetings for decision-making.

Curriculum makers are always in need of funds for the good things they desire for children. Thus, it is not surprising that "the curriculum hobbies of grantors and the sales promotion schemes of businesspeople" have often guided the realignment of curricular priorities. The explosive and erratic growth of knowledge has caused difficulties in determining how knowledges shall be placed within the curriculum. The present concern for evaluation and assessment of the acquisition of these knowledges is very likely to control important curriculum decisions. All four of these prominent factors probably impinge on most curriculum change efforts.

Recommended changes should be based on thorough evaluation and appraisal of the existing objectives of the curriculum, and of the extent to which these curricular objectives are being attained. It is not sufficient to change the objectives, or some of the activities, or certain teaching methods, or to modify testing procedures listed in the course of study, in order to accomplish fundamental curriculum development. By definition, the curriculum is changed only when the actual learning experiences of students are changed. Basic to all curriculum change is the fact that teachers and administrators must change their values and attitudes, and hence their behavior. Changing people is a complex process and usually demands considerable time and effort on the part of those who change and of the leaders who aspire to effect specific changes.

DEFINING CURRICULUM

Definitions that describe *curriculum* as consisting of all experiences conducted under school auspices became established in the 1930s and were not generally questioned until the 1960s.[23] In the 1970s genuine controversy existed concerning the definition of the term. Broadly defined, the school curriculum includes the classroom and laboratory instruction during scheduled classes and also the bus ride to school in the morning, the lunch hour activities, the football game after school, and the conference with the school counselor.

Properly speaking, *curriculum* should be distinguished from *instruction*. *Curriculum* is an educative agency's *plan* for facilitating learning. *Instruction* is the delivery system or the aggregate of educative transactions that constitutes the teaching-learning process for implementing the plan. Macdonald[24] views curriculum as a purposefully selected cultural environment.

> Curriculum . . . is the study of "what should constitute a world of learning and how to go about making this world."

Instruction facilitates learning by persons in the process of becoming. Curriculum tends to focus more on ends, on the *why* and *what* questions; instruction tends to emphasize means, or the *how* questions.

Broadly construed, the physical education program comprises all experiences organized and directed by the physical education staff, including dressing for class, being measured for height and weight, taking a physical fitness test, practicing for varsity basketball, and taking a shower, along with the formal instructional experiences presented during the physical education class period. More specifically, the subject matter of physical education consists of human movement phenomena. Its learning media include such movement forms as individual, dual, and team games; sports and athletics; aquatic activities; various forms of dance; body mechanics activities; and self-testing events. Vigorous movement activities constitute the most conspicuous feature of the physical education program because overt physical responses occur. Out of these observable responses come the desired behavioral modifications, and the accompanying mental, emotional, and social responses that are significant for individual development.

PHYSICAL EDUCATION CURRICULUM DEVELOPMENT

The process of curriculum development is extremely complex. Curriculum specialists in any subject-matter field must begin by clarifying the total educational setting in which they work. The overall educational philosophy of the local school is a starting point; the philosophy of the physical education department must maintain consistency with the overall school philosophy. The objectives of the physical education curriculum and the goals of students are expressed in consonance with this philosophy. The needs of individual students and of groups of learners must be studied and assessed through a variety of techniques in order to state objectives directed toward optimal implementation of local educational philosophy. Given well-defined objectives, the physical education curriculum specialist can then work with the total teaching staff, supported by administrative resources, in consultation with representative students, parents, and community leaders, to plan for (1) scope, (2) sequence, and (3) continuous evaluation of physical education programs.

SCOPE

The total scope of physical education extends to the development and utilization of the individual's movement potential throughout the life span. It includes movement activities and related learnings in non-school as well as school settings. The procedure of selecting activities

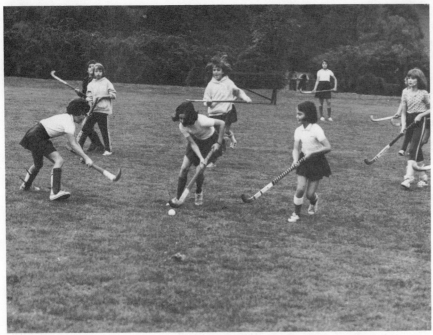

Physical education activities help the student to become a fully functioning adult.

and learning experiences for inclusion in school programs is generally referred to as designating the scope of the physical education curriculum.

What does the discipline of human movement have to offer in the continuing search for knowledge? What movement understandings and skills and which attitudes relating to movement behavior are essential in the pursuit of happiness? These are questions that must be answered in determining the scope of the physical education curriculum.

Voluntary movement is a significant function of human beings. Thus, the school is concerned with how movement functions in an individual's experience and in achieving common human goals. Persons of all ages have the same fundamental purposes for moving. The child needs physical education that will aid in becoming a fully functioning adult; the adult needs movement activities which will permit continuing self-actualization and more nearly complete individual-environment integration. The same key purposes can be used to design programs of movement opportunities for all persons, although specific goals vary and individual experiences must differ. Each individual seeks personal meaning through some unique combination of the shared human movement goals. Each individual *learns to move* to achieve these purposes.

Fitness, Performance, Transcendence. The rationale for physical education in general education is derived from study of its values and potential meanings to the participant. While there are probably 20 or more different meanings to be sought through participation in movement activities, these shared meanings can also be viewed as elements of three value clusters designated as *fitness*, *performance*, and *transcendence*. Fitness includes such standard components as strength, flexibility, and circulorespiratory endurance. Performance identifies all modes of skilled motor behavior in sport, dance, aquatics, gymnastics, and body

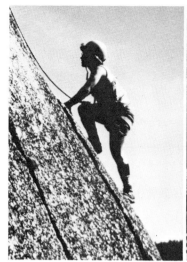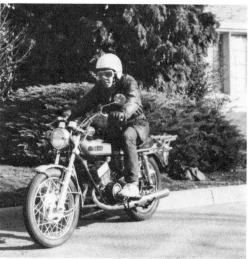

The adult needs movement activities that will permit continuing self-actualization and more complete individual–environment integration.

mechanics activities. Transcendence encompasses, although it is not limited to, self-awareness, inner consciousness, heightened perception, kinesthetic discovery, centering, self-mastery, creative expression, and joy of movement. The scope of physical education can be viewed as extending to include all of these. The curriculum can be structured to encourage the seeking of personal meaning in movement or physical activity through any combination of the many potential shared meanings or any variation of emphasis among fitness, performance, and transcendence.

Expressing Scope. Traditionally, scope is displayed in the form of charts that list instructional units by activity, grade level, and, usually, by number and arrangement of days or weeks assigned to each activity. Other data can be included, such as level of instruction (fundamental, elementary, intermediate, advanced, enrichment), basis of grouping pupils into classes, assignment of teachers, and other relevant factors.

The scope can be described in narrative form in any degree of detail deemed desirable to express the judgment of those charged with responsibility for making curriculum decisions. Scope can be delineated through lists of carefully stated behavioral objectives or by listing statements of desired competencies. We recommend the procedure for determining scope which has been developed through the Physical Education Curriculum Project of the American Alliance for Health, Physical Education, Recreation and Dance.[25]

The Purpose Process Curriculum Framework (PPCF) includes a purpose framework that provides for the selection of curriculum experiences in terms of three key purposes or human movement goals: (1) to fulfill personal developmental potential, (2) to develop movement skills utilized in adapting to and controlling the physical environment, and (3) to assist the individual in relating to other persons. It includes 22 purpose elements for identifying the content of physical education experiences.[26a]

The Purpose Process Curriculum Framework

It is emphasized that a "purpose" in this context identifies a unique way of finding or extending personal meaning through movement activities. The 22 purpose elements are not limited to voluntary goal-setting in physical education classes by either teachers or students. In a broader sense, they identify the various ways in which movement activities have been meaningful to individual persons. Thus, it is hypothesized that these represent potential avenues to other members of the species for enriching their lives through movement activities. It follows that physical education curricula should present to individuals opportunities to become aware of these possibilities and to develop personal abilities appropriate to their realization.

Seven major purposes for describing the scope of the physical education curriculum have been identified through the PPCF. These purpose concepts have been further subdivided into elements which serve as a starting point for local curriculum planners. These purposes are listed and defined below:*

KEY PURPOSE CONCEPT[26b]

I. **INDIVIDUAL DEVELOPMENT**: I move to fulfill my human developmental potential.
  A. **Physiological Efficiency**: I move to improve or maintain my functional capabilities.
      1. *Circulo-Respiratory Efficiency.* I move to develop and maintain circulatory and respiratory functioning.
      2. *Mechanical Efficiency.* I move to develop and maintain range and efficiency of motion.
      3. *Neuro-Muscular Efficiency.* I move to develop and maintain motor functioning.
  B. **Psychic Equilibrium**: I move to achieve personal integration.
      4. *Joy of Movement.* I move to derive pleasure from movement experience.
      5. *Self-Knowledge.* I move to gain self-understanding and appreciation.
      6. *Catharsis.* I move to release tension and frustration.
      7. *Challenge.* I move to test my prowess and courage.
II. **ENVIRONMENTAL COPING**: I move to adapt to and control my physical environment.
  C. **Spatial Orientation**: I move to relate myself in three-dimensional space.
      8. *Awareness.* I move to clarify my conception of my body and my position in space.
      9. *Relocation.* I move in a variety of ways to propel or project myself.
      10. *Relationships.* I move to regulate my body position in relation to the objects or persons in my environment.
  D. **Object Manipulation**: I move to give impetus to and to absorb the force of objects.
      11. *Maneuvering Weight.* I move to support, resist, or transport mass.
      12. *Object Projection.* I move to impart momentum and direction to a variety of objects.
      13. *Object Reception.* I move to intercept a variety of objects by reducing or arresting their momentum.
III. **SOCIAL INTERACTION**: I move to relate to others.
  E. **Communication**: I move to share ideas and feelings with others.
      14. *Expression.* I move to convey my ideas and feelings.
      15. *Clarification.* I move to enhance the meaning of other communication forms.

---

*The key purpose concepts have been rephrased in accordance with current language usage.

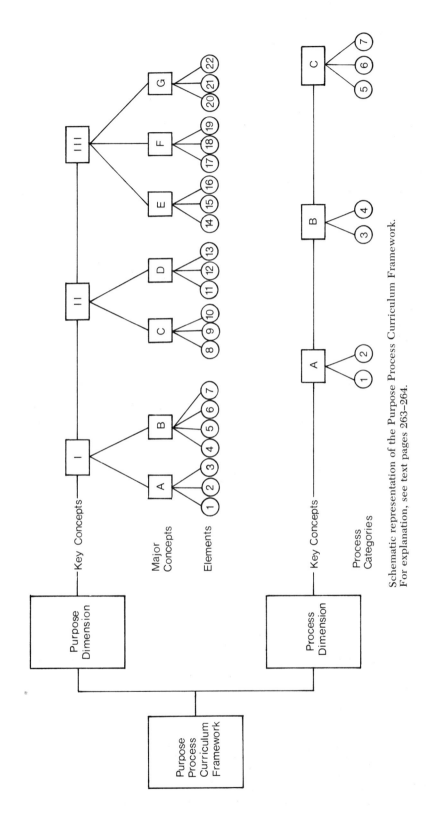

Schematic representation of the Purpose Process Curriculum Framework. For explanation, see text pages 263–264.

16. *Simulation.* I move to create an advantageous image or situation.

F. **Group Interaction:** I move to function in harmony with others.
   17. *Teamwork.* I move to cooperate in pursuit of common goals.
   18. *Competition.* I move to vie for individual or group goals.
   19. *Leadership.* I move to motivate and influence group members to achieve common goals.

G. **Cultural Involvement:** I move to take part in movement activities that constitute an important part of my society.
   20. *Participation.* I move to develop my capabilities for taking part in movement activities of my society.
   21. *Movement Appreciation.* I move to become knowledgeable and appreciative of sports and expressive movement forms.
   22. *Cultural Understanding.* I move to understand, respect, and strengthen the cultural heritage.

Decisions concerning the relative emphasis to be given to particular purposes or elements are based on local educational philosophy and the needs and interests of the appropriate school population. The selection of specific movement activities or learning media depends upon the judgment of the professional staff and upon local conditions and resources. Using this approach a community concerned about the physical fitness status of its young people will give special emphasis to those physical fitness activities in which the current programs show specific deficiencies. If the local school philosophy lends strong support to the life-time sports concept, a popular emphasis in today's schools, curriculum planners will study the participation element of the cultural involvement purpose concept and will establish program goals in terms of variety of sports experience, types of essential "carry-over activity" experiences, and standards for desired proficiency. When a high priority is to be given to the competition element of the larger purpose of group interaction, the scope would reflect this choice in the predominance of skill development activities in the popular competitive sports and the availability of intensive practice opportunities in a wide range of sports to accommodate many students.

SEQUENCE

Curriculum development also requires the sequential organization of selected learning activities and the placement or ordering of planned experiences in designing educational programs for groups and individuals. These processes provide for sequence in a given curriculum. Repetition of a limited few activities from year to year, unthinking seasonal rotation of traditional sports units, and lack of sound sequence are criticisms frequently leveled at physical education.

Limitations to Previous Sequencing Approaches. The usual approach to providing sequence in physical education curricula in the past has been to assign particular activities to specific grade levels on the basis of age standards and the best available knowledge of typical developmental levels for comparable populations. This procedure does not lend itself to individualizing learning and is especially unsatisfactory in non-graded programs and appropriate placement schools. Conscientious physical educators have commonly analyzed sport, gymnastic, and dance activities in terms of complexity of the specific motor skills required, and established recommended *progressions*. While this procedure permits broad classification into beginning, intermediate, and advanced activity units, and can be adapted to a continuous performance or phased curriculum, its limitation is that undue emphasis is placed on the subject matter as traditionally conceived in particular sports and games, thus discouraging the invention of new movement activities, modification of established activities, or the creative design of environments for individual learning.

It is suggested that sequence in physical education can best be facilitated by organizing curricular content in terms of desired movement process outcomes. Movement processes represent one large segment of human behavior. Process learnings are, therefore, essential physical education outcomes. Important learning opportunities include those concerned with the processes by which an individual *moves to learn* — the processes for learning to facilitate, extend, and utilize fully one's unique movement capabilities.

A Movement Process Orientation

We believe that the purposes of movement in prolonging and enriching the quality of life can serve to define the scope of the physical education curriculum and that the processes of self-actualization through movement provide a basis for sequencing potential learning experiences in physical education. The movement classification scheme, developed as the process dimension of the Purpose Process Curriculum Framework, conceptualizes seven movement process categories and offers a taxonomy for the selection and statement of educational objectives.[26c]

MOVEMENT PROCESS CATEGORIES

A. **Generic Movement:** Those movement operations or processes which facilitate the development of characteristic and effective motor patterns. They are typically exploratory operations in which the learner receives or "takes in" data as he or she moves.
   1. *Perceiving:* Awareness of total body relationships and of self in motion. These awarenesses may be evidenced by body positions or motoric acts; they may be sensory in that the mover feels the equilibrium of body weight and the movement of limbs; or they may be evidenced cognitively through identification, recognition, or differentiation.
   2. *Patterning:* Arrangement and use of body parts in successive and harmonious ways to achieve a movement pattern or skill. This process is dependent on recall and performance of a movement previously demonstrated or experienced.
B. **Ordinative Movement:** The processes of organizing, refining, and performing skillful movement. The processes involved are directed toward the organization of perceptual-motor abilities with a view to solving particular movement tasks or requirements.
   3. *Adapting:* Modification of a patterned movement to meet externally imposed task demands. This would include modification of a particular movement to perform it under different conditions.
   4. *Refining:* Acquisition of smooth, efficient control in performing a movement pattern or skill by mastery of spatial and temporal relations. This process deals with the achievement of precision in motor performance and habituation of performance under more complex conditions.

C. **Creative Movement:** Those motor performances which include the processes of inventing or creating movement which will serve the personal (individual) purposes of the learner. The processes employed are directed toward discovery, integration, abstraction, idealization, emotional objectification and composition.

5. *Varying:* Invention or construction of personally unique options in motor performance. These options are limited to different ways of performing specific movement; they are of an immediate situational nature and lack any pre-determined movement behavior which has been externally imposed on the mover.

6. *Improvising:* Extemporaneous origination or initiation of personally novel movement or combination of movement. The processes involved may be stimulated by a situation externally structured, although conscious planning on the part of the performer is not usually required.

7. *Composing:* Combination of learned movement into personally unique motor designs or the invention of movement patterns new to the performer. The performer creates a motor response in terms of a personal interpretation of the movement situation.

In practice, curriculum planners determine the scope of local physical education curricula as described above, making priority decisions concerning major emphases, identifying essential curriculum content, clarifying district-wide agreements, and establishing guidelines for planning within each school and within the various administrative units. Teachers develop instructional objectives using elements of human movement as the content focus and process categories to identify the process toward which instruction is directed. This procedure can be used to generate educational objectives for instructional groups in any learning environment, utilizing a wide variety of learning media encompassing traditional and popular games, stunts, sports and dance activities, innovative movement education challenges, and unfamiliar but potentially satisfying physical recreation opportunities. Even more important, it can be used to identify instructional objectives for individual learners and to guide personalized learning toward different processes for a number of individuals learning in a group environment but not necessarily attempting to achieve the same goal at the same time.

EVALUATION

An important aspect of curriculum development is continuous evaluation of the program as a basis for further improvement. At least once a year an overall appraisal of status is needed in order to review program objectives and modify short-term goals as necessary. In this phase of evaluation it is desirable to involve other members of the school teaching and administrative staff, district office personnel, interested parents, student representatives, and citizens' group representatives, in addition to all department staff members who should be involved in both formal and informal procedures to appraise the physical education program on a continuous basis. Consultation on particular aspects of educational evaluation may also be sought from District Curriculum Department personnel, the State Department of Education, professional associations, and nearby colleges and universities.

Day-to-day evaluation and appraisal of program strengths and weaknesses and the ongoing collection of specific assessment data are responsibilities of the local physical education staff, however. In program areas in which it is feasible to use specific performance objectives, these are developed by the teaching staff, who work directly with students. The concept of formative evaluation is gaining adherents because it permits organized and well-planned instruction to be modified immediately on the basis of information concerning student learning progress.

Certain important educational goals and accomplishments cannot be evaluated satisfactorily by means of specific performance objectives. Learning progress and relative program success in these areas should also be included in appraising the effectiveness and quality of physical education in the local schools. Assessment techniques available include interest preference scales, ratings, attitude inventories, interaction analysis, interviews, structured observation category systems, and audio- and videotape analysis. Evaluation is discussed in greater detail in Chapter 11.

ORGANIZATIONAL PATTERNS

The crucial curriculum decisions are those relating to scope, sequence, and evaluation. If these decisions are soundly based, many organizational patterns can be selected or developed to implement effective educational programs. Many local factors, including geographic and climatic conditions, available instructional areas, available equipment, nature of the total school schedule, class size, teacher loads, and time allotted to physical education, need consideration in planning for the administration and conduct of physical education programs. For purposes of discussion, these are considered in four categories: (1) grouping, (2) scheduling and staffing, (3) learning resources, and (4) individualization and personalization.

Interest in innovative organizational patterns was stimulated in the 1960s by the work and publications of the National Association of Secondary School Principals, particularly its Commission on the Experimental Study of the Utilization of the Staff in Secondary Schools and the more recent Model Schools Project directed by Trump.[27, 28, 29] Although the original impetus related to secondary schools, the key organizational concepts have also been extended to elementary school education. Physical educators have recognized the unique possibilities for similar approaches to improving instruction in their field. The Committee on Organizational Patterns for Physical Education and Recreation, chaired by Heitmann, studied organizational patterns across the nation and reported a variety of innovative patterns and practices. The report of this committee is recommended to all physical educators for helpful descriptions of ways to organize time, students, and staff to facilitate learning in physical education.[30]

GROUPING

Since the function of student grouping is to facilitate learning, any plan for grouping should be flexible and pupils should be able to transfer from one group to another as appropriate. The group environment most conducive to learning will vary with student characteristics, teacher abilities, and learning tasks. Heitmann[31] has identified nine methods of student grouping in physical education: grade level, anthropometric, chronological, social ability, interest, achievement, physical capacity, temperament, and learning characteristics.

Experience and accumulating evidence seem to argue that physical education classes should be grouped on the combined bases of interest and ability. There are secondary schools that have four or five such

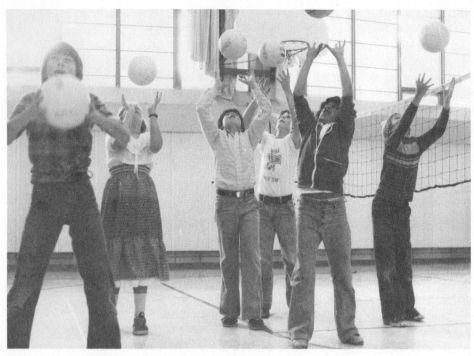

Classes should be grouped on the combined basis of interest and ability.

groupings, each of which has an appropriately different curriculum. These groupings can be achieved by selection of various criteria such as physical performance tests, specific skills tests, teachers' judgments of skills and interests, and pupil expression of interests on inventory forms, questionnaires and free-response instruments. Local staffs should select criteria for grouping after thoughtful consideration of program objectives.

The Non-Graded Elementary School. The non-graded elementary school presents a unique challenge in grouping pupils for physical education. These schools give careful attention to the need for continuity in individual pupil progress. Students proceed through school at individual rates, operating within broad age level ranges. A variety of diagnostic procedures can be used for student placement. A particularly interesting plan used in the University Elementary School, UCLA, is reported by Cunningham.[32] In this situation pupil placement is determined by diagnostic tests in seven major areas of movement: locomotor skills, eye-hand skills, eye-foot skills, body coordination skills, balance skills, sensory motor skills, and rhythm and dance skills. Other procedures for student grouping in non-graded programs are reported by Curtis[33] and Burson.[34]

Prior to about 1930, there was a traditional feeling among professional leaders that boys and girls should be separated for purposes of physical education activities, starting in the fourth grade. This judgment was predicated upon physiological grounds, with particular reference to the safety of girls, and in consideration for the needs and capacities of both sexes. Social customs were a factor also.

For nearly half a century, physical educators debated the pros and cons of coeducational participation in physical education classes. The professional literature from the mid-1930s into the 1970s presented

Coeducational Physical Education

many plans for arranging combinations of single-sex and coeducational instruction and many suggestions for implementing sound programs in which boys and girls were students in the same classes. Most of these guidelines have been made obsolete by recent interpretations of Title IX.

It is now clear that many of the differences frequently observed in physical or motor performances between boys and girls resulted from varied backgrounds of experience rather than sex-related biological potential. There is no question that physical attributes are distributed along a continuum for each sex and that the differences among the girls or among the boys in any one characteristic are apt to be greater than the mean difference in that same factor between the two sexes. The current focus on providing for equality of opportunity has led educators to be more concerned with providing girls and women with educational opportunities of quality equal to those available to boys and men than with measuring sex differences or analyzing the specific reasons for any significant differences observed.

Current standards require that all classes be open on an equitable basis to students of both sexes. This means that bases for grouping other than sex will be the norm in future physical education instruction. Ability groupings will probably be more typical than they have been in the recent past. The use of task contracts and other types of individualized instruction should be stimulated. Students may participate in subgroupings within the class in accordance with a variety of criteria; but students cannot be denied instructional opportunities in dance because they are male nor can they be denied advanced level instruction in an activity such as tennis because they are female.

Intramural programs, sports clubs, and interscholastic and intercollegiate athletic programs must also provide for equity. Separate teams may be organized for male and female students; but the courts have ruled that, if a given activity is not provided for girls, girls are eligible to qualify for participation on the team organized primarily for the boys.

Mainstreaming Handicapped Students

Current educational practice also discourages the organization of special classes for students with handicaps. In the past, many physical education departments have taught special classes in adapted physical education or have arranged for special population groups such as the mentally retarded to have separate classes in physical education. The present trend toward mainstreaming handicapped students in physical education classes with other students is mandated by Public Law 94-142.

SCHEDULING AND STAFFING

Selective and Elective Programs. Recent changes in physical education scheduling have been aimed at minimizing the rigidity which was characteristic until the past decade. Secondary school schedules in particular are opening up options within the physical education program. *Selective programs*, which permit students to select from among several alternative offerings within the requirement, are increasingly popular. Many schools now offer *elective* programs in which participation is optional. Requirements in physical education based on compulsory time spent in activity programs have become more difficult to support in light of the trend toward eliminating all specific subject requirements. Forward-looking physical educators are giving extra thought and attention to strengthening elective programs. Imaginative elective offerings at both secondary and college levels have attracted large enrollments. The physical education activity programs in junior colleges, colleges and universities are now largely elective.

The Intersession Plan. Another innovation in scheduling is the *intersession plan*, which permits intensive study of a particular subject for a brief period of time. Intersessions are usually scheduled during brief vacation periods or other times outside the typical academic calendar. Together with the year-round school concept, intersessions have increased options for student course selection. In physical education, special off-campus opportunities such as skiing, scuba diving, and mountain climbing are very popular. Unfortunately, the rapidly rising costs of liability insurance have led many schools and colleges to restrict or eliminate these "high-risk" activities for fear of possible lawsuits.

Flexible Group Plans and Modular Scheduling. *Flexible group* practices are more feasible now through various forms of modular scheduling which are computer generated. Groups of varying sizes are most appropriate to facilitate the purposes of a particular class on a given day. Although flexible group procedures can also be devised within traditional schedules, many schools are now using modular scheduling as well as flexible grouping arrangements.

Modular scheduling permits the more efficient use of school time to attain educational objectives. A unit of time is selected and the school schedule is built in combinations or multiples of one or more time modules for each subject. Although modules of many different time lengths have been used in the past few years, it appears that twenty-minute modules are in use by a majority. Usually they are scheduled for 21 to 24 modules per day.

Typically, the school schedule repeats itself weekly rather than daily. However, this is not an essential requirement. Other lengths of schedule cycle are possible. The modular schedule is generated by a computer; there are too many combinations and permutations to do it by hand.

Pupils are scheduled into formal classes for 40 to 60 per cent of the total school time available. This time normally includes both small group instruction in groups of 12 to 15 pupils and large group instruction in groups of up to 100 or more. The remaining unscheduled time is available for independent study and for participation in open laboratory work in various subjects, including physical education. Heitmann[35] has provided helpful descriptions of the use of large group instruction, small group instruction, independent study, and open laboratory practice in physical education, and excellent analyses of the advantages, purposes, suggested activities, and operational considerations for establishing each of these four phases of instruction.

Teacher Assignments

Problems involving class size and teacher load have plagued physical educators for years. Appropriate class size depends upon many factors, as suggested by recent innovative plans for grouping, scheduling, and staffing. Where traditional organizational patterns are used, maximum class size should be limited to 25 or whatever figure is used for maximum classroom enrollment in the local school district. Regardless of the particular organizational pattern selected, the individual teacher's load should require regular contact with not more than 200 pupils. The administration should permit lighter class loads for all teachers assigned intramural, sport or dance club, interscholastic, or intercollegiate responsibilities.

Heitmann[36] reviews four methods used in assigning the responsibility of teaching physical education in the primary grades.

> The one preferred by most authors on the subject is the employment of a physical education specialist to handle virtually all phases of the physical education program. The second preference is the employment of a rotating specialist, sometimes called a curriculum associate, to assist classroom teachers by team teaching with them at least once a week, and by providing leadership in program development, equipment and facility planning, and in-service assistance. A third approach is through the exchanging of assignments, whereby one teacher will teach physical education for another teacher, who in turn will instruct in another subject. A different form of this pattern, called "team teaching" by some, requires one teacher to learn and teach dance, for example, another tumbling, and a third ball skills. . . . The fourth and least effective approach is the self-contained classroom where the teacher assumes the complete responsibility without assistance from other teachers.

The Gilmore Study. An unusual analysis of tasks performed by high school teachers of boys' physical education by Gilmore[37] throws light on a basic staff problem of major proportions. He identified 68 tasks these teachers typically perform. He then developed sets of criteria by which each task was evaluated as being professional, semi-professional, or non-professional. A sample of teachers kept daily diaries concerning the amount of time they spent on the 68 tasks. Gilmore found that 46 per cent of their time was devoted to professional tasks, 25 per cent to semi-professional tasks, and 29 per cent to non-professional tasks. If these figures accurately represent the status of male physical education teachers in high schools, there is cause for considerable concern.

Effective Staff Utilization. The obvious basic principle of effective staff utilization is that credentialed teachers primarily should be assigned to perform professional duties. Personnel with varying kinds of preparation and experience should be employed to perform semi-professional and non-professional duties under the supervision of senior credentialed teachers. Accompanying this differentiation of duties would be a differentiated salary schedule. Many physical education departments have realized this problem, and there are examples of schools now assisting teachers by using teacher aides, skill aides, community sports specialists, specialized resource people, volunteers, student teachers, interns, student leaders, community-school directors, custodians, matrons, secretaries, and clerks.

Trump popularized team teaching and differentiated staffing in the 1960s.[38, 39, 40] His recommendations for the nation-wide Model Schools Project sponsored by the National Association of Secondary School Principals are as follows:[41]

> For every 35 pupils enrolled in a school, the instructional staff should include: one teacher, 20 hours per week of instructional assistance, and 5 hours per week of general aides.

He further recommended that the number of teachers assigned to health, physical education, and recreation be one-eighth of the total staff number. Current deemphasis of single-sex classes and separate classes for the handicapped in physical education has stimulated some new variations in team teaching in physical education.

The use of flexible scheduling does not guarantee improvement of instruction; it does permit varying groups and more efficient use of time. Heitmann[42] recommends the following steps in the process for effective utilization of flexible scheduling:

1. The school population must be analyzed to identify the students' needs. . . .
2. The learning tasks that would lead to the desired goal must be determined for each group identified. . . .
3. The most effective methods of presentation for each specific learning task and group must be determined. . . .
4. Determine effective ways to organize instruction. . . .
5. Class sizes appropriate for each learning group must be decided. . . .
6. Designations of time allotments compatible with the students' learning characteristics, planned teaching methods, and learning tasks must be made. . . .
7. Analyze staff requirements and existing staff strengths.

LEARNING RESOURCES

Recent innovations involving the application of computers, television, and other sophisticated forms of technology to educational processes have changed instruction in most school subjects, including physical education. Individualizing each pupil's total program has now become a reality through the capabilities of the computer to generate a flexible or modular schedule. Complex *learning systems* now make it possible for a student to take an entire course on an individual study basis, in a foreign language or in basic biology, for example, with the assistance of a *learning console*.

Uses of Computers. Computer-based instruction has not been used as extensively in physical education as in some other areas, but a number of programs are in operation. Computers are being used in some schools and colleges to schedule pupils into physical education classes, and to schedule complex intramural sport programs. They are used extensively for recording registrations and grades. Some coaches use them to analyze opponents' strategies in football. Physical education researchers have been especially active in utilizing the computer.

Instructional Technology

Educational Television. The potential impact of educational and instructional television is as great in education as that of commercial television in society. Hixson notes that physical education has utilized television at every level of instruction.[43] Series of television lessons such as "Ready? Set . . . Go!" produced by the National Instructional Television Center at Bloomington, Indiana, have been used to provide a major resource for physical education instruction in schools. Single programs have also been used to enrich or supplement instruction.

Microteaching. Instant playback portable television has become very popular in physical education and athletic programs. One of the earliest innovations was in teacher education at Stanford University, where instant playback television has been employed as both a preservice and in-service medium.[44, 45] It is used to tape microteaching episodes by interns in the training program. The camera is transported to the physical education classes of the interns in nearby high schools during the school year. This instrument has proved to be a beneficial source of immediate, accurate feedback information, which contributes significantly to rapid progress in teacher preparation. The instant playback television camera also can be used to project models of excellent teaching, to serve as a selection procedure for the employment of a teacher, and to train student teachers and intern supervisors. The full possibilities of microteaching are still being developed; it seems a particularly promising technique for changing teachers' perception of their own behavior. For a more detailed analysis of the potential and status of microteaching, the reader is referred to Jordan's[46] appraisal of the Stanford program.

Instant playback television is being used extensively as a teaching and coaching aid in physical education classes and with athletic teams. Teachers and coaches are enthusiastic in their support of this assistance. However, very few rigorous experimental research studies have been reported that cite evidence of the efficacy of this instructional instrument in comparison to standard methods of instruction without the camera.

Hixson has provided an excellent summary of the current status of television in physical education, including a list of thirteen additional ways in which television is now being used in physical education.[47] Of particular interest is the establishment by the American Alliance for Health, Physical Education, Recreation, and Dance of a Resource Center on Media in Physical Education, located at the University of South Carolina. The Center maintains a small library of video and audiotapes and is able to provide modest storage, duplication, and distribution services.

Recent Developments. Other forms of technology are finding their way into physical education and sport programs, such as automatic timing devices keyed to the starting signal and the finish line, the finish touch plate at the end of the swimming pool to record the order of finish and the time in hundredths of seconds, an electrical "blanket" placed under the turf of athletic fields, radiotelemetry to study physiological phenomena of athletes in action, use of 8- and 16mm motion pictures, use of tape recorders, and other forms of instructional technology too numerous to recount here.

Advances in Sport Space Development. Recent innovations in facilities make it possible to individualize instruction to a greater extent than previously. Restricted indoor space long has been a source of limitations on programs during inclement weather. Limited shelters[48] provide covered and sheltered space at fractions of the cost of typical gymnasiums and multi-purpose rooms. The Educational Facilities Laboratory at Stanford University has pioneered a new standard school builing construction unit.[49] It is a flexible building module of standard dimensions which can be erected on almost any site. By joining two or more of these building modules together, flexible gymnasium space can be provided at substantially reduced cost. Air-supported shelters are coming into increased use.[50] These are large plastic bubbles, supported by a forced-air generator, which are large enough to cover tennis courts, swimming pools, and outdoor play spaces, thus permitting year-round use of these facilities at low cost.

Synthetic Surfaces. Astro-turf, Tartan, and other synthetic surface materials now cover indoor space, bringing football, baseball, tennis, track, and numerous other activities inside. Elementary schools are covering activity room floors with these materials. Likewise, outdoor football fields, running tracks, and other sports areas are being covered by these products. They have proved to be highly successful and durable. In all of these ways the total physical education and sports programs are

Effective Utilization of Space

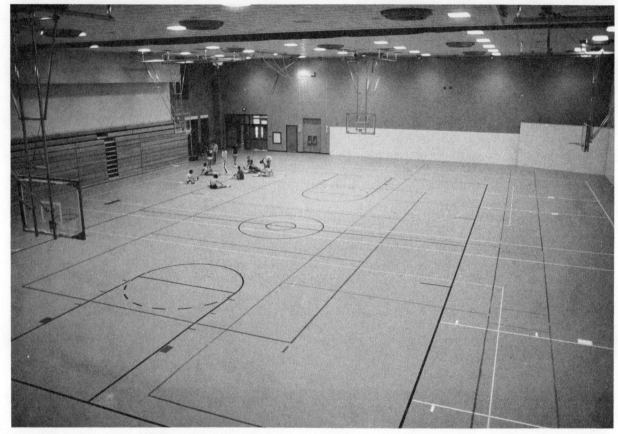

More efficient use of educational facilities is needed.

expanded and made available year-round to larger numbers of students.

Modular Scheduling for Maximum Space Efficiency. School instructional areas can be used more efficiently where modular scheduling has been adopted. Modular time scheduling permits 90 to 100 per cent utilization of available facilities because it allows one class to move into a teaching station almost as soon as the preceding class has left it, rather than to have a 15- to 20-minute period of non-use between classes, as is typical several times each day in traditional scheduling. As much as one and one-half hours of extra time thus is made available for use of physical education facilities each day.

Resource Centers. Schools now are establishing physical education resource centers at all levels. These centers contain a wide selection of instructional aids and relevant literature of value to both pupils and teachers. Audio-visual equipment, bulletin boards, areas for poster display, and similar materials are provided. The center is program-oriented. Sometimes this center is part of the school library or instructional materials center; in other instances it has its own designated area. The latter arrangement is preferable.

Non-School Facilities. Many schools are now using non-school facilities for physical education classes. There is increasing use of such off-campus facilities as community golf courses, driving ranges, bowling lanes, tennis courts, swimming pools, skating rinks, ski slopes, and public playground areas. The open campus concept or the "school-without-walls" suggests many avenues for bringing the community into the school and for extending physical education programs into the community.

By far the biggest challenge facing American education today is to provide a quality program, while at the same time serving large numbers of students. The increasing application of technology to education has led many to express concern about the possibility of "dehumanizing" education. In truth, the many innovations in organization of physical education programs can serve the goals of humanistic education, provided they are used by teachers who are dedicated to the basic goal of meeting individual pupil needs, who interact in a genuinely supportive way with students, and who encourage positive self-concepts and a desire to learn. The primary purpose of contemporary grouping arrangements is to provide a better group environment for individual learning. The real benefits of modular scheduling and differentiated staffing lie in their success in making more possibilities available for personal achievement of different learners. Inventive resources are designed to maximize the learning progress of individual students.

The ascendance of humanism in education increases the concern for individualization in school experiences. Analysis of some of the difficulties resulting from widespread adoption of innovative organizational plans has led some to prefer the term *personalization* to *individualization*. It is possible to individualize learning by adjusting the rate or sequence of planned activities or by isolating a single learner from the group setting. But learning is not necessarily personalized under these conditions. For the humanistic educator concerned with the self-actualization of learners, personalization is what makes learning experiences human.

Accommodating to Medical Assessment

Personalization in physical education should begin with a thorough medical examination before beginning participation in the program. Examinations, given by a family or school physician, are recommended for all students in grades one, four, seven, and ten, for all new pupils entering the district, and for pupils who have extended absence from school due to severe injury or illness. Students with permanent or temporary disabilities should be accommodated in activity situations that provide optimum opportunities for participation appropriate to their needs. They should also be assisted with individual exercise programs designed to help them achieve their maximum individual potentials. Qualified adapted physical education specialists should be available on a consultant basis.

It is the belief of the authors, and of many other physical educators, that no student who is physically able to attend school regularly and carry a normal program of studies should be excused from the physical education requirement. A primary administrative goal in connection with any school program of physical education should be 100 per cent participation. This ideal can be approached in almost every school if individual medical examinations are administered to determine the specific types of activities in which the pupil should engage; if the program is varied enough to offer activities appropriate to the needs and conditions represented in the entire group of students; if the *why* of physical education is clarified for students and others involved; if the physical education department wins the confidence and cooperative interest of school administrators, officials, parents, medical examiners, and students through good communications; and if students are grouped, scheduled, and guided in ways that truly facilitate personalized learning.

Current thought is that by the end of the age of compulsory educa- *Meeting Personal* tion all youth should be well-grounded in a broad, liberal education, and *Needs Consonant* should have the motivation to continue it throughout life by assuming *with Student Goals* responsibility for maximum self-direction in learning, both in formal school situations and informally. Not only should the schools provide broad, liberal education for all pupils, but by the time of high school graduation or school-leaving age, students should have begun specialized study along lines of their individual abilities and interests.

Individualized or personalized instruction in physical education is an aspiration in consonance with this challenge. Physical education has been remiss in helping pupils to develop self-responsibility and the skills of personal decision making. In general, teaching has been quite authoritarian in nature, and too often topics have been taught in what Mosston calls a "command style."[51]

Schools committed to this viewpoint now provide opportunities for pupil responsibility and decision-making experiences in several ways:

1. Each student assesses his or her physical education needs at the beginning of each year. This process includes a physical fitness test, a self-rating of skill levels in the various sports in which instruction is available, and a self-report of other goals that he or she chooses to pursue through an activity program.

2. With the help of a physical education advisor, the student selects from among the available offerings those best suited to his or her purposes, and tests and evaluates present skills and knowledges in each of the content areas selected. The results of this assessment are recorded in an individual physical education cumulative file.

3. At the start of each unit, the student sets and records personal goals to guide work during that unit. Student responsibility extends to the selection of learning experiences, proposals for practice routines, and planning schedules to be followed during the unit. In pursuing these plans the student seeks assistance from classmates and teachers; students interact among themselves and help each other to achieve individual goals.

4. Progress is evaluated both formally and informally as the student recognizes a need, periodically as guided by the teacher, and at the end of each unit. Summative evaluation procedures are conducted with the assistance of peers and teachers and recorded in individual student folders. The student considers progress in the unit in relation to long-range goals clarified at the beginning of the year, and discusses progress, feelings, remaining problems, and hopes for future experiences and accomplishments with the teacher.

The role of the teacher in humanistic physical education is in **HIDDEN** marked contrast to the assumptions underlying the "mass instruction" **CURRICULUM** methodology characteristic of traditional programs. The teacher becomes an encourager, a facilitator, a diagnostician, a prescriber, a consultant, and a resource agent. To an important degree, the teacher is also the creator and manipulator of the educational environment. The teacher is one element in the student's personal environment, functioning as a key factor in determining the extent to which the environment is supportive and conducive to the achievement of desired learnings.

Educators are becoming increasingly aware of previously unstudied aspects of the process of schooling. The term *hidden curriculum* appears frequently in the literature, defined by some as the unintended outcomes of schooling[52] and by others as attitudes and values implicitly represented in the education environment.[53] Knowledge about the hidden curriculum is accumulating. Philip Jackson[54] holds that the key elements in the hidden curriculum are praise, or the teacher's use of rewards or punishments; crowds, or the quality of life in a crowded group; and the teacher's power. Lawrence Kohlberg[55] takes the position that the hidden curriculum should be approached from a theory of moral education and defines six stages of moral development. Kohlberg claims that our schools are Stage 4 — law, order, and authority institutions — while our Constitutional government aspires to social contract democracy and human rights, which he has defined as Stage 5.

Bain[56] has studied and reported on values implicit in physical education class environments. It is becoming increasingly apparent that physical educators must be aware of the significance of the hidden curriculum. Arrangements for grouping students, decisions concerning scheduling and staffing, the selection and utilization of particular learning resources, and the degree of individualization or personalization inherent in the instructional procedures used are all factors contributing to the physical education "hidden" curriculum. Hopefully, a humanistic philosophy of education will more frequently determine organizational patterns and will guide more physical education programs throughout the country.

PHYSICAL EDUCATION CURRICULUM MODELS

Issues relating to national standards or exemplary models in education are difficult to resolve. For generations physical educators have recognized uneven quality in local curricula. Many have sought models of ideal curricula to provide guides toward upgrading programs. A similar situation pertains to all subject-field areas. It is probably inevitable in a country in which the major curriculum decisions are made on the local district level, while important educational regulations are legislated at the state level, and federal grants, subsidies, and affirmative action programs also have significant impact on certain aspects of local curriculum development. The problem of supporting high quality educational opportunities for all in a democratic society without unduly restricting local autonomy is exceedingly complex. When this problem is studied in the context of differing local and individual educational needs, the appropriate use of educational models becomes an important question.

FAMILIES OF PHYSICAL EDUCATION MODELS

A large number of educational models have been developed over the years. Probably the best recent analysis is that reported by Joyce, Weil, and Wald,[57] in which they state that educational models can be used in three ways: as a basis for curriculum plans, as guidelines for teacher interaction with students, and as specifications for instructional materials. They classify 16 models of teaching by "family" and mission. The selection of an educational model from among those that have been developed depends upon one's view of humankind and the universe and the expression of one's view of reality as a philosophy of education. The choice of an educational model, in turn, determines the roles of teacher and learner, the function of subject matter, the selection of methodologies, and specifications for learning environments and instructional materials.

Models for physical education programs can be grouped into three broad families in terms of the prevailing orientation:

Disciplinary models are subject-matter oriented. Knowledge and understanding of human movement phenomena and development of fitness and movement skill are top priorities. The teacher is a performer, a model, an information dispenser, even a taskmaster; the learner's role is to receive instruction, to emulate the teacher's model, and to strive to master the knowledge and skill exemplified. The focus is on learning to move; subject matter is of primary importance.

Social-interaction models are society-oriented. They are concerned with environments that facilitate social processes. The teacher is the source of authority and a guide to the accumulated group wisdom, a facilitator of group activity and an environmental manager. The learner is viewed as an immature and relatively inexperienced group member whose goal is to become socialized into the prevailing customs, mores, ideals, and skills of the group. Subject matter is regarded as the context for group interaction. The physical education class or the athletic contest is society in microcosm and the focus is on learning movement activities as a means of growth toward optimum contribution to social betterment.

Personalized models are learner-oriented. The teacher, as well as the pupil, is a learner; he or she is a stimulator, a reflector, a counselor, a resource. Learners are self-directed, responsible for identifying their own goals. Each develops his or her own uniqueness. Subject content becomes the medium for fulfillment of individual human potential. The focus is on moving to learn and upon the processes of personal self-actualization.

These three broad families of physical education models are selectively adapted to fill academic, social, and personal missions of different educational programs. Many variations within each broad family as well as hybrid models combining elements of more than one basic model are in use. The individual physical educator chooses a role, methodologies, and instructional materials in accordance with the model best adapted to a personal educational philosophy and individual professional competencies.

The use of any educational model presupposes that the curriculum planner is working within a framework which defines the scope of operations. It is now generally accepted, in physical education as in other educational specializations, that any particular curriculum should be developed within a conceptual framework. Many professionals are concerned about the need for an adequate conceptual framework for physical education; a number of proposals have been offered.

PHYSICAL EDUCATION CONCEPTUAL FRAMEWORKS

LaPlante[58] has reviewed those frameworks that provide a conceptual network for curriculum development in physical education and evaluated them according to four criteria: (1) the important concepts of the body of knowledge are represented; (2) the concepts are relevant to the individual's total development; (3) the processes of knowledge acquisition receive attention; and (4) the framework is dynamic and flexible so as to reflect societal change and to allow for the inclusion of new knowledge. She found that while many structures are used for organization of content she was able to identify only eight which qualified as demonstrating development from a conceptual framework.

Frameworks Based on Movement Analysis. The Stanley[59] and Tillotson[60] frameworks are each based on analysis of movement elements. The Stanley framework grows directly from Laban principles and is definitely suggestive of a movement education approach. The Tillotson framework was a result of the Title III Project ME conducted in Plattsburgh, New York, which developed an innovative elementary school program with a movement education focus.

Framework Emphasizing Scientific Concepts. The Battle Creek[61] framework was also initiated as a Title III project. It was developed for use in Battle Creek, Michigan, and was one of the first systematic approaches to planning a physical education curriculum emphasizing carefully selected scientific concepts.

Framework for Development of Kinesiology Curriculum. The Mackenzie[62] framework offers guidelines for the development of the "kinesiology" curriculum from preschool through undergraduate professional education. This framework is distinctive in the breadth of purposes offered, the humanistic philosophical orientation, and its specific suggestions for organizing experiences at five stages of learning.

Framework Emphasizing Fitness as a Way of Life. The Pye and Alexander[63] framework was developed as a teaching-learning guide for the college physical education program at the University of Florida. It is rooted in an overall philosophy that physical fitness is a way of life that is individually related to one's potential and performance.

Frameworks Based on Movement in Total Development. The Austin[64] framework, the Brown and Cassidy[65, 66] frameworks, and the Purpose Process Curriculum Framework[67] build on concepts of the role of movement in total development. The premise of the Austin framework is that physical activity is a unifying life force which makes operational the whole person by integrating and extending all resources as he or she moves in relation to other objects in various environments. The Brown and Cassidy frameworks describe movement behavior in terms of both individual and environmental variables and postulate three categories of movement possibilities: development, coping, and expression and communication. The Purpose Process Curriculum Framework originates from individual purposes for moving.

Purpose Process Curriculum Framework. The Purpose Process Curriculum Framework was developed under the auspices of the Curriculum Project of the Physical Education Division of AAHPERD. The project was part of a large-scale long-term effort to clarify the theoretical structure of physical education, to generate curriculum theory appropriate to human movement knowledge, to apply theoretical insights to exemplary curricular practices, and to provide guidelines for improving physical education programs throughout the country.

The Purpose Process Curriculum Framework is based on the assumption that the primary concern of physical education is the individual human being moving in interaction with the environment. The functions of human movement in achieving the human goals have been logically analyzed and organized as the three key concepts of individual development, environmental coping, and social interaction, encompassing seven major purposes that are used to define the scope of the physical education curriculum and to select program content. The twenty-two subpurposes or purpose elements identify unique ways of finding or extending personal meaning through movement activities. Each individual person may seek personal meaning through any combination of the shared human movement goals; individual learning within a class group may be guided in accordance with many diverse combinations of desired personal meanings.

Instructional planning requires a second or process dimension in the model. The process dimension has been developed in the form of a classification scheme for identifying major types of movement operations, by describing seven processes by which a human being learns to move. The focus is on learning processes and the attempt has been to differentiate important learning operations in order to facilitate improvement of instruction. Summaries of both purpose concepts and process categories of the Purpose Process Curriculum Framework appear in earlier sections of this chapter (see pp. 245–250).

The individual curriculum planner selects a conceptual framework within which to develop local physical education curricula. Using this framework to clarify educational objectives and a teaching model chosen in terms of a personal educational philosophy, the planner develops programs appropriate to societal conditions and goals and the personal needs and goals of learners.

PROGRAM EMPHASES

Although general guidelines can be helpful, local curricula must be developed in accordance with local considerations and with the participation of those persons who implement them in particular school programs. The suggestions for program emphases which follow reflect our own orientation, experience, and convictions. Both authors have been involved in the development of the Purpose Process Curriculum Framework; the programs envisioned in the succeeding paragraphs illustrate curricular decision-making using this framework. A more detailed description and analysis of the PPCF is available in a recent AAHPERD publication, *Curriculum Design: Purposes and Processes in Physical Education Teaching-Learning*.[68]

Preschool Programs

The concept that the responsibility of physical education begins with children in their fifth or sixth year and ends with persons reaching legal maturity at eighteen to twenty-one years of age is definitely obsolete. Organized preschool education programs are increasing rapidly. In the expansion of this important phase of organized education, it is vital that the role of physical education be recognized and that the priorities in learning in and through motor performance activities be established for persons of all ages and degrees of health.

Physical educators should work with early childhood educators to provide movement exploration and perceptual-motor development programs for three- and four-year olds, guided by knowledgeable and sensitive adults. Guided movement experiences and planned perceptual-motor challenges need not be limited to school environments but should be included in the services of day care centers, pediatric clinics, and varied social agency programs.

"Head Start" programs must be available for those with unusual movement education or motor development needs. Enrollment should not be restricted to children from welfare families or those with multiple disadvantages, but encouraged for every child whose daily environment lacks the stimulation of novel and varied movement tasks, or whose responses to such tasks suggest the need for more intensive or extensive movement experience.

Elementary School Programs

The youngest school learners should certainly have daily opportunities for movement experiences. Elementary school children may be programmed as classroom groups for some phases of physical education. However, some of the time allotted to physical education should be used to encourage the children to come to various movement learning centers, individually or in small groups, for self-directed individual learning projects, teacher-assisted supplementary practice of movement performance skills, or movement activities designed for groups of children from several different classrooms.

Elementary school physical education is highly individualized and personalized. Although children frequently participate in groups, they can be guided within these groups toward self-awareness, consciousness of position in time-space, and identification of a dynamic self in an environment of moving objects and other persons. Teachers of elementary school children in America's third century capitalize on the best that we have learned from each of the many advocates of Movement Education — guided exploration and discovery in a wide variety of activities with and without equipment; systematic and progressive experiences in fundamental locomotor skills and ball-handling skills; strenuous physical activity, involvement, and success for everyone; unique responses, creative expression, and dance for each child. Adults provide innovative equipment; children invent their own ways of moving over, under, and through it. Games as well as dances are created by the children.

Early Elementary School Curriculum. Much of the child's movement curriculum is organized to focus on moving in space. Curriculum content for the youngest school learners is designed to achieve purposes of body awareness, locomotion, object manipulation, and movement expression. Movement exploration techniques can be used to develop concepts of general body awareness, movement capabilities of various body parts, relationships of different body parts to each other, personal size relative to the external physical environment, and voluntary modification of individual body shape and size.

Basic *locomotor patterns* of walking, running, sliding, and jumping are the introductory content in the area of relocation and are learned, adapted, and refined through imitation, experimentation, solving movement tasks set by teachers, and performing such skills in self-testing, chasing, and rhythmic games. More complex locomotor patterns are introduced as the children demonstrate their readiness.

Ball- and *object-handling* activities involving throwing, catching, kicking, and striking also receive major attention. Primary grade children enjoy rolling, tossing, bouncing, and catching rubber balls, balloons, plastic balls, bean bags, beach balls, and yarn balls. They should participate in striking activities requiring *foot-eye coordination* as well as *hand-eye coordination*. They can develop object *reception skills* by catching parachutes or other objects dropped from a height; by intercepting rolled balls with feet, hands, or paddles; and by striking tossed objects with or without implements.

Communication-Based Curriculum. The elementary schools now view communication as a legitimate core around which to plan the curriculum, so that the various areas of study may contribute to each child's unique ability to cope with the world. Movement experiences in schools have come into their own in the last decade as educators have recognized the crucial role played by movement in self-expression and communication. Elementary learnings in using movement to relate to others are achieved through creative rhythms, folk dance, and games. Every child should have opportunities in physical education to express personal ideas and feelings through self-directed movement.

Learning Sequences. Learning sequences appropriate for most seven-, eight-, and nine-year-olds emphasize body projection, spatial relationships, object manipulation, and teamwork. In addition to the more complex locomotor skills such as galloping, hopping, leaping, and skipping, the child learns more advanced forms of propulsion on hanging and climbing apparatus, on poles, ropes, ladders, and stegels. Students develop more sophisticated concepts of directionality and spatial relationships and better body movement control through games emphasizing dodging, guarding stationary and moving objects, chasing, and tagging; and through stunts, tumbling, trampoline, and other kinds of gymnastic activities.

The teacher plans object-manipulation challenges using hoops, ropes, wands, batons, and many types of balls and striking implements. Games are selected and designed to provide practice in the particular movement skills already identified and to stimulate the development of elementary concepts of cooperation, competition, leadership, and the functioning of rules in group activities. Although concepts of body projection, spatial relationships, object manipulation, and teamwork generally determine learning progressions at this level, teachers are also alert to opportunities to emphasize self-knowledge, challenge, and movement expression.

Intermediate Level Elementary Physical Education. Purposes emphasized at the intermediate level are those of physiological efficiency, spatial orientation, object manipulation, and group interaction. Together with continuing attention to increasing efficiency in skill performance, learning sequences are designed for progressive development of strength, balance, agility, flexibility, and circulo-respiratory endurance. Elementary concepts of effective body mechanics are included. Modified track and field events are popular with both girls and boys.

Skills Integration. A major goal of the physical education program at this level is to help the student to integrate skills that involve coping with the physical environment and to guide the development of more sophisticated concepts of moving in space. Gymnastics are stressed; skating and basic swimming instruction are recommended. Students learn to maneuver weight with simple combatives such as handwrestling and in a variety of weight training activities using circuit training designs. Object projection activities focus on more advanced ball and stick skills and on competitive throwing events.

Group Interaction. Concepts of group interaction are stressed through group and team games, relays, and folk dance. Concepts of offense and defense and position play are introduced and the roles of partner, opponent, teammate, captain, squad leader, coach, official, and spectator are experienced and analyzed. Each child is encouraged to compete with himself or herself as well as to vie with others to achieve group and individual goals.

Cultural Involvement. Learning sequences are also structured to provide basic concepts and skills required for cultural involvement of preadolescents. For these purposes children learn rope-jumping, tether ball, hop-scotch, four-square, marbles, jacks, skating, swimming, kick-ball, dodgeball, prisoner's base, and other popular games. Many of these skills are learned and practiced by children in small groups as they select their own movement learning activites; often they learn these movements from classmates or older children rather than by formal teacher instruction.

Joy Through Movement. Popular games are introduced; but boys and girls are not separated to play them. Everyone is expected to feel pleasure in dancing, just as everyone is expected to run as fast as possible and to throw a ball as efficiently as the pupil's level of motor development will permit. Perhaps most important, teachers provide frequent guidance in individual awareness of the body in motion and of personal response to this inner being that compels the student to actively fight to retain and extend the feeling of human joy in physically demanding and psychologically exhilarating movement.

Physical education experiences throughout the elementary school are designed to assist the individual child in self-mastery, through development of an acceptable body image and a positive self-concept in movement settings. Each child should have ample opportunities for knowing personal joy in movement. Physical activities already discussed (movement exploration, fundamental locomotor movements, body management activities, ball and object handling practice, rhythms and dances, traditional and creative games) provide the learning media for reaching these goals.

Open Facilities. Open gymnasiums blend with open classrooms and the wide open space of the outdoor world to make it possible for children to learn, as whole persons, key concepts that often have more meaning when experienced in a bigger universe. True, some of the most important knowledges will begin to have meaning in the gymnasium; but certain motor concepts gain richer meanings when extended to outdoor education and survival camping. Personal awareness and self-direction need consistent supportive environments in school classrooms, laboratories, corridors, and playgrounds.

The middle school offers a unique challenge to the physical educator. Emphasis on extending the child's sensory perceptions should continue. It is more important that the pupil be aware of the feeling qualities of a successful physical performance than of the result as measured by a performance score. The child increases self-knowledge and self-confidence in experiencing gymnastic activities of all kinds; stunts which test balance and flexibility as well as strength; and dances which permit free and expressive movement as well as those which require precision, control, and endurance.

Middle School Programs

Middle schools are using modular scheduling, team teaching, ability grouping, large group instruction, small group instruction, and open laboratory plans effectively. The curriculum in middle school physical education should emphasize two major elements, expanding understanding of movement through refining personal skills, and greater depth of social understanding through experiences in movement activities of the student's own and other cultures.

Self-Mastery and Skill Achievement. Concepts of self-mastery are strengthened through achievement of higher levels of skill in familiar activities and by successfully meeting the challenges of learning new skills. Venturesome activities requiring more personal courage should be included. Students should attain a growing understanding of movement principles in situations emphasizing modifications of environmental media. Attention should be given to enriching the environment, to making the surroundings for physical activity pleasant. Much of the programmed activity should be conducted outdoors in the natural environment which will be available when the gymnasium doors are locked. Games played on the sand, in the snow, on the ice, on a grassy slope, or in the woods have special challenge and unique satisfaction. Track activities which have universal appeal — running, jumping, vaulting, throwing — can be given more prominence. Cross-country running can be added. Skiing may be introduced.

Swimming is a high priority. Aquatic experiences may comprise from 20 to 35 per cent of individual programs. All students should learn principles of buoyancy and adaptations of biomechanics, balance, and breathing appropriate to propulsion in the water. Instruction can include specific water survival techniques, elementary forms of rescue, standard stroke patterns, diving, water stunts, and electives for those students qualified for more advanced aquatic activities.

Tumbling, gymnastics, and trampolining are emphasized to extend concepts of spatial awareness, relocation and balance, and to encourage the development of body projection skills utilizing limited ground contact. Basic gymnastic skills acquired during elementary school years serve as a foundation for learning standard stunts required in competition on all pieces of apparatus. Capsule programs have been developed to assist students at a wide range of individual performance levels to work independently in large group instructional settings with minimum supervision. Creative exercise routines offer opportunities for fun and novelty as well as for the satisfaction of skill achievement.

New Games Movement.   The "new games movement" is attracting the attention of physical educators as "movement education" did in the 1960s. The concept of creating new games is appropriate to all age levels but might receive special emphasis in middle school programs. Every generation of middle school children enjoys its own innovations in play. The hula hoop, the scooter, the parachute, the whiffleball, and the skateboard are all examples. But the new games concept goes beyond acquiring new equipment and modifying the old games as in playing frisbee softball. As stated by the New Games Foundation:[69]

> When we play New Games, our goal is to have fun together. We want the players to enjoy the games they're playing—all of the players, not just some of them. And we want everyone to play who wants to.
> Sometimes, the search leads to remembering old games. Sometimes, to changing rules, or even creating games.... And the next step, after changing the rules, is to design new games.... Rather than replace competition with cooperation, we look for the right combination of competitive and cooperative games for a group of players....
> When no one is left out, when players can all use their different skills, when everyone feels recognized by the group, and can share in determining the rules, then players feel more trusting of each other. They become willing to become more involved, to play harder, and to suggest both games and ways to change games. It's easier for players to stand back at times, too, to wait and see where others will take the group. Eventually, a New Games play group becomes a play community, with everyone playing to their limits, and everyone taking part in making the playing fun.
> In other words, New Games is a process. It's not what you play, be it Earthball or baseball, but how you play. This process begins with

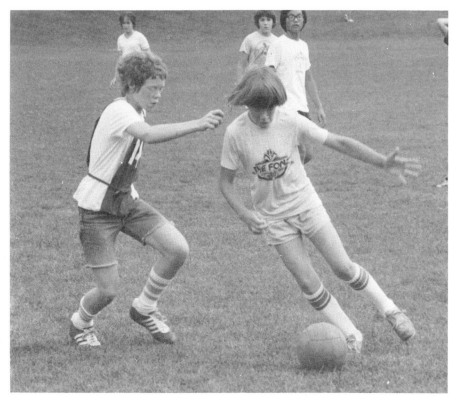

In middle schools, teamwork concepts are highlighted through instruction in such sports as soccer.

your own enjoyment, extends to an awareness of the other players, and eventually results in creating some altogether new ways to have fun.

Socialization and Cultural Understanding. Middle school organization offers unparalleled opportunities for socialization through the development of team sports and social dance skills. Skill development and team strategy are stressed in popular team games. Teamwork concepts are highlighted through instruction in soccer, touch football, basketball, volleyball, hockey, and softball. Group games which reflect the recreational interests of young people in other societies also should be introduced. Students from differing subcultures can share such aspects of their heritage with each other. Exchange students from other countries and local citizens or foreign visitors who have lived in regions where other games are popular can provide key resources. Social dance offerings may include traditional dances, American square dance, folk dances of many lands, and current popular dance forms. Opportunities for healthful competitive sport and for recreational dance should be varied and extensive in middle school extraclass programs.

Team activities and skills of the popular team sports clearly have a place in middle school physical education. However, the middle school curriculum planner must break away from the domination of high school athletics and the limitations of activities and drills selected to develop the specific skills of three or four competitive team games. At this age, there are still many sport and athletic possibilities to explore. The development of new games should be a goal of every teacher and every physical education class. Each child should have opportunities for self-testing in a physically demanding activity as well as to find satisfaction in self-mastery. For every body type, there is some physical activity which makes it possible to surpass physical limitations and become a more integrated part of the universe.

The physical education curriculum in the modern American high school has been modified by changing concepts of education and schooling and by the introduction of more flexible graduation requirements, and more options in course offerings; wider use of modular scheduling, team teaching, flexible grouping, and open campus organization; more student responsibility, more open laboratory and independent study programs; increasing demands for accountability; and greater student involvement in decision-making. The major goals of high school physical education curricula should include understanding and appreciation of human movement, physical fitness, and lifetime sports competence. Student assessment and program evaluation should be concerned with each of these areas; student learning progress should be guided according to demonstrated achievement in each of these areas.

Secondary School Programs

Biomechanics Principles and Movement as Communication. Understanding and appreciation of human movement should include knowledge of principles of human movement and the ability to apply these principles in sound body mechanics in daily movements, in participation in physical recreation activities, and in learning new work or leisure skills. It encompasses abilities to use movement as an expressive and communicative medium. Secondary school students can develop these abilities through choreographic experiences in dance, water ballet, or free exercise, or through developing new games or movement forms. Student projects have included designing movement sequences for musical and theatrical productions, staging physical education demonstrations, programming movement for film or television showing, and planning novelty events for local track and field days, archery meets, or aquatic fun nights.

Discovering Roles of Movement and Sport. Physical education learnings in movement understanding and appreciation should also include introduction to the role of human movement activities in society. Movement appreciation offerings can provide analysis of the historical role of sport in various cultures; explore the critical role of movement in child development; highlight basic concepts of sociology of sport and of sport psychology; and identify contemporary social problems relating to sport locally, nationally, and internationally. Student participation experiences in guiding movement activities of children, leading neighborhood activity programs, planning family recreation activities, or engaging in movement activities of other societies or particular subcultures are especially desirable.

Physical Fitness. The development of physical fitness is discussed in detail in Chapter 5. As a goal in the high school curriculum, it is reasonable that students demonstrate individually appropriate levels of muscular strength, circulo-respiratory endurance, and survival aquatics. Adequate assessment techniques are available and adapted programs should be provided for students with unusual needs in this area, in secondary school as at all other educational levels. Students should have several options for achieving desired levels of fitness, including participation in vigorous sports of their choice, as well as such fitness activities as weight training, jogging, circuit training, and developmental exercise programs.

Lifetime Sports Competence. More and more schools are adopting competence in lifetime sports as a physical education program requirement. Numbers, types, and participation levels for identifying "lifetime sports" goals must be determined at the local level. Competence standards should be practical tests of ability to participate at a personally satisfying level, since the intent is to provide instruction in procedures for planning personal activity programs and to encourage voluntary participation throughout life. The secondary school student should be free to select from among many elective sport offerings at beginning, intermediate, or advanced levels.

Developing the "Ultimate Athlete." Humanistic educators are urging a shift of emphasis in secondary school physical education. They are insisting that true understanding and appreciation of human movement, and a total education, should go beyond the typical goals of even our best current programs, and focus on the personal search for what Leonard[70] has termed the *ultimate athlete*. According to Leonard's definition, there is no single ultimate athlete. Each of our students has unsuspected human potential; each could become the ultimate athlete. If we, as educators, are to effectively aid the search, we must remember that changes in the nature of what is satisfying and rewarding to human individuals are bound to accompany significant social reforms.

Awareness Activities and Risk Sports. Activities that might receive greater emphasis in the secondary school include running, aquatics, dance, dual sports, and "risk" sports. Running is the essence of most sports. It is the best test of all-around conditioning. It can also be a varied, fascinating, demanding, keenly satisfying activity. Youth who are out of touch with their own feelings and the realities of the environment can be guided through "run for awareness" programs to discover, as even middle-aged persons have, that running is its own reward.

Aquatics brings the athlete in touch with a relatively unknown realm as mastery of the mysteries of propulsion through water opens up such worlds as diving, surfing, and scuba diving. Dance can be openness to existence and full awareness, an attitude toward life which restores perspective. Dual sports in the secondary school are refined as a cooperative enterprise of two participants, providing the strongest possible defense as a stimulus for an ever-more-skillful offense, initiating each new action as a variation in the rhythmic flow of vigorous human activity.

The growth of "risk" sports during the past 30 years has been phenomenal. Rock-climbing, sky-diving, skiing, skin-diving, hang-gliding are a few examples. Perhaps one reason for the increasing popularity of "risk" sports is the opportunity afforded for integration with the universe. Evidence has been reported that regular participation in risk sports makes us more efficient, more creative, and more productive persons. Perhaps it is

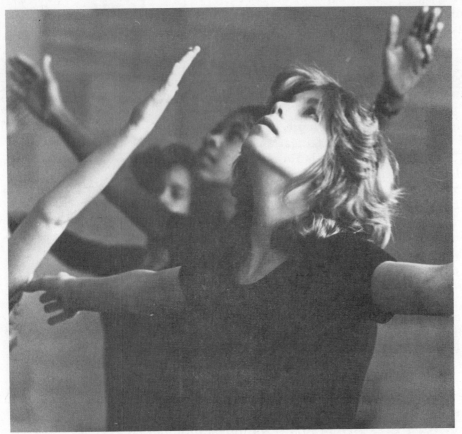

Dance can be openness to existence and full awareness, an attitude toward life which restores perspective.

because these sports share not only an element of risk, but also aspects of boundaries crossed, limitations transcended, and perceptions gained.[71]

These suggested activities all provide possible contexts for learning balance and centering, for developing greater conscious awareness and body balance, for strengthening the motivation and willingness to push beyond previous physical limitations. All of these should be among the goals of school physical education. Our programs should also help every young person to find his or her own game. If our present games do not offer the right choices, new games can be invented. It is time to create new games with new rules more in tune with the times, especially games with no spectators and no second-string players.

Compulsory College Physical Education. While physical educators are practically unanimous in their endorsement of a required program in elementary and secondary schools, there exists a wide variety of opinion regarding the requirement in colleges and universities. Probably all physical educators agree that it would be well to have every college student

COLLEGE PROGRAMS

CHAPTER SEVEN

engaged in appropriate and enjoyable activities, but many are unwilling to support a compulsory program. Actual practices in colleges illustrate this diversity of opinion. Because of rapidly expanding enrollment on limited campus space, decreasing specific requirements in higher education generally, and increasing pressures toward fiscal economy, the recent trend is toward reduction or elimination of physical education requirements.

Community colleges enrolling large numbers of youth for post-secondary education need to give particular attention to changing the focus of physical education programs from repetition of traditional secondary school courses to innovative programs designed to have genuine relevance for young adults. Four-year colleges and universities should give similar attention to "basic instruction" programs designed primarily for entering freshman students; their major contribution probably should be made through expanding elective programs to all undergraduate and graduate students. Analysis of the college physical education curriculum using the Purpose Process Curriculum Framework suggests that the purposes which provide soundest direction are physiological efficiency, psychic equilibrium, communication, and cultural involvement, and that the processes to be emphasized are perceiving, refining, varying, improvising, and composing.

Personal Physical Conditioning and Fulfillment. Many of today's college students are genuinely interested in personalized physical conditioning regimens. Designing program offerings attractive to college students seeking to improve and maintain their functional capabilities would result in courses of instruction in aerobic training, weight training, and neuromuscular relaxation. It would provide the rationale for adding class sections in scuba diving, judo, and orienteering. It would require laboratories equipped for student self-assessment of conditioning levels and individual self-directed exercise routines. It would support requests for jogging trails, bicycle traffic lanes, expanded swimming facilities, and all-season orienteering courses.

The college student who looks to the physical education department for opportunities to achieve personal integration may be seeking joy of movement, self-knowledge, catharsis, challenge, or any combination of these. Some haven't experienced genuine pleasure in strenuous physical activity since early childhood and have forgotten the pure joy inherent in vigorous human motion. As young adults, one may find joy in simple running, another in dance, a third in springboard diving. Others prefer the sensations of movement characteristic of gymnastics, swimming, or physical combat sports.

Self-knowledge can be gained through basic movement instruction (often remedial in nature); but it can also be enhanced through participation in any one or several of a multitude of activities that permit the individual to determine what he or she, as a functioning organism, is capable of doing and becoming. Successful learning may increase self-appreciation as one extends physical capabilities beyond limits previously accepted. College youth may experience catharsis in conditioning exercises, running, dance, skating, sailing, handball, tennis, wrestling, karate, volleyball, or softball. An individual may test prowess and courage in a wide spectrum of activities; those that offer great challenge to many college-age individuals certainly include skiing, surfing, fencing, riding, mountain climbing, and sky diving.

Today's typical undergraduate is preoccupied with the search for identity. A wide variety of appropriate physical education experiences can be structured to support the human quest for personal integration or transcendence. College and university students need continuing opportunities for physical activity programs emphasizing personal fitness development, participation in lifetime sports, and body experience focused in a personal becoming. Those still seeking a "fit" in an activity medium might be guided into inner tennis, awareness running, yoga, orienteering, or zen archery.

Communication and Social Involvement. Communication is a fundamental human activity. It is a prime concern of this generation of college and university students. Physical education classes could become more nearly exemplary in providing an environment for healthful interpersonal communication, and extra-class programs could be conducted in ways that would facilitate more open communications among students and faculty members. It is recommended that greater emphasis be given to opportunities within our programs for the development of personal movement communications skills. Words do not represent the only means of communication any more than they represent the only means of learning. Among common purposes of human movement, one moves to share ideas and feelings with others. College programs in dance and other forms of expressive movement should maximize opportunities for enhancing individual communicative movement skill.

A major contribution of physical education to cultural involvement concerns the individual's desire for participation in social movement activities. Sport is a cultural universal. The popularity of specific activities varies cross-culturally, but participation in sport is a phenomenon which exists in all societies. Physical recreation programs in college and university communities should provide opportunities for ethnic subgroups to enjoy and extend interest in movement activities which lend uniqueness to a particular cultural heritage. Instructional electives should provide for the development of advanced skills in these activities as well as for skill development in currently popular adult physical recreation activities.

Influence of Local Interests and Campus Environment. College students all over the United States are interested in being able to participate in tennis, golf, bowling, handball, volleyball, and social dancing. Local interests and facilities determine whether students seek opportunities to learn sailing, judo, orienteering, mountain climbing, curling, fencing, ballet, casting, skiing, scuba, surfing, or white water canoeing. General college programs in physical education should be directed toward helping the young adult to become an educated and more appreciative observer of sports and expressive movement forms as well as a more skillful participant in chosen activities. Full participation in society includes both direct involvement in sport and dance and the intellectual, aesthetic, and emotional involvement of indirect participation in movement activities.

The scope of a college or university physical education curriculum is determined by the common purposes of human movement sought by selected young adults in a particular campus environment. Important

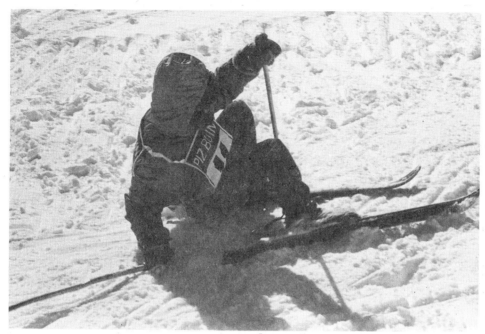

Local interests and facilities determine where students seek opportunities to learn.

curricular decisions must also be made relative to the process orientation of teaching-learning opportunities. The most typical movement process needs of American college and university students are perceiving, refining, varying, improvising, and composing.

Kinesthetic Perception.   The movement process of perceiving is usually associated with preschool or elementary school learning. However, many freshmen still enter our colleges and universities without having experienced quality foundational elementary and secondary school physical education; as long as this circumstance continues, remedial instruction should be provided in basic movement, movement fundamentals, or foundations of human movement. Specialized laboratory offerings in posture, relaxation, object projection, and rhythmic training may also be needed. In addition to remedial work directed toward perceiving movement, college-level physical education should be concerned with increasing levels of sophistication in perceiving. Regardless of the level of physical performance skill, the college student can profit from greater kinesthetic awareness, keener sensitivity to personal perceptual-motor responses, and deeper understanding of the integrated perceptual-motor act.

Refining Skills.   While the learning of new sports or physical activities selected by the college student necessitates learning and adapting movement patterns, the focus in much of our sports instruction should be on the ordinative processes of refining learned movement patterns. We need to offer more courses designed to help participants achieve intermediate or advanced levels of skill. Instruction should aim toward the acquisition of smooth, efficient control of performance through the elimination of extraneous movements, the mastery of spatial and temporal relations resulting in precision timing, and habitual skillful performance under more complex conditions.

Cultivating Creativity. It is generally agreed that our civilization must find better ways to encourage and nurture creativity. The very least physical educators can do is to permit freedom for the generation of possibilities and to offer guidance in the development of creative movement potential. Although many college students today have almost no prior physical education experience with creative movement processes, they can be encouraged to construct unique or novel options in performing movement patterns or skills. Variations in techniques for returning a badminton serve, putting a golf ball, negotiating a slalom course, or drawing a fencing opponent off balance may serve the individual's purpose more effectively than the "correct" style as the instructor learned it. Classes can be structured to maximize opportunities for extemporaneous origination or initiation of novel movements or combinations of movements and thus give students more experience and skill in improvising. Courses in choreography or composing movement can be designed to achieve advanced competency in dance, aquatic arts, or gymnastics. They can be planned as independent study options to challenge students capable of creating new games or movement forms, or as interdisciplinary courses integrating the creativity resources of more than one department.

Continuing Physical Education Programs

Physical education can no longer neglect its responsibility to the adult who is not seeking a high school diploma or a college or university degree. Seeking personal well-being and harmony through physical activity is a lifelong pursuit. Continuing education in this field of knowledge is as vital to individual physical and mental health, adult personal development, and societal advancement as continuing education in any other broad subject area. Opportunity for participation and educational guidance in the quest for fitness, sport performance ability, and self-actualization through physical activity is a right of the adults who outnumber the full-time student population in this country.

Developing the Adult "Inner Athlete." Continuing education programs sponsored by local public school districts, colleges and universities, and public and private agencies should build in physical education offerings which focus on fitness for life. They should provide instruction in how to evaluate one's own level of fitness, how to set individual and realistic goals for improving fitness status, and how to plan personal exercise and activity programs to maintain the level of individual fitness desired. They should seek to develop in adults commitment to schedules which build in a continuing search for the "inner athlete." Schools, colleges, and public service agencies should extend instructional opportunities to encourage adults to develop active recreation participation knowledges and skills selected from a wide range of potential lifetime sports. Considerable emphasis should be placed on safety knowledges and attitudes, especially those relating to essential conditioning and preparation for such activities

CHAPTER SEVEN

as marathon running, minimizing hazards in such popular sports as aquatics, and wise selection of sports clothing and equipment. The relationships of exercise to such health concerns as diet and drug usage should also be included. Education of parents and future parents concerning the facilitation of normal motor development and the guidance of children in sport and physical activity programs is essential.

The general public needs to be more informed about the importance of supporting programs of continuing physical education and active recreation. Taxpayers' demands for economy must not result in short-sighted savings through cuts in essential educational and recreational facilities and services. This nation needs more public lands where jogging trails provide access to beautiful surroundings, where orienteering courses can be set for athletes of varying abilities, where adults and children together can discover new games. Expansions, not cuts, are needed in most public park and recreation programs. Neighborhoods, housing developments, public institutions, corporate complexes, and retirement areas need facilities for exercise and physical activity and educational services to stimulate their effective use.

Public programs should complement and extend the growing adult physical education opportunities in the private sector and ensure that such opportunities are available to all adults. We need more clubs and social groups, public and private, with common interest in tennis, golf, racquetball, camping, aquatics, skiing, hiking and climbing. We need more programs in which we can choose to learn the "inner game" of tennis or other selected activity, as well as perpetually popular approaches to sports instruction. The importance of continuing education for adults is widely recognized. Americans need to be more alert to the significance of continuing physical education as an essential component of this total concept.

SUMMARY

The challenges still confronting all teachers and administrators of physical education are the need for constant curriculum improvement, better selection of activities, development of new activities that can provide even more desirable learning experiences for students, improvement of instructional methods and organization procedures, and more effective appraisal techniques.

Physical education, like all other curricular areas, seeks "frontier thinkers," leaders with vision who, through creative thought, are willing to experiment with new ideas in curriculum development. The authors argue that the greater current challenge lies in clarification of the essentially human variables in physical education curricular decision making — the purposes and processes of human movement. What any one of us achieves as a moving being will always depend upon human purposes. What meaning an individual finds in movement experiences will always be a function of how appropriate the processes are to his or her unique needs. The opportunities are unlimited.

[1]Elliot W. Eisner and Elizabeth Vallance, *Conflicting Conceptions of Curriculum*. Berkeley: McCutchan, 1974. p. 10.

[2]Lesley H. Browder, Jr., *Emerging Patterns of Administrative Accountability*. Berkeley: McCutchan Publishing Corporation, 1971.

[3]Chris Pipho, "Minimum Competency Testing in 1978: A Look at State Standards," *Phi Delta Kappan*, 59:585–588 (May, 1978).

[4]Walter Sandefur and Douglas Westbrook, "Involvement of AACTE Institutions in CBTE: A Follow-up Study," *Phi Delta Kappan*, 59:633–634 (May, 1978).

[5]Henry M. Brickell, "Seven Key Notes on Minimum Competency Testing," *Phi Delta Kappan*, 59:589–592 (May, 1978).

[6]Arthur E. Wise, "Minimum Competency Testing: Another Case of Hyper-Rationalization," *Phi Delta Kappan*, 59:596–598 (May, 1978).

[7]Morril J. Clute, "Humanistic Education: Goals and Objectives," *Humanistic Education: Objectives and Assessment*. Washington, D.C.: Association for Supervision and Curriculum Development, 1978. p. 9.

[8]Donald E. Orlosky and B. Othanel Smith. *Curriculum Development: Issues and Insights*. Chicago: Rand McNally, 1978. (Chapter 3.)

[9]William Bridges, "The Three Faces of Humanistic Education," *Liberal Education*, 59:325–335 (October, 1973).

[10]Association for Supervision and Curriculum Development. *Humanistic Education: Objectives and Assessment*. Washington, D.C.: ASCD, 1978, pp. 9–10.

[11]Association for Supervision and Curriculum Development. *Humanistic Education: Objectives and Assessment*. Washington, D.C.: ASCD, 1978, pp. 52–55.

[12]Arthur W. Foshay, "Curriculum Design for the Humane School," *Theory Into Practice*, 10:204–207 (June, 1971).

[13]J. Bronowski, *The Identity of Man*. Garden City, N.Y.: Natural History Press, 1971.

[14]Harold A. Linstone, and W. H. Clive Simmonds, *Futures Research: New Directions*. Reading, Mass.: Addison-Wesley, 1977.

[15]Harold G. Shane, "America's Educational Futures 1976–2001, *The Futurist*, X:252–257 (October, 1976).

[16]Harold G. Shane, *The Educational Significance of the Future*. Bloomington, Indiana. Phi Delta Kappa Educational Foundation, 1973, pp. 68–91.

[17]Bruce R. Joyce, Marsha Weil, and Rhoada Wald, "The Training of Educators: A Structure for Pluralism." *Teachers College Record*, 73:371–391 (February, 1972).

[18]Roger A. Kaufman, *Educational System Planning*. Englewood Cliffs, N.J.: Prentice-Hall, Inc., 1972.

[19]Margaret Gill Hein, "Planning and Organizing for Improved Instruction," *Curriculum Handbook for School Executives*. Arlington, Va.: American Association for School Administrators, 1973, p. 366.

[20]*Career Education*. U.S. Department of Health, Education, and Welfare Publication No. (OE) 72–39.

[21]Arthur W. Foshay, "Curriculum." From Robert L. Ebel, (ed.), *Encyclopedia of Educational Research*. (4th ed.) London: Macmillan, 1969.

[22]Ronald C. Doll, "The Multiple Forces Affecting Curriculum Change," *Phi Delta Kappan*, 51:382–384 (March, 1970).

[23]Arthur W. Foshay, "Curriculum." From Robert L. Ebel, (ed.), *Encyclopedia of Educational Research* (4th ed.). London: Macmillan, 1969.

[24]James B. Macdonald, "Values Bases and Issues for Curriculum," *Curriculum Theory* (Alex Molnar and John A. Zahorik, eds.). Washinton, D.C.: Association for Supervision and Curriculum Development, 1977. p. 11.

[25]Ann E. Jewett and Marie R. Mullan, *Curriculum Design: Purposes and Processes in Physical Education Teaching-Learning*. Washington, D.C.: American Alliance for Health, Physical Education, Recreation and Dance, 1977.

[26a]Ibid., p. 4.

[26b]Ibid., pp. 4–5.

[26c]Ibid., pp. 9–10.

[27]J. Lloyd Trump, *Images of the Future*. Washington, D.C.: National Association of Secondary School Principals, 1961.

[28]J. Lloyd Trump, "The NASSP Model Schools Program for Health, Physical Education, Recreation." From Helen M. Heitmann, (ed.), *Organizational Patterns for Instruction in Physical Education*. Washington, D.C.: American Alliance for Health, Physical Education, Recreation and Dance, 1971.

[29]J. Lloyd Trump and Dorsey Baynham, *Focus on Change: Guide to Better Schools*. Chicago: Rand McNally and Co., 1961.

[30]American Association for Health, Physical Education, Recreation and Dance. *Organizational Patterns for Instruction in Physical Education*, Helen M. Meitmann (ed.), Washington, D.C.: AAHPERD, 1971.

[31]Helen M. Heitmann, "Rationale for Change." From Helen M. Heitmann (ed.), *Organizational Patterns for Instruction in Physical Education.* Washington, D.C.: American Association for Health, Physical Education, Recreation and Dance, 1971.

[32]Craig Cunningham, "Movement Education at the University Elementary School." From Helen M. Heitmann (ed.), *Organizational Patterns for Instruction in Physical Education.* Washington, D.C.: American Association for Health, Physical Education, Recreation and Dance, 1971.

[33]Delores M. Curtis, "Bringing about Change in Organizational Patterns in Elementary Schools." From Helen M. Heitmann (ed.), *Organizational Patterns for Instruction in Physical Education.* Washington, D.C.: American Association for Health, Physical Education, Recreation and Dance, 1971.

[34]Robert Burson, "Nongraded Curriculum and Modular Scheduling." From Helen M. Heitmann (ed.), *Organizational Patterns for Instruction in Physical Education and Recreation.* Washington, D.C.: American Association for Health, Physical Education, Recreation and Dance, 1971.

[35]Helen M. Heitmann, op. cit.

[36]Ibid., pp. 30–31.

[37]John C. Gilmore, *The Professional Levels of Tasks of Teachers of Boys' Physical Education.* Unpublished Ed.D. dissertation, Stanford, Calif.: School of Education, Stanford University, 1967.

[38]J. Lloyd Trump, *New Horizons for Secondary School Teachers.* Urbana, Ill.: Commission on the Experimental Study of the Utilization of the Staff in the Secondary School, 1957.

[39]J. Lloyd Trump, *Images of the Future.* Washington, D.C.: National Association of Secondary School Principals, 1961.

[40]J. Lloyd Trump and Dorsey Baynham. *Focus on Change: Guide to Better Schools.* Chicago: Rand McNally and Co., 1961.

[41]J. Lloyd Trump, "The NASSP Model Schools Program for Health, Physical Education, Recreation." From Helen M. Heitmann (ed.), *Organizational Patterns for Instruction in Physical Education.* Washington, D.C.: American Association for Health, Physical Education, Recreation and Dance, 1971.

[42]Helen M. Heitmann, op cit., pp. 8–13.

[43]Chalmer G. Hixson, "Television in Physical Education," *Quest,* XV:58–66 (January, 1971).

[44]T. C. Jordan, "Micro-Teaching: A Reappraisal of Its Value in Teacher Education," *Quest,* XV:17–21 (January, 1971).

[45]John E. Nixon, "Innovations in Teacher Education," *J. Phys. Educ-Rec.,* 37:55–57 (September, 1966).

[46]T. C. Jordan, op. cit.

[47]Chalmer G. Hixson, op. cit.

[48]*Shelter for Physical Education.* College Station, Texas: Texas A & M College, Texas Engineering Experiment Station, 1961.

[49]*School Construction Systems Development: The Project and the Schools.* New York: Educational Facilities Laboratories, Inc., 1967.

[50]*Air Structures for School Sports.* New York: Educational Facilities Laboratory, 1966.

[51]Muska Mosston, *The Teaching of Physical Education: From Command to Discovery.* Columbus, Ohio: Charles E. Merrill Publishing Co., 1966.

[52]Association for Supervision and Curriculum Development. *The Unstudied Curriculum.* Washington, D.C.: ASCD, 1971.

[53]Michael Apple, "The Hidden Curriculum and the Nature of Conflict," *Interchange,* 2:27–43 (1971).

[54]Philip Jackson, *Life in Classrooms.* New York: Holt, Rinehart, and Winston, 1968.

[55]Lawrence Kohlberg, "Moral Education for a Society in Transition," *Educational Leadership,* 33:46–54 (October, 1975).

[56]Linda L. Bain, "Description of the Hidden Curriculum in Secondary Physical Education," *Research Quarterly* 47:154–160 (May, 1976).

[57]Bruce R. Joyce, Marsha Weil, and Rhoada Wald, op. cit.

[58]Marilyn LaPlante, *Evaluation of a Selected List of Purposes of Physical Education Utilizing a Modified Delphi Technique.* Unpublished doctoral dissertation, University of Wisconsin, Madison, 1973.

[59]Sheila Stanley, *Physical Education: A Movement Orientation.* Toronto: McGraw-Hill Book Co., 1969.

[60]Joan Tillotson, *A Program of Movement Education for the Plattsburgh Elementary Schools.* Final report of Title III Elementary and Secondary Education Program, 1969.

[61]Paul Vogel, "Battle Creek Physical Education Project," *J. Phys. Educ. Rec.,* 40:25–29 (September, 1969).

[62]Marlin M. Mackenzie, *Toward A New Curriculum in Physical Education.* New York: McGraw-Hill Book Co., 1969.

[63]Ruby Lee Pye, and Ruth Hammock Alexander, *Physical Education Concepts: A Teaching-Learning Guide*. Middleton, KY.: Maxwell Co., 1971.

[64]Patricia L. Austin, "A Conceptual Structure of Physical Education for the School Program." Unpublished doctoral dissertation, Michigan State University, 1965.

[65]Camille Brown, "The Structure of Knowledge in Physical Education." *Quest* IX:53–67 (December, 1967).

[66]Camille Brown, and Rosalind Cassidy, *Theory in Physical Education: A Guide to Program Change*. Philadelphia: Lea and Febiger, 1963.

[67]Ann E. Jewett, and Marie R. Mullan, op. cit.

[68]Ibid.

[69]New Games Foundation, *New Games Resource Catalog*. San Francisco: 1979, i.

[70]George Leonard, *The Ultimate Athlete*. New York: Viking Press, 1975.

[71]Ibid.

American Association for Health, Physical Education and Recreation. *TV: Production and Utilization in Physical Education*, Washington, D.C.: AAHPER, 1971.

American Association for Health, Physical Education and Recreation. *College Physical Education— The General Program*, Washington, D.C.: AAHPER, 1973.

American Alliance for Health, Physical Education, Recreation and Dance, *Planning Facilities for Athletics, Physical Education and Recreation*. Washington, D.C.: AAHPERD, 1979.

American Alliance for Health, Physical Education and Recreation, *Adapted Physical Education Guidelines; Theory and Practices for 70's and 80's*. Washington, D.C.: AAHPER, 1976.

American Alliance for Health, Physical Education and Recreation, *Complying with Title IX in Physical Education and Sports*. Washington, D.C.: AAHPER, 1976.

American Alliance for Health, Physical Education and Recreation, *Ideas for Secondary School Physical Education*. Washington, D.C.: AAHPER, 1976.

American Alliance for Health, Physical Education and Recreation, *Personalized Learning in Physical Education*. Washington, D.C.: AAHPER, 1976.

American Alliance for Health, Physical Education and Recreation, *Echoes of Influence for Elementary School Physical Education*. Washington, D.C.: AAHPER, 1977.

American Alliance for Health, Physical Education and Recreation, *Programs That Work - Title IX*. Washington, D.C.: AAHPER, 1978.

American Educational Research Association, *Perspectives of Curriculum Evaluation*. Monograph Series on Curriculum Evaluation. Smith, B. Othanel (ed.). Chicago: Rand McNally and Co., 1967.

Berman, Louise M. and Roderick, Jessie A., *Feeling, Valuing and the Art of Growing: Insights into the Affective*. Washington, D.C.: ASCD, 1977.

Brandwein, Paul F., *The Permanent Agenda of Man: The Humanities*. New York: Harcourt, Brace, Jovanovich, 1971.

Brown, George I., *Human Teaching for Human Learning: An Introduction to Confluent Education*. New York: The Viking Press, Inc., 1971.

Cheffers, John and Evaul, Tom, *Introduction to Physical Education: Concepts of Human Movement*. Englewood Cliffs, N.J.: Prentice-Hall, 1978.

Eisner, Elliot W., and Vallance, Elizabeth (eds.), *Conflicting Conceptions of Curriculum*. Berkeley: McCutchan, 1974.

Goodlad, John I., The Development of a Conceptual System for Dealing with Problems of Curriculum and Instruction. ERIC Report Resume ED# 010–064. Washington, D.C.: USOE, 1966.

Haag, Herbert, *Sport Pedagogy: Content and Methodology*. Baltimore: University Park Press, 1978.

Heitmann, H. M. and Kneer, M. E., *Physical Education Instructional Techniques*. Englewood Cliffs, N.J.: Prentice-Hall, 1976.

Humanistic Education: Objectives and Assessment. Washington, D.C.: Association for Supervision and Curriculum Development, 1978.

Jewett, Ann E., "Key Concepts in Program Development with Proposed Taxonomy of Educational Objectives," *Sport for All*. Tehran, Iran: Michael Rice and Company, 1973.

Jewett, Ann E., "Relationships in Physical Education: A Curriculum Viewpoint," *The Academy Papers*. Washington, D.C.: American Academy of Physical Education, 1977.

Jewett, Ann E. and Mullan, Marie R., *Curriculum Design: Purposes and Processes in Physical Education Teaching-Learning*. Washington, D.C.: American Alliance for Health, Physical Education, Recreation and Dance, 1977.

Journal of Physical Education and Recreation, "Focus on Community Recreation Facilities," *JOPER* 48:9 (Nov.-Dec., 1977). pp. 33–46.

Journal of Physical Education and Recreation, "What's Happening in Facilities," *JOPERD* 49:6. (June, 1978). pp. 33–48.

Leonard, George, *The Ultimate Athlete*. New York: Viking Press, 1975.

Linstone, Harold A. and Simmonds, W. H. Clive, *Futures Research: New Directions*. Reading, Mass.: Addison-Wesley, 1977.

Macdonald, James B., Wolfson, Bernice J. and Esther Zaret, *Reschooling Society: A Conceptual Model*. Washington, D.C.: ASCD, 1973.

Molnar, Alex, and Zahorik, John A. (eds.), *Curriculum Theory*, Washington, D.C.: ASCD, 1977.

Nixon, John E., and Locke, Lawrence F., "Research on Teaching Physical Education." From Travers, R.M.W. (ed.), *Second Handbook of Research on Teaching*. Chicago: Rand McNally, 1973. pp. 1210–1242.

Pinar, William (ed.), *Curriculum Theorizing*. Berkeley: McCutchan, 1975.

Pipho, Chris, "Minimum Competency Testing in 1978: A Look at State Standards," *Phi Delta Kappan*, 59:585–588 (May, 1978).

Siedentop, Daryl, *Developing Teaching Skills in Physical Education*. Boston: Houghton Mifflin, 1976.

Travers, Robert M. W. (ed.), *Second Handbook of Research on Teaching*. Chicago: Rand McNally and Co., 1973.

Ulrich, Celeste, and John E. Nixon (eds.), *Tones of Theory*. Washington, D.C.: AAHPERD, 1972.

Unruh, Glenys C., *Responsive Curriculum Development: Theory and Action*. Berkeley, Calif.: McCutchan, 1978.

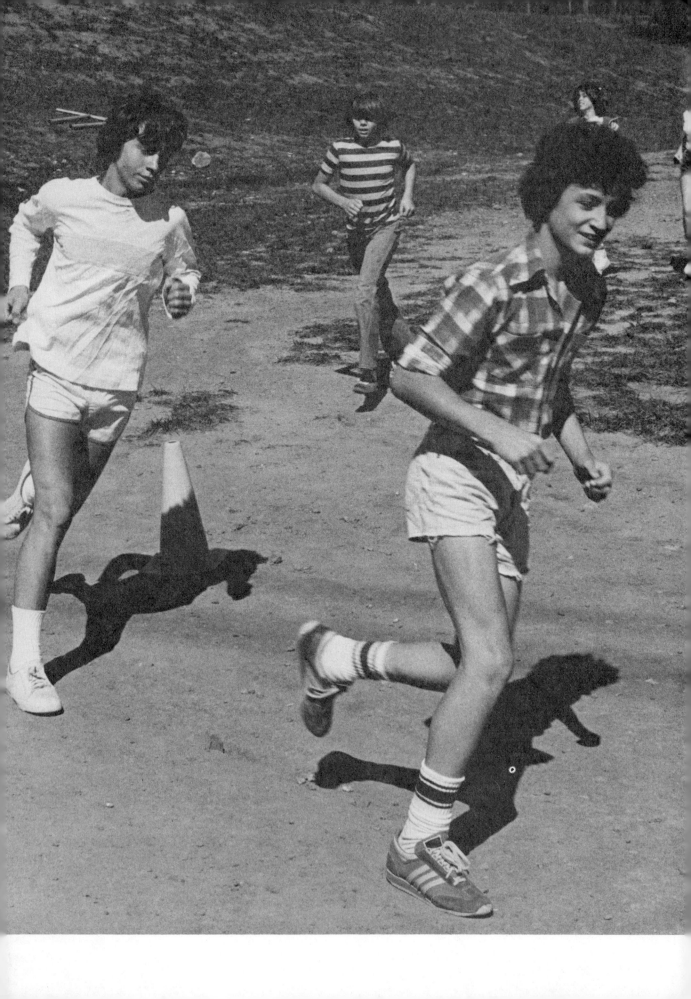

8

TEACHING PHYSICAL ——————— ——————— EDUCATION

Teaching children, youth, and adults to participate with skill and enjoyment in sport, dance, and gymnastic exercises is a professional occupation freely engaged in by hundreds of thousands of teachers, coaches, sport leaders, and others in the United States and around the world. *Coaching* is a specialized area of teaching that usually involves the formal instruction of organized sport team members requiring qualified assistance in order to perform skillfully for personal and organizational purposes. Teaching and coaching occur in physical education and sport settings of many types — schools, colleges, universities, private clubs, commercial clubs, voluntary groups, community recreation programs, youth organizations, industrial groups, governmental organizations, professional sport teams, dance performance groups, and so on. It would be very difficult to estimate accurately the number of persons who teach and coach participants of all ages in sport, dance, and gymnastic exercises in the United States.

We may assume that most teachers and coaches are motivated by an intrinsic desire to assist others in learning and performing sports, dance, and exercises and to help make these experiences pleasurable and fulfilling. Of course, involvement with professional athletes and dancers is accompanied by the primary motivation of financial gain.

This book is designed mainly for the purpose of discussing physical education, dance, and exercise in formal school settings; therefore, its main emphasis is on the students, teachers, coaches, and administrators who learn and work within the academic community. This chapter focuses on the phenomenon of teaching. We will review selected terms used often in this text and present models of teaching; a discussion concerning effective teaching will then follow, accompanied with an outline of selected approaches to teaching in physical education.

Teaching. Teaching occurs when one individual deliberately attempts to assist another individual, or a group of persons, in performing or

283

learning a specific activity or concept. The key to the definition is the *intent* on the part of the teacher to provide assistance to another person or persons in learning. When the teacher directs the students to engage in specific behaviors with the intention of producing definite outcomes, the procedure is called "product" teaching. The teacher may also attempt to create an environment in which the student will experience a specific emotion, a skill in action, or a sense of appreciation; although no tangible or identifiable product comes from such a procedure, it involves intentional teaching nonetheless. In sum, the deliberate attempt by one person to assist others in performing, learning, or experiencing is the fundamental concept in the definition of teaching.

Teaching does not always result in learning. There can be incidents of teaching with no learning, and examples of learning with no other person involved in a teaching role. Teaching is only one of several important variables that can influence pupil learning.

Gage[1] defines teaching as "any kind of interpersonal influence aimed at improving the learning of another person." We believe that teaching occurs when the teacher and the student are in direct personal interaction with each other. Siedentop[2] says that the purpose of teaching is "to help students learn and grow, to design environments where changes in the cognitive, social, affective, and the motor behavior of students can be accomplished efficiently, and to do it all in a manner that enables the students to enjoy the learning experience and to learn to enjoy the activity or subject matter being studied."

Management. The teacher is continually engaged in other duties and responsibilities not included in the previous definition of teaching. In fact, classroom studies have demonstrated that teachers spend less time in formal teaching and more time in *classroom management* than is generally realized. Teachers may spend as little as 30 percent of their total time in the classroom (including physical education instructional areas such as gymnasium, basketball and tennis courts, baseball fields, swimming pools, and similar areas) teaching the students. Much of the remaining time of the entire day at school is devoted to management activities and responsibilities. Planning the lesson, accumulating and preparing instructional facilities, equipment, and supplies, planning evaluation instruments, controlling and disciplining the students, and doing various other tasks that must be performed to set up and control the educational environment and the activities of the students — all fall in the category of classroom management. Although informal, or incidental learning may occur on the part of some or all of the pupils at any given time while the teacher is engaged in management responsibility (including negative learning), these teacher functions are not being undertaken for the express purpose of eliciting pupil learning. Therefore, these teacher activities are classified as management functions rather than teaching behaviors.

Instruction. The terms teaching and instruction often are used synonymously but such usage is incorrect and should be avoided. *Instruction* refers to the combination of teaching and classroom management. Both are the primary responsiblity of the teacher but their functions and purposes are distinct; too often teachers confuse these concepts when they should be differentiated. Student teachers and inexperienced teachers are more likely to suffer this confusion to the detriment of their ability to plan and teach effectively. Therefore, it is essential for teaching success that teachers conceptually and behaviorally distinguish when they

CHAPTER EIGHT

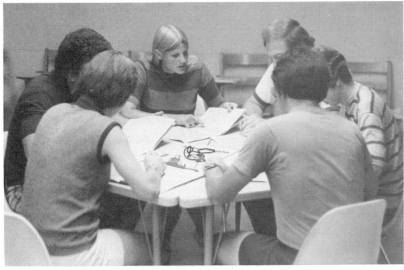

"Classroom management" includes such duties as lesson planning and preparing evaluation instruments, as well as other assorted tasks.

are engaging in teaching acts, and when they are performing management responsibilities.

Coaching. Obviously, this term is frequently used in schools and colleges, and in the public media, as a generic category to identify persons who are responsible for the instruction of institutional and associational sport teams. In our view the *coach* is a teacher who has teaching responsibilities similar to those described for physical education teachers. The only difference is that, by long tradition, the teachers assigned to instruct institutional sport teams have been more publicized. Presumably they have been carefully selected and appointed to coaching duties because of their formal educational qualifications, experiences, and character and personal traits, and therefore fulfill the criteria of qualified teachers. While some coaches work with teams that are composed of beginning level student aspirants or teams that exist purposely for the players with low skills, most coaches are involved with the more athletically talented

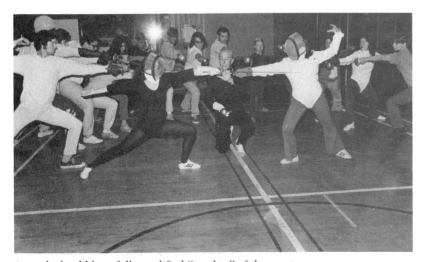

A coach should be a fully qualified "teacher" of the sport.

students. In either case, the point remains: the coach in any sport team should be a fully qualified *teacher* of the sport.

Curriculum. Although there is a separate chapter in this book devoted to physical education curriculum it is important to define this term briefly now so that its interrelationship with instruction and teaching will be clearly understood.

Succinctly stated, the formal *curriculum* of the school refers to learning opportunities that are planned and organized for the pupils to experience under the direction of the teachers for the purpose of achieving as completely as possible the stated educational objectives. The curriculum is a *plan of possible and potential learning opportunities*. How the curriculum is planned and developed is explained in detail in another chapter. Once the pupil undergoes actual class experiences, based on the *curriculum plan* and completes the lessons or the course of study, it can be said that the student *engaged* in learning experiences. Since each student's curriculum differs, even in highly structured, authoritarian schools, for any one student we refer to the curriculum had or experienced by that individual. This probably will not be precisely the curriculum that was planned.

Scheffler[3] defines three types of teaching, namely: *teaching that, teaching to,* and *teaching how to*. When a teacher "teaches a pupil that . . .," there is either a fact or a norm-statement involved. To "teach someone to" implies the idea of "ought." To "teach someone how to" refers to the area of teaching technical behaviors and elements of improved skilled performances, as in sports. A pupil might well learn how to behave in a certain situation and may desire to behave in that way, but may not necessarily "know how to." There is common agreement that teaching is primarily an art rather than a science and that it is in its earliest stages of scientific development.

Skill and Style. Other dimensions of teaching include teaching *skill* and teaching *style*. *Skill* refers to the degree of excellence with which the teacher performs the arts of teaching. *Style* refers to the unique and personal teacher behaviors revealed as the teacher assists students in learning.

ELEMENTS OF TEACHING

Types of Teaching

Another perspective of teaching is that it is essentially *interactive*. Teaching involves (1) the act of teaching, and (2) the act of receiving instruction. A logical analysis of the teaching/learning situation indicates that the teacher has determined the present state of the pupil or pupils, that is, he has diagnosed how the pupils are feeling, what their interests are, and how much comprehension or skill they possess about the topic or behavior under consideration. The teacher then decides the course of action to be taken in teaching those students with respect to the stated objectives. The students, on the other hand, receive the teaching and in so doing perceive the teacher's behaviors, make a judgment about them, and then react in some way or another. This process is repeated over and over again, and when enough learning conditions and the practice cycles are processed by the pupils, achievement performance or learning can result.

It is well known that successful teachers have the ability and experience to accurately perceive and understand behavioral signals being

TEACHING: AN INTERACTIVE PROCESS

emitted by their pupils with respect to their interests, their readiness for learning, and their motivational states at particular moments. Excellent teachers are not only able to estimate students' behavioral conditions, but also can relate the content and style of their teaching to the specific classroom climate at a given time. The above conditions, although very briefly described, indicate why teaching is called an *interactive* process. It is obvious that the teacher must be able not only to "size up" his students at any given moment, but also to decide and react appropriately in a short time period. Appropriate types of teacher reactions and their timing are crucial to successful teaching. Obviously, teachers must be most flexible and responsive in their reactions to their pupils; that is, they must have a variety of alternative ways in which they can respond to student actions and attitudes.

Contingencies in Teaching. Also, teachers must be prepared for "contingencies in teaching." This phrase refers to interruptions, diversions, unexpected events in the classroom, and other influences that cannot be predicted in advance or fully planned for prior to the teaching episode. This is an area of weakness of many novice teachers. They tend to place too much concentration and attention on the subject matter and neglect the behavior cues being emitted by the students in the class. Teachers must learn as rapidly as possible to assess accurately, and then to respond appropriately, to the interests and motivational states of their students.

Five Views of Teaching. Finally, Gage[4] indicates that there are several views of teaching, such as (1) the effects of teacher recruitment, selection, and retention; (2) teaching as human interaction; (3) teaching as skilled performance; (4) teaching as a linguistic process in a cultural setting; and (5) teaching as clinical information processing.

Teaching Variables

There are four types of variables involved in teaching. In their book, *The Study of Teaching*, Dunkin and Biddle[5] have a detailed discussion of these categories and the specific variables within them.

Presage variables concern information about the teacher such as age, sex, years of experience, social class background, major subjects in college, and types of practice teaching experiences. Also, they include teacher characteristics, skills, intelligence, motivation, attitudes, and personality traits.

Context variables describe the classroom, school environment, and conditions in which the teacher works. Included is information about the teacher's pupils, their age, sex, previous educational background, parents' social class, and so on. Also, test information about the pupils concerning educational skills, knowledge of subject matter, and attitudes are included. Other elements of this category are school and community characteristics, the ethnicity of the student body, the population of the school, and whether or not busing is involved. Information about classrooms is also important, such as the availability of textbooks, the number of pupils in the class, the provision of audio-visual aids, seat arrangement, the location of aisles, whether or not it is an open classroom, and so forth.

Process variables refer to individual behaviors that are exhibited in the classroom by the students and the teacher. The interactions between the students and the teacher are very important. What are the verbal and nonverbal interactions? How much of the interaction involves academic or nonacademic material? What are the teacher aims with respect to student achievement? Do the aims include cognitive, psychomotor, and affective objectives?

The *product* variable involves changes in student performance. Examples are students' scores on teacher prepared examinations concerning knowledge of subject matter or skill performance just studied or performed. Also, long range retention of knowledge skills by students is included. Changes in student attitudes over time is another aspect.

Various types of research in teaching can be organized within each of these classes of variables.

Joyce and Weil[6] propose four models of teaching: *Models of Teaching*

1. *Information Processing.* The focus of attention is on the learning processes. The student's learning capacity, ability to process information, and effectiveness in retrieving information accurately are fundamental. Concern for processing detailed information, accumulating verbal information, developing verbal skills, improving in the recall of verbal materials, encouragement of problem-solving behaviors, and urging student creativity are teacher responsibilities.

2. *Social Interaction.* Emphasis is on social interaction, the social-personal development of each student, and student interaction. The teacher provides many experiences and interactions in human relations, human communications, and interpersonal understanding.

3. *Personal Resources.* The teacher encourages and enhances pupil opportunities to improve in problem-solving skills and in learning to be original and creative. Also emphasized is self-development, personal development, self-image, self-concept, and total personality develop-

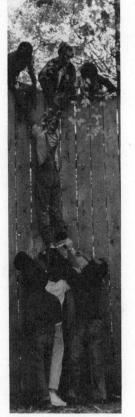

The social interaction model emphasizes student interaction.

ment. Likewise, the teacher encourages nonverbal expression and physical skills. Instructors assist students in increasing self-discovery, in realizing individual potentialities and in being realistic about their limitations.

4. Behavior Modification. Emphasis is on the effects of the environments of human beings and the ways people behave. Learning principles that effect behavioral changes are implemented through formal instructional procedures. The teacher frequently uses *reinforcement* by means of a reward or recognition when students demonstrate acceptable behavior, increased educational attainment, or the final fulfillment of stated educational goals. Positive reinforcement is emphasized while negative reinforcement is used seldom, if at all. Programmed instruction, a method of presenting new material through a sequence of steps at the student's individual pace, is an important mode in this model.

RESEARCH STUDIES OF TEACHER EFFECTIVENESS

In recent years many research studies have attempted to measure teacher effectiveness by reference to, or by correlation with, pupil achievement. Research studies have focused on teacher behaviors, personal characteristics of teachers, and the technical skills of teaching that seem to be closely related to, and have causal effect on, pupil achievement and learning. Teaching is still regarded as an art. Research has yet to produce very much valid evidence that teaches teachers "how to teach." However, in the long run, research on teaching effectiveness appears to have potentiality for bringing a clearer understanding of how teachers can be more effective in assisting pupils to learn in formal education settings (schools). The literature on this topic is proliferating rapidly. Interested readers should refer to it for further information and guidance. Several recent studies are briefly described in this section.

MEASURING TEACHER EFFECTIVENESS

Product versus Process and Presage Criteria. An interesting study by Jenkins and Bausell[7] surprisingly indicates that teachers do *not* view student learning as the major criterion for the determination of effective teaching. Two hundred sixty-four teachers in the State of Delaware replied to a survey instrument expressing their views on this topic.

The teachers evaluated *product* criteria such as student growth in skills, increase in knowledge of subject matter, and attitudes attributed to the teacher's influence in producing learning.

Second, *process* criteria were evaluated involving teachers' classroom behaviors such as the verbal methods used, classroom control, and individualization of instruction. Students were also rated for their attentiveness and conformity. Teacher-student interactions were judged for rapport and climate.

The third group of criteria rated included *presage* variables. Factors involved were the teacher's personality, intellectual attributes, undergraduate gradepoint average, grade received in student teaching, score made in a national teacher examination in the subject matter field, and certain in-service status characteristics such as number of years experience, officerships held in professional organizations, and similar criteria.

The findings of the Jenkins and Bausell study reveal that the criterion of effective teaching rated most highly by the teachers was "relationship with his class," a process criterion. The second highest rating was for teacher flexibility, a presage criterion. Teachers did not rate a product criterion in their first five choices. They did rate "his influence on students' behavior" as their sixth choice. Another major finding was that among 16 criteria the one labeled "amount students learn" ranked 11th in teachers' judgments about teaching effectiveness.

In summary, in this study teachers believed that "what one does in the classroom counts at least as much as the effects or outcomes of the doing."[8] It is evident that leaders of the movement for the accountability of teachers must coordinate their efforts and come to a closer agreement with the teachers who are being held accountable for pupil learnings than is the case at the present time.

The Gage Study: Variables for Successful Teaching. Gage[9] presents a summary of research findings that he believes most accurately inform us about conditions in classrooms that tend to improve student achievement.

The first variable he mentions is *enthusiasm*. There is considerable evidence that teachers who are enthusiastic affect student learning more favorably than less enthusiastic teachers.

A second variable is *acceptance of students' ideas*.

The *organization* of the teacher's lesson and its presentation is another variable that has shown positive relationship to student achievement.

The *ability of a teacher to ask higher order questions* also is related positively to student achievement.

Another teacher characteristic is called *warmth*, which means that the teacher acts approvingly and supportively. The teacher speaks well of the students and appears to like people in general. The teacher takes a positive attitude toward others, showing trust rather than fear or suspicion.

Gage designates a sixth teacher characteristic as *indirectness*. These teachers do not depend entirely upon autocratic, command-style teaching. They offer suggestions, present alternatives for pupils to evaluate and select from, vary the options for carrying out assignments, and so forth. Another characteristic of successful teachers is that they reinforce student ideas and opinions by approving them, making use of them in and out of class, and by letting students know their ideas are, indeed, valued. Finally, Gage indicates appropriate use of the teaching techniques of guided discovery as being desirable. Again, the student is encouraged to "find his own way" through the learning materials to seek a learning goal.

Dunkin and Biddle: A Research Summary. Dunkin and Biddle,[10] a year later than Gage, summarized research studies on teacher behaviors that are related to increased pupil achievement as follows: (1) humanistic attitudes toward students; (2) expectation of positive achievement from the students; (3) knowledge of what is going on in class, which the authors call "with-it-ness"; (4) ability to keep the learning activities moving along toward a specific goal, a characteristic called "smoothness" or "momentum"; (5) management or control of two or more objects or items or ideas at one time, which is called "overlappingness"; (6) ability to hold students responsible or accountable for completing a classroom task during the period, rather than allowing them to delay it or to have an incomplete performance; and (7) enthusiasm for and cultivation of student involvement and curiosity, called "teacher valence." Although the studies reviewed do not involve physical education classes, their conclusions have strong implications for the teaching and coaching of complex motor skills to pupils in physical education classes and to members of athletic teams.

Costa: Three Categories of Teaching Behavior.   Costa[11] indicates there are three broad categories of teaching behaviors, namely, (1) initiating, (2) responding, and (3) modeling. Costa says:

> These research studies indicate that teachers' behaviors are a key factor in effective classrooms. A teacher who consciously formulates questions that correspond to desired levels of cognitive thought; who structures the classroom with clarity and precision; who accepts, extends, and clarifies students' ideas; and who models the same behaviors desired in students can create a classroom learning condition in which maximum student growth will most likely occur.
>
> Teachers who master the information from these research studies can come to use their own behaviors as tools to enhance instruction and learning.

The Smith Study: Effective Teaching Behaviors.   Smith[12] is a strong proponent of the notion that the teacher's attitudes toward his pupils will have a strong influence on the degree of achievement. The students will perform in the direction of a teacher's expectations. Obviously, the teacher's personality is a very important factor in this assessment. So far, research on teaching has not revealed the extent to which teacher personality traits directly relate to pupil achievement and attitude.

In a review of more than fifty "process-product" studies, Smith[13] summarizes the findings concerning teacher behaviors that were shown to have the strongest effect on pupil achievement in a variety of classrooms and in several different subject matter fields. The following five teacher behaviors received the strongest support from the research:

1. *Clarity,* the teacher's ability to present the subject matter clearly
2. *Variability,* the different types of instructional materials or teaching devices that were used
3. *Enthusiasm,* including physical movement, gestures, and voice inflection
4. *Task-oriented or business-like behavior*
5. *Opportunities* presented to the students to learn the key materials in the lesson

Six other behaviors of teachers that were related to pupil achievement included use of student ideas and a general indirectness, criticism or control, use of structuring comments, types of questions asked, encouragement of further student response, and presentation of instructional material at the appropriate level of difficulty for optimum student understanding.

Smith[14] reminds us that:

> Teaching, one aspect of educating, is an interaction between a teacher, a person who can induce intelligent behaving, and a learner, a person who is to acquire intelligent behavior.
>
> Teaching is limited to those instructional interactions in which the behavior of the teacher is a necessary and sufficient condition for producing learning.
>
> Heuristic teaching is an infinite-state information-processing model designed to produce effective procedures or heuristics in a learner so that he may solve problems or acquire intelligent behavior.

Evans: Investigating Teacher Effectiveness. Evans[15] says there are three major categories for investigating teacher effectiveness: the personal characteristics of the teacher, the attributes of the instructional process, and the teacher impact on pupil behavior.

In general, Evans believes that summaries of research concerning teacher effectiveness lead to the following conclusions: (1) teacher warmth and praise do not relate strongly to pupil achievement; (2) there is strong evidence that negative teacher reactions and criticisms, if strong, may lead to poor pupil performance; (3) the degree and type of pupil activities may not be strongly related to pupil achievement; (4) too much teacher talk is not as effective as a minimum essential amount of talk required to provide explanations and give directions; (5) effective teachers do make extensive use of the ideas and judgments offered by the pupils thereby communicating to the student that the teacher is listening and believes that what the students are saying is important; (6) teacher enthusiasm including body movement, eye contact, and spontaneity and enthusiasm definitely are related to pupil achievement; (7) teacher "with-it-ness" appears to be related to pupil achievement because the teacher is aware at all times of what is going on in the classroom, provides a positive attitude of support for the pupils, acts promptly to prevent disruptive student behaviors, and in general applies sound group management strategies.

Teachers as Self-Researchers. In an interesting set of experiments Clark, Snow, and Shavelson[16] attempted to determine the extent to which teachers could improve their teaching effectiveness in the subject of physics. Concerning the teachers in this study the investigators concluded that practice in teaching a particular lesson did not assist the teachers in increasing student achievement. The investigators suggest that teachers should be provided with more formal opportunities to observe in a systematic way the effects of their teaching on students. In effect, the recommendation is that teachers receive a training program that would help them to become researchers concerning their own teaching effec-

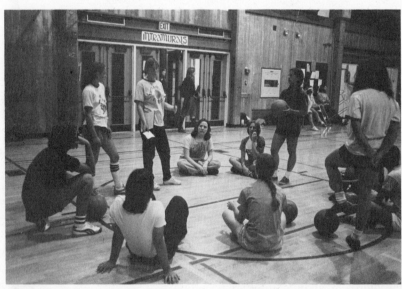

Effective teachers communicate better with students through the use of ideas and judgments offered by the pupils.

CHAPTER EIGHT

tiveness. There is more likelihood that teaching effectiveness will increase when teachers learn to define and solve instructional problems in terms of the uniqueness of the complex teaching situations they face on their own.

Rodin: Toward Relevant Evaluation Techniques. Miriam Rodin[17] raises some provocative questions about the use of student learning as the major criterion for assessing teacher effectiveness.

What is the effect on students that we want most to accomplish? Is the amount of information assimilated by the students, and their ability to remember it in a paper and pencil test, the main criterion? Are there other possibilities that might be enumerated, such as depth of understanding, increased sensitivity and sensibilities, greater acceptance of novel ideas, an inner appreciation of learning for a lifetime, the ability to tolerate ambiguity and diversity in others, the realization that asking relevant questions is as important as their answers, and the development of habits of rational thinking?

Perhaps the reason so much emphasis currently is being placed on student learning (knowledge) is because it is easy to measure compared with the learning outcomes listed above. Also, the above factors are mostly accumulated through experience or have delayed effects and are not learned only in the formal classroom.

Rodin concludes that probably no one accountability instrument will adequately measure teacher effectiveness; rather, a combination of several relevant evaluation techniques will be required in the long run.

Vittetoe: Success and Failure of First-Year Teachers. Vittetoe[18] studied the reasons for success and failure of first-year teachers as judged by their supervisors.

The leading characteristics of superior first-year teachers included rapport with students, staff, and parents; personality; knowledge of subject matter; personal attitude and enthusiasm; and professional attitude and manners.

The characteristics cited most frequently as exhibited by inadequate teachers were lack of discipline and control of the class; an ineffective personality; lack of willingness to take advice and assume responsibility; inflexibility; and lack of rapport with parents, staff, and students.

Tikunoff: Teaching Dimensions. Selected findings on teacher effectiveness from the Tikunoff[19] study are as follows: Twenty-one dimensions (factors) were found to be generic across both grade levels and subject matter areas. Under the category *classroom climate* were (1) adult involvement, (2) conviviality, (3) cooperation, (4) defiance (a negative dimension), (5) engagements, and (6) promoting self-sufficiency. These factors represent a warm, positive environment in which students and teachers share a common, convivial spirit and cooperate with each other.

There are eight generic dimensions in the category of *teacher instructional moves:* (1) abruptness, (2) attending, (3) filling time, (4) illogical statements, (5) monitoring learning, (6) pacing, (7) spontaneity, and (8) structuring. The effective teachers exhibited a greater number of dimensions that were viewed as positive (2, 5, 6, 7, 8), and fewer of those dimensions which were viewed as negative (1, 3, 4).

Under the category of teacher behaviors called *control moves* were (1) belittling, (2) consistency of message (control), and (3) oneness. The more effective teachers more frequently were observed to display consistency of message. They less frequently displayed belittling and oneness (negative dimensions).

Also, more effective teachers were found to be more accepting, more optimistic; they possessed a greater knowledge of subject matter, and they displayed less recognition-seeking behavior.

The Videotape Data Bank Project. William G. Anderson[20] and his graduate students have engaged in the Videotape Data Bank Project since 1971. The primary purpose of the project is to employ descriptive-analytic research to record and analyze activities and events that occur in naturalistic physical education class settings so as to better understand the teaching processes and the teacher-student interactions that occur in these classes on a day-to-day basis. A classification of physical education activities was developed and the amount of time each activity was included in the program was recorded.

Teacher-Student Interactions

A second purpose was to identify and describe all occasions when teachers presented augmented feedback to students. On the average, these teachers provided this feedback 54 times per class period. Feedback was divided into 56 per cent negative, 43 per cent positive, and 2 per cent neutral. Ninety-five per cent of this feedback was auditory, 4 per cent auditory-visual, and 1 per cent auditory-tactile.

A category system of student behaviors in physical education classes was developed and the per cent of time the students were engaged in each behavior was charted. The most time was spent in "awaiting" (18.8 per cent), "playing a game" (18.7 per cent), and "receiving information" (15.8 per cent). Ten other behaviors were identified and recorded.

Another segment of the study recorded the amount of time pupils were active or inactive in physical education classes (moving, or not moving). Fifty-three per cent of the time students were inactive, 35 per cent of the time they were involved in movements directed toward physical education class objectives, and 12 per cent of the time they were engaged in other movement tasks.

How teachers spent their time in physical education classes revealed many interesting results. About 95 per cent of their time was spent interacting with students, helping students prepare for participation, guiding them while playing, and observing student performances. Obviously, a very small amount of time was spent on administrative and related responsibilities.

Another interesting finding was that teachers talked almost continuously during the class; furthermore, they spent only 2 or 3 per cent of their time listening to what the students said.

Teachers determine to a large extent the type of activities pupils will engage in and the amount of time they will spend in each activity. In 83 per cent of the cases of activity selection, the teachers prescribed what students would do. In 5 per cent of the cases teachers provided some alternatives from which pupils would choose. In 12 per cent of the time, the students had "free choice."

The basic question raised by these studies was the extent to which teachers were appropriately providing students with shared and individual responsibility in arranging important conditions of learning in physical education classes.

Obviously, there are crucial implications for the improvement of teacher education in physical education, and for the in-service education of experienced teachers. This type of study ultimately will have as its most beneficial contribution the development of sophisticated teacher self-analytic systems for the improvement of teaching effectiveness.

Teacher Time

The Portland Time Study. How teachers spend their time undoubtedly is related to effective teaching. One study[21] of how elementary school teachers spent their time during a typical school day revealed some surprising findings. The study was made in Portland, Oregon, and involved teachers in grades one through four. Forty-seven teachers were observed for a full day and a detailed account was kept of the time they spent on different activities or tasks.

The major finding was that these teachers spent 30 per cent of their time in activities which were directly concerned with academic instruction and pupil learning — an average of 100 minutes during a five-and-one-half-hour school day. Seventy-five minutes were given to language-arts, eighteen minutes to math, and no more than one or two minutes daily were involved with any other subject in the curriculum.

These teachers spent 40 per cent of the time each day in routine activities such as clerical work, housekeeping, disciplining children, and other non-professional or management activities. Another ten per cent of the time involved making announcements, participating in ceremonies, and other management activities.

The remaining 20 per cent of teacher time was spent on miscellaneous personal and professional activities and functions that vary daily and do not fit into prescribed categories.

The study did show that each teacher with an average of 25 children was indeed very busy. There was virtually no time for relaxation or what might be called free time for the teacher.

The central conclusion was that these teachers were made responsible for a large variety of professional and non-professional tasks, and that they had to spend more time on the latter type of tasks and not enough time on direct teaching.

It seems obvious that significant changes in this situation are required. One suggestion is to make extended use of non-professionals and paraprofessionals to take over many of the non-instructional activities noted in this study.

*Teacher
Expectations of
Pupil Achievement*

A very important principle of teaching that all young teachers, as well as experienced ones, should learn as soon as possible has to do with the effect of teacher expectation upon pupil achievement. Studies have shown that frequently the expectations teachers hold toward the capabilities of a student to perform learning tasks at a specified level of achievement become self-fulfilling. That is, the pupil performs at the expected level, or in some cases, lower, even though the pupil may have the ability to perform at a higher level. It has also been shown that teachers are more likely to discuss a part of the lesson with the brighter students, to ask them questions more frequently, and to call on them for comments when their hands are up. Teachers also direct more praise toward the better students.

When labels are attached to clusters of students such as the "slow" group, the "average achievers," or the "gifted" students, the amount of learning by each group usually is influenced by the psychological effect of these labels on the teacher. This situation is more likely to occur when teachers are given information about their pupils that is indeed accurate rather than false, as has been done in some studies. Teachers will not believe labels that are too divergent from their everyday observations of their pupils.

Some studies indicate that there are teachers who expect girls to perform better than boys. Also, there is a common belief that the intelligence levels and aptitudes for learning are higher for girls than for boys whereas, in fact, tests disproved this.

Briefly, it can be concluded that teachers' expectations can become self-fulfilling; however, this is not necessarily the situation in many classrooms and with many teachers. It is cited here to help teachers to be well aware of and to seek to prevent such premature conclusions about students at any time in their teaching. Some teacher training programs appear to reinforce the possibility of this phenomenon. Also, teachers who lack confidence in themselves and who are rated low on a teaching ability scale are more likely to be guilty of this maltreatment of children.

Rapport and Pupil Evaluation.   Finally, it has been shown[22] that children who are friendly, active, and more relaxed generally are able to develop satisfactory personal relationships with their teachers, which in turn means that the teachers have more information from which to draw accurate conclusions about their pupils. On the other hand, the quiet, withdrawn pupil who seldom speaks up and attracts little attention from the teacher is more likely to be judged incorrectly by the teacher with respect to learning aptitude and abilities.

Thelen,[23] who is noted for his work on teacher-pupil compatibility, says,

Teacher-Pupil Compatibility

> The central proposition is that a teacher does a better job with some pupils than with others, and that therefore it makes sense to assign him a class composed of the sorts of students with whom he has been found to do a better job. An obvious corollary is that the students assigned to each teacher must be determined in some way that takes each teacher into account.

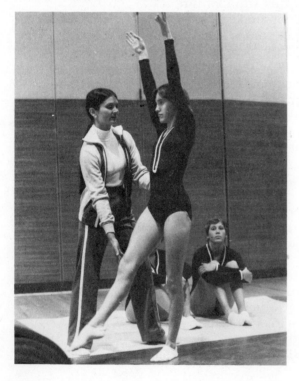

Some studies indicate that there are teachers who expect girls to perform better than boys.

The rationale for this recommendation seems obvious, yet seldom is followed even today in American public schools. Some teachers interact more effectively with certain students than with others. Selected students are attracted to, and learn more from, some teachers than others. Therefore, why should there not be a system developed to match pupils with compatible teachers? Thelen's research in classrooms suggests how such an administrative policy might be carried out.

This proposal does not imply that certain teachers teach correctly while others are poor teachers. It focuses on the notion of *how* teachers teach, *what* their idiosyncrasies in teaching style are, and *which* pupils would benefit most from each of the teachers. The teachers should have the major decision-making power with respect to implementing this type of grouping. Thelen's research has shown that there are fewer management problems in what he calls the "teachable groups."[24] We frequently observe teachers reassigning pupils in their classes to other teachers on an informal exchange basis. Sometimes administrators will transfer a pupil from one teacher to another for some identifiable cause. However, the wide scale implementation of the notion of assigning pupils to teachers on the basis of compatibility is seldom carried out in schools today. Thelen's suggestions for how to put this system into action demand attention.

Teaching the Individual

Cronbach and Snow[25] in a recent monumental book describe years of intensive effort to provide more enlightened research evidence concerning the problem of individual differences of pupils in school and how they may be most effectively taught. The focus of this work is called *aptitude-treatment interactions*. The overall thrust is to seek "an integrated understanding of the nature of individual differences in ability to learn." The research concentrates on attempting to identify the most effective methods of instruction relevant to the learning characteristics of individual pupils. As Cronbach and Snow say, "The scientific problem is to locate interaction of individual differences among learners with instructional treatments, that is, Aptitude × Treatment interactions." What are the types of learning aptitudes that are accrued by each student in each school subject? What instructional treatments are most appropriate for and relevant to student aptitudes for learning?

Cronbach and Snow have not only carried on their own investigations, but also critiqued many research studies done with students in various subject matter fields and at differing educational levels. Unfortunately, no research in physical education per se is recorded in this book. However, teachers in any field of learning will be aided by the study of this classic volume. We strongly urge interested physical educators to become engaged in this type of teaching-learning research.

TECHNICAL SKILLS OF TEACHING

Bush and Allen[26] provide a list and description of what they call technical skills of teaching, which have been widely adopted throughout the country. Briefly they are:

1. *Establish set.* Development of rapport (cognitive) between teacher and pupil, which should be initiated early in the sequence of lessons.

2. *Establish appropriate frames of reference.* Teach the lesson from two or more viewpoints.
3. *Achieve closure.* Help students relate new learnings to old ones. Provide students with a psychological feeling of accomplishment.
4. *Recognize and attend behaviors.* Be able to recognize behavioral evidence of pupil boredom or interest. Then change the pace, alter the learning activities, introduce new materials, and ask questions.
5. *Feedback.* Provide information about results and performances. Encourage student questions and comments. Provide visual cues. Hold informal quizzes and provide for rehearsals.
6. *Rewards and punishment.* Emphasize positive rewards that are tangible. Provide positive reinforcement. Deemphasize the use of punishment.
7. *Control participation.* Observe type and degree of participation of as many pupils as possible at all times. Provide encouragement for those who need it. Move around to various positions so as to observe most of the students most of the time.
8. *Redundancy and repetition.* Clarify and reinforce major ideas, concepts, and skills. Show different examples and applications and demonstrate skills. Use metaphors and analogies, similes, gestures, and audio-visual aids.
9. *Provide examples and demonstrations.* Clarify, verify, substantiate, illustrate. Use inductive and deductive approaches.
10. *Ask stimulating questions.* Learn how and when to ask questions. Vary the level of difficulty and types of questions.
11. *Ask higher order questions.* Require students to develop a concept or locate a principle not available on recall.
12. *Ask probing questions.* Request additional information. Ask for a justification or rationalization. Have students state a different viewpoint. Have a second student supplement the comment of the first student.
13. *Ask a divergent question.* Urge students to ask alternative questions. Ask questions that elicit one or more possible answers.
14. *Utilize teacher silence and non-cues.* Pause after an introductory statement. Pause after a question to a student and after an answer from a student.
15. *Encourage student questions.* Encourage or provoke students into asking questions.
16. *Seek completeness of communication.* Ask for clarification by student. Ask student to state the idea in his own words. Ask the student to demonstrate.
17. *Lecture clearly and interestingly.*
18. *Demonstrate a skill correctly.*

After reviewing several studies on how teachers employ the technical skills of teaching in order to produce desirable cognitive responses, Shavelson[27] concludes that "any teaching act is the result of a decision, whether conscious or unconscious, that the teacher makes after the complex cognitive processing of available information. This reasoning led to the hypothesis that *the* basic teaching skill is decision-making." Not only should teachers be taught how to use the various technical skills of teaching effectiveness, but they should also be taught how to decide *when* to use them in each instance with each pupil or group of students.

This section discusses recent developments in the teaching of physical education. Selected instructional programs that exemplify the latest theories and practices designed to improve teaching in physical education are cited. Basic principles of organizing and implementing effective teaching in physical education are emphasized.

HUMANISTIC PHYSICAL EDUCATION

In recent years physical education has seen a rapid increase in the number of programs that espouse what the teachers call "humanistic physical education." This movement has gained strength all over the country as teachers realize that under the so-called traditional programs physical education has been conducted in ways that were quite militaristic, formal, teacher dominated, and controlled by a large number of laws, rules and administrative policies to which all pupils had to conform. One set curriculum has governed this area of teaching to the neglect of students' individual needs, interests, and abilities; and other policies and procedures existed that did not fully recognize the inherent uniqueness of each individual.

This humanistic movement is not completely new to physical education. Several leaders in the field have been conducting programs of this type in their own schools and colleges for years and have expressed their dissatisfaction with traditional programs along with interpreting the values of the humanistic programs.

Humanistic educators emphasize such individual goals of students as self-realization, self-fulfillment, self-actualization, and a positive self-concept. It is beyond the scope of this text to delve into the details of the

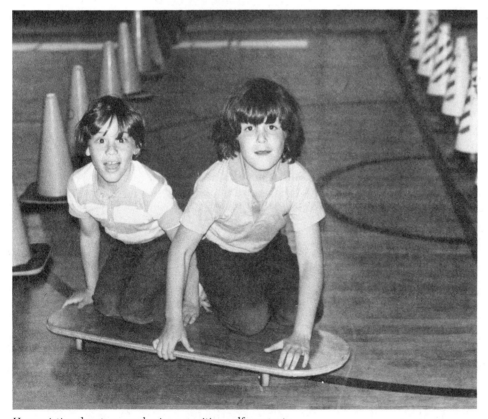

Humanistic educators emphasize a positive self-concept.

philosophy of these viewpoints. The works of Abraham H. Maslow[28] and Carl R. Rogers[29] should be consulted for in-depth analysis. George B. Leonard's[30] visions of schools in the future provides a prominent place for physical education in the humanistic philosophy.

Traditionally, physical education across the country has been taught in a militaristic and authoritarian manner. Children have been lined up and identified by numbers for roll call purposes, and they have been asked to stand at attention while attendance is being taken. Instructions by teachers have been issued primarily in the form of commands to engage in some performance that is highly prescribed. A strict behavior code has been stipulated and announced orally and posted on the bulletin board to be followed by all concerned throughout the physical education period or the practice of the athletic team. Point systems have been devised that the teacher applies arbitrarily and records in a grade book when a pupil has apparently violated one of the provisions of the code of conduct. Sometimes the system permits the earning of credit points for positive behavior, but most systems that monitor attendance and grade pupils in physical education are weighted in a negative point direction. Individuals frequently are treated as anonymous names in a grade book rather than as unique, valued persons. We are all familiar with this traditional type of physical education atmosphere and environment. Much dissatisfaction and unrest has arisen in recent years, and perceptive and concerned teachers now are developing programs in an environment that can be described as humanistic.

In humanistic physical education, the basic concern is for the unique identity of each individual. Teachers attempt to bring out the best of the potentialities in each student. The atmosphere is positive and teacher support is apparent at all times. Pupils are reinforced positively for their successes; they are recognized as significant individuals; their progress is evaluated in terms of individual development rather than against class norms; and they are allowed and encouraged to exhibit more personal freedom and responsibility than under the traditional system.

Combs: Treating the Pupil as a Valued Individual. Combs[31] has an excellent chapter on humanistic education with emphasis on treating each pupil as a unique and valued individual. Some of his ideas are as follows: First, learning should be viewed as the personal discovery of meaning. Combs says, "Any information will affect a person's behavior only in the degree to which he had discovered the personal meaning of that information for him." This view opposes stimulus-response conditioning and behavior modification techniques. Teachers and other school personnel should be "effective helpers," and should provide a facilitating atmosphere. Emphasis should be placed on discovering personal meaning throughout all learning stages.

Teachers should aid students to become self-actualized persons. A positive self-concept is essential in this frame of reference. Pupils should be taught to view themselves and their environment in an open manner.

Self-actualized individuals identify positively with others. There is an atmosphere of trust and mutual encouragement. Friendly interactions are stimulated.

Education must be future oriented. Perceptive, problem-solving individuals can best cope with a rapidly changing world. Creativity should be fostered and rewarded.

Cassidy and Caldwell. Cassidy and Caldwell[32] are among the leading advocates of humanistic physical education. They state their fundamental premise for humanistic physical education as follows:

> We deeply believe in and are committed to a philosophy of modern humanism: a way of looking at individuals in their world which supremely values the dignity and worth of all human beings; a way of looking at individuals valuing freedom of choice, the open individual in the open society; a way of looking at the uniqueness of each individual person; a way of looking at the humanitarian person as a freer facilitator, encourager, and a guide in the process of liberation of the human spirit and actualization of human capabilities and potential.

Hellison: Three Major Concepts in the Search for Self. Don Hellison[33] is one of the leading advocates of what is frequently called "humanistic physical education." Briefly, Hellison observes that he is primarily involved in a "search" for his students' self and his own self. Hellison emphasizes three major concepts which describe his view as a physical education teacher.

The first concept he calls *nonpossessive warmth*. It is concerned with caring about the student as a person and as a unique human being in a "communicative way." The teacher "feels good about himself and therefore can devote major attention to the student instead of to self."

The second teacher characteristic he calls *empathetic capacity*. Such a teacher is acutely aware of the feelings of each student, is sensitive to his perceptions, and is almost able to change places with the student in terms of being able to understand and feel what the student is feeling.

The third factor he calls *genuineness*, which means that the teacher acts honestly, is always open, and behaves in a truthful way with the students without projecting blame or criticism on them. Hellison provides suggestions about strategies teachers can employ to fulfill these qualifications of the humanistic teacher.

Hellison[34] summarizes his strong faith in the humanistic approach by stating "I believe the artistry of the teacher-student relationship is crucial to the student's search for self in a physical education setting, from gaining some sense of personal worth to becoming more aware and more creative and spontaneous."

Problem Areas and Ways to Seek Change

The problem with some of the major objectives of humanistic physical education such as self-actualization, self-fulfillment, and positive self-concepts is that they provide little guidance in specifying the curriculum and teaching methodologies that best lead to the attainment of these ends. There are no objective measurements of these lofty ideals, so one cannot accurately assess the extent to which each student is making educational and personal progress toward them.

Teachers and coaches, if properly self-motivated, can change their teaching styles and behaviors to interact with the pupils in ways that are most effective in assisting the students in developing in the general direction indicated by these humanistic concepts. Beginning teachers who desire to teach in the humanistic mode, as well as experienced teachers motivated to change toward a more humanistic orientation, must undergo intense self-analysis, be analytical of the reactions of their students to the teacher's changing behaviors, talk with other teachers who have similar goals, and in all of these ways attempt to assess the extent to which success is being achieved as revealed by changing attitudes, improved skills, and more pleasant inter-relationships between teachers and pupils over time.

Selected references at the end of this chapter provide additional information, insights, curriculum examples, and other information to assist interested individuals in learning more about what humanistic physical education is, its philosophical basis, its program implementation, and how students and programs are evaluated in this type of setting.

In summary, humanistic physical education is highly personalized. It is a human relationship that includes the teacher, the pupil, and pupil peers in the class. Its major purpose is to *free the pupil to learn*. The humanistic teacher is authentic, genuine, empathetic, and holds pupils in respect. Affective and cognitive components of learning in physical education are as important as skills.

TEACHING STYLES

Mosston's Spectrum of Styles. Mosston's[35] book on teaching is indeed a classic in physical education literature. His pioneer work in developing and describing a variety of teaching styles has been adopted as a basis for teacher education programs in many colleges and universities in the United States.

Mosston has created what he calls a "spectrum of teaching styles." This spectrum includes teaching by command, teaching by task, reciprocal teaching (the use of the partner), the use of small group, the individual program, guided discovery, and problem-solving. The major premise of Mosston's spectrum of styles is that by learning to use each of these styles in appropriate circumstances, teachers can assist students to develop individuality and originality in physical performances, social interactions, emotional control, and intellectual power. The teacher and the

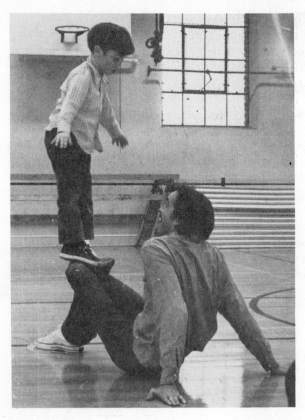

Humanistic physical education is highly personalized.

students move along the spectrum in a gradual manner. The teaching styles take into account what Mosston calls the physical channel, social channel, emotional channel, and intellectual channel of each pupil, encouraging and promoting growth and development in each channel simultaneously throughout the child's physical education experience. Moving along the continuum of styles, the student gradually assumes more self-responsibility and progresses in a positive direction in each of the channels. The Mosston spectrum is an individualized instruction model; the teacher gradually relinquishes direct control over the pupil and continually encourages the pupil's self-reliance and self-responsibility with the ultimate goal being a "free student."

Mosston urges that the final goal of the teacher be to increase the student's capabilities for creative behaviors. A person can learn to learn in novel ways and become more creative through the Mosston spectrum of styles of teaching physical education under the guidance of qualified teachers.

A Systems-Approach Model of Teaching. Singer and Dick[36] advocate a model of teaching physical education that combines aspects of information processing and behavior modification. The major steps in the systems-approach to teaching are:

1. Identify instructional goals that become student terminal objectives.
2. Conduct an instructional analysis of the goals. Identify the prerequisite skills and knowledges required of the student to progress to the successful accomplishment of the goals.
3. Evaluate the student's entry skills, knowledge, and characteristics.
4. Develop performance objectives.
5. Develop criterion-referenced evaluation instruments.
6. Design instructional strategies.
7. Select instructional media.
8. Develop or select instructional materials, supplies, and equipment.
9. Relate evidence from the formative evaluation to the instructional analysis and to the description of entry skills, knowledge, and characteristics through feedback.

This approach is another example of individualized instruction and emphasizes the following components:

Instructional Goals
Instructional Analysis
Entry Skills, Knowledge, and Characteristics
Performance Objectives
Criterion-Referenced Evaluation
Instructional Strategies
Media Selection
Instructional Materials
Formative Evaluation

Singer and Dick[37] summarize:

What has been presented is clearly a new role model of the teacher. It will require him to be an analyst in terms of what is being taught and somewhat of a researcher in terms of collecting data on student performance and relating it to the instructional setting. At the same time it requires him to become more of a humanist in terms of recognizing the vast array of individual differences among children and trying to provide instruction which will accommodate these differences.

Annarino: Individualized Sport Instruction. A series of instructional manuals by Annarino[38] is available for individualized instruction in selected sports. Each manual provides the following sections of information for student understanding and application for self-practice, self-study, and self-evaluation. Each manual provides individualized programmed instruction. Sport skills and knowledge are emphasized. Mastery learning is a central focus.

Student Information
Introduction
Behavior Objectives
Practice Procedures
Equipment
Time Element
Safety Factors
Independent Skill Assignment Procedures
Independent Reading Assignment Procedures
Student Progress Record
Sports Theory Concepts
Resource Materials

Siedentop: Physical Education Teaching Skills. Siedentop[39] has made a major contribution to the improvement of teaching physical education. The use of "a systematic data collection format to improve teaching skills" is a notable research contribution.

Siedentop defines teaching as follows:

> The basic task of teaching is to find ways to help students learn and grow, to design environments where changes in the cognitive, social, affective, and motor behavior of students can be accomplished efficiently, and to do it all in a manner that enables the students to enjoy the learning experience and to learn to enjoy the activity or subject matter being studied.

Siedentop presents many suggestions and principles concerning teacher roles, classroom management, interpersonal relations between teachers and students, planning for instruction, carrying out effective instruction, implementing school policies, and the professional development of the teacher. This book provides a variety of activities and instruments that teachers can utilize to become more effective.

Healey and Healey: A Problem-Solving Approach. In a recent book, Healey and Healey[40] have taken the approach of describing the teaching of physical education from a problem-centered perspective. Major problems in physical education are identified. Fundamental concepts of problem-solving procedures are described. The physical education teacher, the coach, and the administrator are instructed how to apply problem-solving methods to critical problems existing in physical education and sports.

The case study approach is used with actual examples from various schools serving as the problems to be analyzed and studied. The authors then propose methods for solving the problems presented and report the outcome of effective problem-solving in each instance. Some of the problems presented are administrative in nature rather than instructional. Others are involved in the responsibility of physical education teachers during the instructional phase of their duties. Seventy-one varied problems in physical education are presented. We recommend the formal study of these problems and the problem-solving processes, which should provide a basis for improved problem-solving behaviors on the part of individuals who undergo these exercises seriously.

There is little doubt that physical education teachers and athletic coaches face a formidable array of problems all day long involving a large number of pupils. Being responsible for as many as 200 to 250 pupils per day in four or five periods of physical education teaching, plus coaching the after school sport teams means that the physical educator is constantly "solving problems." The Healey and Healey book should make a valuable contribution to the teacher's problem-solving abilities both in the instructional aspects and the managerial roles of the teacher's assignment.

Heitmann and Kneer: An Individualized Humanistic Approach. Heitmann and Kneer[41] recently produced a book that emphasizes an individualized humanistic approach. These teachers, experienced in both high school and university, present modern concepts of humanistic physical education, joined with a variety of techniques for individualizing instruction.

The authors contend that the students they have taught through individualized instruction with the humanistic approach have made achievement gains equivalent to those attained by pupils in traditional highly directed, teacher-dominated classes. In addition, it is affirmed that the students in the individualized humanistic program demonstrated significantly improved satisfaction with the results of this type of teaching and that they progressed further in their abilities to learn how to learn through accepting greater self-responsibility.

Heitmann and Kneer[42] say, "We believe that through individualized learning the student will find more relevant motivation and success in education."

Among other valuable items, the book presents:
— a comprehensive rationale for individualized humanistic instruction;
— a description of the characteristics of students in physical education classes;
— definitions of the roles, competencies, and professional responsibilities of teachers;
— a review of modern theories of learning most applicable to the physical education situation;
— a chapter on how to develop a unit lesson plan;
— an explanation of how to plan and conduct individualized instruction.

Other discussions involve how to prepare "learning transactions" for the teaching of specific activity skills (the word "transactions" used here refers to pupil interactions with the learning environment); how to plan and develop formative and summative types of evaluations of pupil performances; how to motivate student learning; how to evaluate the total program of individualized humanistic physical education; and how teachers can change from traditional modes of teaching to individualized humanistic teaching. Also explored are teacher decisions and pupil decisions in the context of individualized humanistic learning, and teacher assistance for pupils with learning difficulties. The book concludes with a presentation of samples of individualized instructional units and modules.

Locke and Lambdin: Cohort versus Personalized Instruction. Locke and Lambdin[43] describe individualized instruction as the attention the teacher gives to the most important learning characteristics in the lesson at hand. The teacher deliberately helps each pupil to find relevant objectives, specific and suitable content, variations in instruction and methods of practice, and other aspects of teaching and learning that will ensure progress at an optimum rate to accomplish the learnings set forth. With the student's help, the teacher attempts to mold educational processes and goals to student interests and needs.

A basic assumption underlying individualized instruction is that a teacher can work with most if not all of the students as individuals who have unique needs and interests, and that this can be done while maintaining and improving educational efficiency on the part of each child. It is a safe guess that most teachers who move to a system of individualized instruction do so to escape what Locke and Lambdin call "cohort instruction" and the evils it promotes.

Cohort instruction, as used by Locke and Lambdin, refers to the traditional and long-standing method of teaching that involves presenting the same lesson and experience to all the students in the class at the same time, employing the same methodology for all students, requiring the same type of practice on the same schedule, and judging each student by the same standards and criteria. No doubt most of the readers of this book will recognize this mode of instruction from their own past educational experiences.

Locke and Lambdin favor *personalized instruction*, which they see as represented by two distinct types: The first type refers to all forms of instruction in which students and teachers try to adjust the goals of learning to the needs and interests of each learner. This is a *product* definition, exemplified by the contract system of learning.

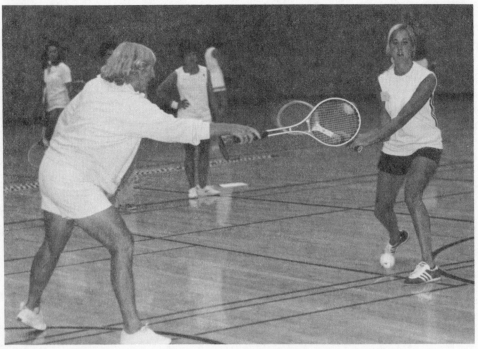

The teacher deliberately helps each student to progress at an optimum rate.

The second type of personalized instruction is any type of individual instruction that involves the learner with others in the educational atmosphere. One student may serve as a tutor to another student; the teacher may interact with the learner; or resource persons can be utilized to assist the students. Note that this type of learning is different from independent study, in which the students work entirely on their own.

Locke and Lambdin describe this type of instruction as having a strong element of social interaction. Also, it is fundamentally concerned with each student's personal feelings and affective goals. Such long-range aims as self-actualization and personal awareness are prominent. Students are encouraged to engage in self-examination as well as to be as open as possible in their communication with others. This method stresses active participation, self-responsibility, and the opportunity to *elect* curricular experiences and learning methodologies.

Of course, this philosophy requires teachers who believe in it and have a complete respect for the individuality and unique capabilities of each student. Its basic assumption is that pupils are capable of rational self-direction in learning.

Conclusion. In conclusion, we may state that research concerning categories and variables relating to teaching physical education is in its infancy. No scientific laws of teaching have been evolved from this evidence. The findings are tentative. They may suggest possible ways for a teacher to improve in selected aspects of teaching, but there has been little integration of the findings into a comprehensive theory from which principles of teaching can be derived on a generalized basis. There is an increment in the number of qualified researchers engaging in theory formulation and classroom research so that we expect significant advances in research findings and in application to effective teaching in the years ahead.

A note of caution: Few studies have been undertaken in physical education classes in naturalistic settings. Most if not all of the research reported above does not involve actual physical education classes and pupils. Therefore, there is a danger in improperly generalizing much of the available research evidence on teaching effectiveness from classrooms in English, social studies, mathematics, reading, and spelling to teacher effectiveness in physical education classes.

SUMMARY

Teaching occurs when one individual deliberately attempts to assist another individual, or group of persons, to perform or to learn a specific activity or concept.

Research has yet to produce very much valid evidence which teaches teachers "how to teach." However, research on teaching effectiveness appears to have potentiality for bringing a clearer understanding of how teachers can be more effective in assisting pupils to learn in formal educational settings (schools).

Humanistic educators emphasize such individual goals of students as self-realization, self-fulfillment, self-actualization, and a positive self-concept.

Humanistic physical education teaching is highly personalized. It is a human relationship including the teacher, the pupil, and pupil peers in the class.

Singer and Dick advocate a model of teaching physical education which combines aspects of information processing and behavior modification called the systems-approach model.

Heitmann and Kneer contend that the students they have taught through individualized instruction with the humanistic approach have made achievement gains equivalent to those attained by pupils in traditional, highly directed, teacher-dominated classes.

[1]Nathaniel L. Gage, *The Scientific Basis of the Art of Teaching*. New York: Teachers College Press, 1978, p. 1.

[2]Daryl Siedentop, *Developing Teaching Skills in Physical Education*. Boston: Houghton-Mifflin Company, 1976, p. 5.

[3]Israel Scheffler, *The Language of Education*. Springfield, Ill.: Charles C. Thomas, Publisher, 1964.

[4]Nathaniel L. Gage, op. cit.

[5]Michael J. Dunkin and Bruce J. Biddle, *The Study of Teaching*. New York: Holt, Rinehart and Winston, 1974.

[6]Bruce R. Joyce and Marsha Weil, *Models of Teaching*. Englewood Cliffs, N.J.: Prentice Hall, Inc., 1972.

[7]Joseph R. Jenkins and R. Barker Bausell, "How Teachers View the Effective Teacher: Student Learning Is Not the Top Criterion," *Phi Delta Kappan*, 55:572–573 (April, 1974).

[8]Ibid., p. 573.

[9]Nathaniel L. Gage, op. cit.

[10]Michael J. Dunkin and Bruce J. Biddle, op. cit.

[11]Arthur L. Costa, "Recent Research on the Analysis of Instruction," "News, Notes, and Quotes," Newsletter of *Phi Delta Kappan*, XXI:3. (May/June, 1977), p. 3.

[12]Othaniel B. Smith, *Research and Teacher Education – A Symposium*. Englewood Cliffs, N.J.: Prentice-Hall, Inc., 1971.

[13]Ibid., pp. 43, 49–54

[14]Ibid., pp. 73, 79

[15]Ellis D. Evans, *Transition to Teaching*. New York: Holt, Rinehart and Winston, 1976, pp. 84, 89–95.

[16]Christopher M. Clark, Richard E. Snow, and Richard J. Shavelson, "Three Experiments on Learning to Teach." Research and Development Memorandum No. 140, School of Education, Stanford University, Stanford, California (December, 1975).

[17]Miriam Rodin, "Rating the Teachers," *The Center Magazine*, Center for the Study of the Democratic Institutions. Santa Barbara, California, VIII, 55–60 (September/October, 1975.

[18]Jack O. Vittetoe, "Why First-Year Teachers Fail," *Phi Delta Kappan*, 58:429–430 (January, 1977).

[19]William J. Tikunoff, D. B. Berliner, and R. C. Rist, *Special Study A: An Ethnographic Study of the Forty Classrooms of the Beginning Teacher Evaluation Study Known Sample*. San Francisco: Far West Laboratory for Educational Research and Development, 1975.

[20]William G. Anderson, "Videotape Data Bank," *Journal of Physical Education and Recreation*, 31–34 (September 1975).

[21]*New York Times*, May 21, 1974, p. 4.

[22]Jere E. Brophy and Thomas L. Good, "Teacher Expectations: Beyond the Pygmalion Controversy," *Phi Delta Kappan*, 54:276–278 (December, 1972).

[23]Herbert A. Thelen, *Classroom Grouping for Teachability*. New York: John Wiley & Sons, Inc., 1967, p. 191.

[24]Ibid., p. 192

[25]Lee J. Cronbach and Richard E. Snow, *Aptitudes and Instructional Methods: A Handbook for Research on Interactions*. New York: Irvington Publishers, 1977, pp. 1, 2.

CHAPTER EIGHT

[26]Robert N. Bush and Dwight W. Allen, *A New Design for High School Education: Assuming a Flexible Schedule.* New York: McGraw-Hill, 1964.

[27]Richard J. Shavelson, "A Basic Teaching Skill: Decision-Making." Research and Development Memorandum No. 104, School of Education, Stanford University, Stanford, CA., 1973.

[28]Abraham H. Maslow, *Toward a Psychology of Being* (2nd ed), Princeton, N.J.: D. Van Nostrand Co., Inc., 1968.

[29]Carl R. Rogers, *Freedom to Learn: A View of what Education Might Become.* Columbus, Ohio: Charles E. Merrill Publishing Co., 1969.

[30]George B. Leonard, *Education and Ecstasy.* New York: Delacorte Press, 1968.

[31]Arthur W. Combs, "Fostering Maximum Development of the Individual," *Issues in Secondary Education,* Seventy-fifth Yearbook of the National Society for the Study of Education, Part II. Chicago: University of Chicago Press, 1976, pp. 65–87.

[32]Rosalind Cassidy and Stratton F. Caldwell, *Humanizing Physical Education – Methods for the Secondary School Movement Program,* Fifth Edition. Dubuque, Iowa: William C. Brown Company, 1974. p. ix.

[33]Donald Hellison, *Humanistic Physical Education.* Englewood Cliffs, N.J.: Prentice-Hall, Inc. 1973.

[34]Ibid, p. 28.

[35]Muska Mosston, *The Teaching of Physical Education: From Command to Discovery.* Columbus, Ohio: Charles E. Merrill Publishing Co., 1966.

[36]Robert N. Singer and Walter Dick, Instructor's Manual, *Teaching Physical Education: A Systems Approach.* Boston: Houghton-Mifflin Co., 1974, p. 55.

[37]Ibid., p. 75

[38]Anthony Annarino, *Tennis: Individualized Instruction Programs.* Englewood Cliffs, N.J.: Prentice-Hall, Inc., 1973.

[39]Daryl Siedentop, op. cit., pp. 1, 5.

[40]John Healey and William A. Healey, *Physical Education Teaching Problems for Analysis and Solution.* Springfield, Ill.: Charles C. Thomas, 1975.

[41]Helen M. Heitmann and Marian E. Kneer, *Physical Education Instructional Techniques.* Englewood Cliffs, N.J.: Prentice-Hall, Inc., 1976.

[42]Ibid., p. xiv.

[43]Lawrence F. Locke and Dolly Lambdin, "Personalized Learning in Physical Education," *Journal of Physical Education and Recreation,* 47:32–35 June, 1976.

SELECTED REFERENCES

Anderson, William, "Descriptive Analytic Research on Teaching," *Quest,* 15:1–8 (January 1971).

Borich, Gary D., *The Appraisal of Teaching: Concepts and Process.* Reading, MA: Addison-Wesley Publishing Co., 1977.

Brophy, Jere E., and Good, Thomas L., *Teacher-Student Relationships: Causes and Consequences.* New York: Holt, Rinehart and Winston, 1974.

Burdin, Joel, "The Changing World and Its Implications for Teacher Education," In Kevin Ryan (Ed.), *Teacher Education,* Seventy-fourth Yearbook of the National Society for the Study of Education. Chicago: University of Chicago Press, 1975.

Cheffers, John, and Evaul, Thomas, *Introduction to Physical Education: Concepts of Human Movement.* Englewood Cliffs, N.J.: Prentice-Hall, Inc., 1978.

Churcher, Barbara, *Physical Education for Teaching.* Reading , MA: Allen & Unwin, Inc., 1977.

Cronbach, Lee J., "How Can Instruction Be Adapted to Individual Differences? In Robert M. Gagné, (Ed.), *Learning and Individual Differences.* New York: Merrill Publishing Company, 1967.

Dougherty, Greyson, and Bonanno, Diane, *Contemporary Approaches to Teaching Physical Education.* Minneapolis, MN: Burgess Publishing Company, 1979.

Dougherty, Greyson, and Lewis, Clifford G., *Effective Teaching Strategies in Secondary Physical Education* (3rd Ed.). Philadelphia: W. B. Saunders Co., 1979.

Dowell, Linus, J., *Strategies for Teaching Physical Education.* Englewood Cliffs, N.J.:Prentice-Hall, Inc., 1975.

Eisner, Elliot, "On the Uses of Educational Connoisseurship and Criticism for Evaluation of Classroom Life." *Teacher College Record*, 78:345–358 (February 1977).

Freeman, William H., "Competency-based Teacher Education: The Other Side," *Journal of Physical Education and Recreation*, 26–27 (January 1977).

Gage, Nathaniel L., "Models for Research on Teaching." Occasional Paper No. 9, Stanford Center for Research and Development in Teaching, School of Education, Stanford University, 1976.

Gage, Nathaniel L. (Ed.), *The Psychology of Teaching Methods*. Seventyfifth Yearbook of the National Society for the Study of Education. Chicago: University of Chicago Press, 1976.

Gage, Nathaniel L., "Should Research on Teaching be Generic or Specified? Unpublished paper, Center for Educational Research at Stanford, School of Education, Stanford University, 1977.

Gage, Nathaniel, L., *The Scientific Basis of the Art of Teaching*. New York: Teachers College Press, 1978.

Gagné, Robert M., and Briggs, Leslie J., *Principles of Instructional Design*. New York: Holt, Rinehart and Winston, 1974.

Hawley, Robert C., *Evaluating Teaching: A Handbook of Positive Approaches*. Amherst, MA: Education Research Association, 1976.

Hellison, Donald R., "Teaching Physical Eduction and a Search for Self." In Dorothy J. Allen and Brian W. Fahey (Eds.) *Being Human in Sports*. Philadelphia: Lea and Febiger, 1977.

Jewett, Ann E., and Mullan, Marie, R., "A Conceptual Model for Teacher Education." *Quest*, XVIII:76–87 (June, 1972).

Jewett, Ann E., and Mullan, Marie R., *Curriculum Design: Purposes and Processes in Physical Education Teaching-Learning*. Washington, D.C.: American Alliance for Health, Physical Education and Recreation, 1977.

Kneer, Marian (Ed.), "Curriculum Theory into Practice," *Journal of Physical Education and Recreation*, 49:24–37 (March 1978).

Lindeburg, Franklin A., *Teaching Physical Education in the Secondary School*. New York: John Wiley & Sons, Inc., 1978.

Logsdon, B. J., Barrett, K. R., Ammons, M., Broer, M. R., Halverson, L. E., McGee, R., and Roberton, M.A., *Physical Education for Children: A Focus on the Teaching* Process. Philadelphia: Lea & Febiger, 1977.

Nixon, John E., and Locke, Lawrence F., "*Research on Teaching Physical Education*." In Robert M. W. Travers (Ed.), *Second Handbook of Research on Teaching*, AERA. Chicago: Rand McNally & Company, 1973.

Pease, Dean A., and Taber, Terry R., "Teaching for Skill Acquisition: A Competency-based Teacher Education Model," *Competency-based Teacher Education Briefings*. National Association for Physical Education of College Women and National College Physical Education Association for Men, 1975.

Popham, W. James, and Baker, Eva I., *Systematic Instruction*. Englewood Cliffs, N.J.: Prentice-Hall, Inc., 1970.

Rarick, G. L., Dobbins, D. A. "A Motor Performance Typology of Boys and Girls in the Age Range 6 to 10 Years." *Journal of Motor Behavior*, 1975, 7, 37.

Robb, M. *The Dynamics of Motor-Skill Acquisition*. Englewood Cliffs, N.J.: Prentice-Hall, Inc., 1972.

Roper, Susan S., and Nolan, Robert R., "Down from the Ivory Tower: A Model for Collaborative In-Service Education." Occasional Paper No. 16, Stanford Center for Research and Development in Teaching, School of Education, Stanford University, 1977.

Ryan, Kevin (Ed.), *Teacher Education*. Seventy-fourth Yearbook of the National Society for the Study of Education. Chicago: University of Chicago Press, 1975.

Schmidt, R. *Motor Skills*. New York: Harper and Row, 1975.

Stelmach, G. (Ed.) *Information Processing in Motor Control and Learning*. New York: Academic Press, 1978.

Stelmach, G. (Ed.) *Motor Control*. New York: Academic Press, 1976.

"Teacher Expectations: Beyond the Pygmalion Controversy," *Phi Delta Kappan*, 54:276–278 (December 1972).

Ulrich, Celeste, and Nixon, John E., *Tones of Theory*. Washington, D.C.: American Association for Health, Physical Education and Recreation, 1972.

Vannier, Maryhelen, and Fait, Hollis F., *Teaching Physical Education in Secondary Schools* (4th Ed.). Philadelphia: W. B. Saunders Co., 1975.

Vannier, Maryhelen, and Gallahue, David L., *Teaching Physical Education in Elementary Schools* (New 6th Ed.). Philadelphia: W. B. Saunders Co., 1978.

Weil, Marsha, and Joyce, Bruce, *Information-Processing Models of Teaching.* Englewood Cliffs, N.J.: Prentice-Hall, Inc., 1978.

Weil, Marsha, Joyce, Bruce, and Kluwin, Bridget, *Personal Models of Teaching.* Englewood Cliffs, N.J.: Prentice-Hall, Inc., 1978.

Whiting, H. T. A., *Concepts in Skill Learning.* London: Lepus Books, 1975.

Whiting, H. T. A., *Readings in Human Performance.* London: Lepus Books, 1975.

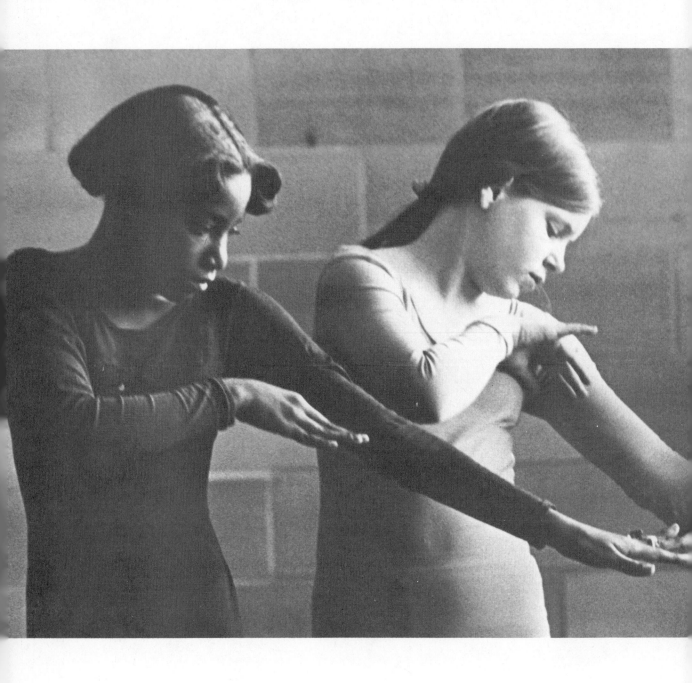

SOCIETAL ROLES OF THE MOVEMENT ARTS AND SPORT SCIENCES

9

Introduction

A field of knowledge is significant for human beings through its potential for contributions to individual and societal survival and its ability to enhance one's personal life and to enrich group life. Philosophers through the ages have asked, "What knowledge is of most worth?" School curricula have always been based on what we perceive to be the answers to this question. School subjects find their way into the organized courses of study because their knowledge is judged to be of value in a broad social context; thus the movement arts and sport sciences, usually termed "physical education" in the curriculum, developed in response to human needs and common interests.

Movement is essential to life. The movement arts and sport sciences have developed in response to human needs and common interests. Therefore, it is essential that their key concepts be included in the curriculum. Typically, the school program termed "physical education" provides for learnings in this field of knowledge.

The ways in which individuals seek personal meaning in movement activities were discussed in Chapter 7 as a framework for determining curriculum goals and selecting physical education content. These purposes are paralleled, in many instances, by societal roles assigned to the movement arts and sport sciences.

We believe that the movement arts and sport sciences have many roles in our society. The most important roles are in education, health and fitness, social service, communications, leisure and recreation, and business and economics. These will be discussed in this chapter. Each role is viewed from the perspectives of its cultural significance, its relationships to the foundations reviewed in Chapters 3 through 6, its relationships to school physical education programs discussed in Chapters 7 and 8, and its organizational leadership and professional ramifications.

We are convinced that through these roles the movement arts and sport sciences have much potential for enriching the quality of human life. As researchers provide more information about humans in social groups, and as leaders at all levels of government become more aware of the needs of citizens in relation to the movement arts and sport sciences, opportunity for professionals in these fields will be dramatically increased.

EDUCATION

Schooling is just one area of our lives in which the movement arts and sciences are important; yet the educational role is crucial and basic to effective performance in the other societal roles. The educational role of the movement arts and sport sciences has been discussed previously as providing guidance in the search for personal meaning in movement activities. Individuals learn to move in various ways and to perform particular movements in order to develop their movement abilities for daily living, and participate in recreational sports. Conditioning and training programs guide learners through vigorous activities to achieve fitness and to learn how to develop and maintain it. Modern physical education programs also provide experiences that can be self-directed toward the personal integration of the individual.

School programs also fulfill the educational role of the movement arts and sport sciences through employment of movement activities for other learnings. Participants learn more about themselves as moving beings and whole functioning persons. Through movement activities, physical education provides understanding of motion as a universal phenomenon and of how to cope with motion in the environment. The curriculum also provides for learning from interaction with others in the social environment.

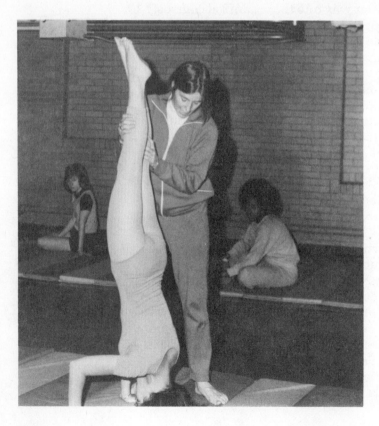

Learners are guided in various activities to achieve fitness.

The educational goals and objectives of physical education have been discussed in considerable detail in previous chapters. Ways of achieving these goals through the planned curriculum and through instruction in physical education have also been identified, described, and analyzed. Effective application of the educational role of the movement arts and sport sciences provides a foundation for the satisfaction of individuals in all areas of living.

A majority of the people of the United States are most fortunate in that they enjoy one of the highest standards of living in the world. From a medical standpoint, in spite of certain significant problem areas, we are probably healthier as a total population today than at any time in our history. We live in a world that considers optimum health and fitness more important than ever; yet these very real gains of our modern civilization have created new health problems. Automation and television have contributed to sedentary lifestyles. High levels of personal anxiety and stress and difficulties in interpersonal communication are common in many segments of the population. Alcoholism, drug abuse, and forms of psychological imbalance ranging from phobias to suicidal tendencies are serious social problems. Clearly our standard of individual health leaves much to be desired.

Ours is a world in which the health of the people must be a continuing concern. Solutions to problems of environmental pollution are not yet in sight. Technological advances may have side effects dangerous to health. The pressures of increasing population and anticipated changes in lifestyles are unlikely to reverse the trend of less physical activity required in daily living.

HEALTH AND FITNESS

The relationship of exercise to health is well established. With regular exercise, the heart rate becomes lower at all levels of submaximal effort; the stroke volume becomes larger with each beat of the heart. Recent studies support the now widely accepted view that strenuous physical exercise on a regular basis results in a definite protective effect on the cardiovascular system, and that regular exercise habits may contribute to satisfactorily coping with, and even reducing, stress. Many doctors now prescribe regular vigorous exercise for their patients. As noted, the Assistant Secretary for Health, Dr. Theodore Cooper, of the Department of Health, Education, and Welfare, reported in 1977 a 14 per cent decrease among Americans in the incidence of fatal heart disease. He attributed improved heart health to better dietary habits, less smoking, and more exercise, pointing out that the most significant change was in exercise habits.

The societal role of physical education in helping to maintain and improve health and fitness reflects the relationship of exercise to health; in other words, the more effective the movement activity program, the better the physical well-being of the general public. With increasing recognition of the vital nature of this relationship, public interest in fitness programs, movement therapy services, and preventive medicine is growing rapidly. Biological research has clarified key concepts of exercise physiology, helped us to understand the important relationship of exercise to health, and taught us how to assess physical fitness. The scientists in these fields are attempting to find out more about the processes of aging and to learn more about the role of the movement arts and sport sciences

The Role of Movement and Sport

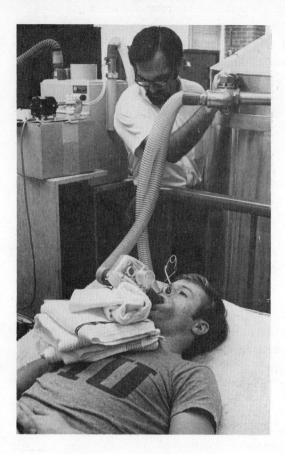
More doctors are now prescribing regular vigorous exercise for their patients.

in improving the quality of living among our increasing numbers of senior citizens. Behavioral scientists are compiling more and more evidence of positive relationships between exercise and mental health. Social scientists are stressing the need for improving attitudes toward positive health practices, for public programs focusing on the abilities, rather than the disabilities, of the handicapped, and for extending more preventive medical and national health care to all our citizens.

School physical education programs have long supported the health and fitness role of the movement arts and sport sciences in our society. Educating for the understanding, development and maintenance of physical fitness has always been a major goal. Although research data have been scant, sports participation has been viewed as a channel toward psychological and emotional well-being, as well as physiological health. More recently, physical education programs have begun to emphasize the role of physical activities and related instruction in achieving personal integration and total fitness as a whole human being.

Health and fitness are of primary importance to any society, since its survival depends upon achieving minimal health standards and its advancement is directly related to upgrading the fitness, in the broadest sense, of its total citizenry. The movement arts and sport sciences will always play a significant role in the health and fitness of the American people. The major current manifestations of this role, beyond school programs, are the expanding fitness programs, burgeoning therapeutic uses, and new emphases in preventive medicine.

Exercise has become fashionable for adults in our contemporary world. Popular magazines and professional journals express concern for the "weekend warriors of sport," "cycling nuts," former "armchair athletes" who have taken up racket sports with such fervor, to the neglect of all else, that they appear to suffer from "an acute case of simplemindedness." Jogging has attracted so many participants that it is frequently described as a fad, craze, or addiction. There is no doubt that a staggering number of adults now participate in fitness activities. Many persons are motivated to consider seriously commitment to exercise. The fact that more Americans have come to recognize the desirability of personal involvement in fitness activities is truly encouraging; but even those who understand *why* they should exercise need further education on *how* to exercise safely and healthfully.

Agency Programs. The need for sound fitness programs, led by responsible and knowledgeable exercise leaders, is great, and the demand is growing rapidly. Good programs have been available through local Young Men's and Women's Christian Associations (YMCA, YWCA), Young Men's and Women's Hebrew Associations (YMHA, YWHA), Catholic Youth Organizations (CYO) and Junior Chambers of Commerce (JCC) for years. Fitness programs offered through community public recreation and continuing education agencies are expanding to meet the demands. These programs need increased tax support and contributions from the private sector to meet constantly growing needs and to ensure competent leadership in the best interests of the exercising public.

Corporate Health Centers. Corporate health centers have shown promise of contributing toward positive health and fitness for adults employed by large industries. Insurance companies and other large corporations that have provided exercise and sport facilities within the industrial complex, permitted their employees exercise breaks during the working day, and hired qualified educational and health service personnel to operate the health center have found that absenteeism is reduced and that costs for sickness benefits are decreased. It seems shortsighted that more corporations have not taken the initiative in establishing employee health and fitness centers. It is surprising that unions have not pressed more agressively for such facilities in negotiations for better health benefits.

Health Clubs and Spas. It is abundantly clear that Americans in increasing numbers want extended opportunities for participation in fitness programs. If attractive, well-managed, low-cost programs are not provided by public agencies, by non-profit organizations, or by their employers, people will engage in unscientific and potentially hazardous physical activity without qualified leadership — or they will support the "health spa industry" with their membership and service fees. An estimated 1000 health spas or health clubs are now operating very lucrative enterprises across the United States. Although health spas can indeed provide needed health services for those who can afford to pay the price, commercial health clubs have been much criticized.

Most of the knowledgeable criticism of the health spa industry is directed toward the alleged failure to utilize current scientific knowledge of adult physical fitness in planning and administering fitness programs. In the early 1970s many journalists published articles describing questionable practices in health club operations. A 1972 feature in *Today's Health*,[1] entitled "What You'd Better Know Before Joining a Health Club," was one of the early reports that stimulated considerable public concern. The lack of competent instructors to work with adult fitness programs, insufficient attention to necessary medical clearance, and poorly designed exercise programs have been noted. Too often health clubs promote passive exercise and spot reducing rather than scientifically based exercise programs, or the clubs overemphasize weight reduction and neglect cardiovascular fitness and aerobic exercises.

Fortunately, many commercial health clubs do offer needed services to the public, operating reputable businesses and providing sound scientific exercise programs. It behooves the physical education profession and leaders in the health service occupations to accept some responsibility for protecting the public interest through the regulation and upgrading of the health spa industry. Licensing of exercise leaders should certainly be required. Henschen[2] has suggested some key objectives for making the most of the positive aspects of the health club business:

1. Exercise programs offered to adults must be of the type, frequency, duration and intensity that will be most effective in producing the levels of fitness the public so desperately needs and desires. . . .

2. Spas should adopt a standard approach to testing, evaluation and medical clearance prior to program participation. . . .

3. Instructional staff . . . should have at least some college training and preferably a college degree in physical education to be working with a commodity as precious as another person's health. . . .

4. Although fitness programs, like other products and services in the business world, need to be marketed, standardized procedures and acceptable techniques should be utilized. . . .

5. Fitness companies should commit themselves to ongoing programs for improvement and quality control of personnel and services. . . .

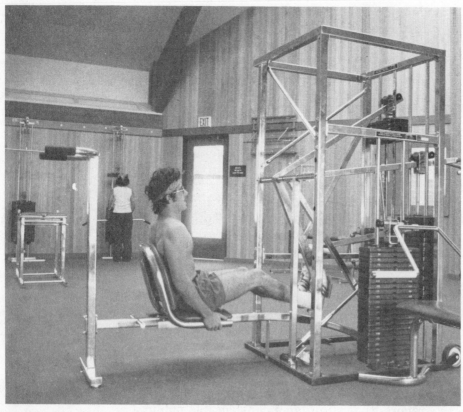

Many health clubs offer needed services to the public.

Henschen[3] has described a "Health Spa Certification" program through the physical education curriculum at the University of Utah that could prepare qualified leadership to assist in the effort to realize the positive potential of commercial health clubs. We believe that more colleges and universities engaged in professional preparation in physical education should consider offering such programs. Now that the concept of "physical fitness" is generally viewed positively, physical education professionals should do everything possible to ensure that exercise is recognized as a lifetime pursuit, that fitness motivation is maintained beyond the initial enthusiastic participation, and, above all, that adult citizens have ample opportunities for soundly designed programs guided by qualified personnel.

As a civilized society increases its concern for individual human **THERAPY** rights and equality of opportunity, greater attention is focused on the persons within that society who may be disadvantaged in any aspect of living through genetic limitation, illness, accident, or environmental or social circumstances. Physical activity has been found to be an effective therapeutic modality for many disabled, disadvantaged, and exceptional children, youths, and adults. Professionals with special expertise in the movement arts and sport sciences are needed as therapists in a wide variety of career fields.

Physical Therapy. Rehabilitative medicine and physical therapy are well-established professional specializations. All hospitals, clinics, veterans facilities, and public health departments make provision for physical therapy services on an inpatient and outpatient basis. Physical therapy is often an essential phase of treatment for patients recovering from surgery or accidents, for regaining maximum range of joint action following an injury, for relieving pain or speeding the healing process. Physicians frequently prescribe physical therapy on a regular basis, directing the therapist to supplement medical procedures with massage, exercise, mechanical apparatuses, heat and cold, light, radiation, water, and various forms of electricity.

Corrective Therapy. Significant growth and development of corrective therapy as a professional field has occurred during the period of marked expansion in physical and mental rehabilitation since World War II. Corrective therapy is defined as the application of medically prescribed therapeutic exercises and activities in the treatment of the mentally and physically ill. The therapy is aimed not only at the physical disability, but also at the psychological and sociological needs resulting from disease and illness. The corrective therapist is a member of a team of medical, paramedical, and behavioral specialists, applying some of the teaching methods and activities of physical education in working *with* the client rather than *on* the patient in solving an individual's physical or mental problems.

Occupational Therapy. Occupational therapy is another health-serving profession concerned with helping the victims of serious illness, accidents, or developmental disabilities find their way back into the mainstream of society. The occupational therapist also works as a member of a team of rehabilitation specialists, focusing on self-help skills essential for gaining personal independence and on basic psychomotor skills needed for employment in a competitive labor market. Therapists working in this area of rehabilitation frequently use physical activities as a medium of communication and restoration.

Dance Therapy. One of the fastest growing of the movement professions is the field of dance therapy. The dance therapist works with children and adults, using dance and expressive movement as another medium of communication and guidance. Inherently pleasurable and successful, dance has certain unique values as a therapeutic tool. Because of the freedom of movement the patient can avoid anxiety-provoking situations. Schmais[4] describes the role of the dance therapist, who assists patients in creating "dances that are based on the subtle interplay of moods and feelings."

> These dances help to clarify, broaden, control, or intensify the patient's movements. Through these movement dialogues, patients start to build a sense of self, to express their feelings, to gain insight, to touch others, and to be in touch with themselves. The therapist plays many parts in this dance, such as director, leader, follower, catalyst, target, etc. All the parts played and the motions made are in the interest of the patient's health.

Recreation Therapy. Recreation therapy is another rather recently established specialization. The demand for recreation therapy is growing rapidly and a current upswing in the number of individuals desiring to qualify as therapists is supported by federal programs funding professional preparation in therapeutic recreation. As with dance therapy, recreation therapy involves a medium that is inherently pleasurable. The scope of activities is far broader in recreation, however, since any form of leisure activity, including many that are not primarily physical in nature, can be employed. Because play is ordinarily a nonthreatening aspect of life, recreational activities have a high potential for creating an environment in which patients with either mental or physical illness can relax, receive positive emotional stimulation, and feel joy in living. Individuals needing therapy can discover themselves, improve communication and appreciate others, and establish lasting feelings of significance and self-worth.

Historically, the medical profession has been primarily concerned with helping individuals to recover from illness, disease, and accidents. In recent decades health has been increasingly defined as a positive concept, encompassing much more than the absence of disease. Paralleling this view, medical practice has reflected increasing concern for preventive medicine, with development of medical specialties and health care plans that place major attention on maintaining optimum individual and societal health.

PREVENTIVE MEDICINE

Movement Counseling. Clinics specializing in preventive medicine employ nutritionists, leisure counselors, social workers, and health educators to work with physicians and therapists in providing preventive health services. Movement specialists should also have a role on the preventive medicine team, although not many are yet recognized as essential members of these cooperative working groups. More and more physicians are prescribing exercise as a treatment, however, and much illness and many injuries could be avoided if movement specialists were called upon to help identify potential problem areas in lack of physical conditioning, decreasing joint flexibility, inappropriate body alignment, and inability to initiate conscious neuromuscular relaxation techniques. Clients should have access to the services of movement counselors who

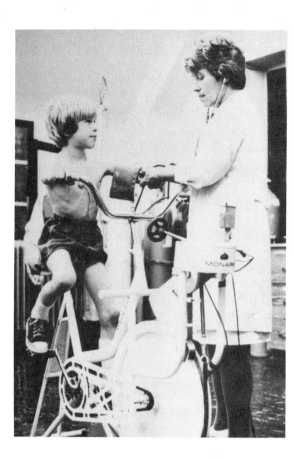

Emphasis in medicine has shifted to preventive medicine and health maintenance.

are qualified to educate them in fitness assessment procedures, to guide the planning of individual exercise programs, and to be resource persons for discovering physical recreation activities appropriate to individual interests and lifestyles.

Sports Medicine. Sports medicine should be viewed not as a medical subspecialty but as a cooperative, positive health endeavor with a major responsibility for preventing and treating sport injuries. Today sports-medicine clinics are in operation all over the United States. Clients seek treatment for tennis elbows; stress fractures; tendinitis; dislocated shoulders, hips and fingers; strains and sprains; and all manner of bruises, abrasions, lacerations, and concussions. The vast majority of injuries result from the "overuse syndrome"—trying to push an out-of-condition body too far too fast. It is estimated that during 1977, 20 million Americans were hurt in recreational athletics, and that 80 per cent of such injuries could have been avoided with some simple precautions.[5] The best sports-medicine clinics are staffed by orthopedists, internists, cardiologists, nutrition experts, clinical psychologists, exercise physiologists, and athletic trainers. In addition to treating injuries, they conduct research and provide counsel as coaches and equipment advisers.

The American College of Sports Medicine. The American College of Sports Medicine was founded in 1954 by a group of physicians, physical educators, and physiologists. The following purposes were identified: (1) to promote and advance scientific studies dealing with the effect of sports and other motor activities on the health of human beings at various stages of life; (2) to cooperate with other organizations concerned with various aspects of human fitness; (3) to sponsor meetings of physicians, educators, and other scientists whose work is relevant to sports medicine; (4) to make available postgraduate education in fields related to the objectives of the College; (5) to initiate, encourage, and correlate research; and (6) to publish a journal dealing with scientific aspects of activity and their relationship to human fitness. The College is affiliated with the American Alliance for Health, Physical Education, Recreation and Dance and the Fédération Internationale de Médecine Sportive. It holds an annual national convention, and the College's regional chapters conduct scientific meetings. It publishes a regular newsletter and a quarterly journal, and published the first edition of *The Encyclopedia of Sport Sciences and Medicine* in 1972.

SOCIAL SERVICE

Most analysts of the human condition agree that today's people face difficult problems in all areas of living. While Western civilization can point with considerable pride toward great progress in extending the frontiers of agrarian cultures, in industrializing large human societies, and in advancing technology, progress in improving human social arrangements has been less impressive. The world's people have not yet learned to live together happily, either within national boundaries or as a global community. Philosophers urge attention to the clarification of personal and social values in the pursuit of common human goals. Scientists express concern for the ethical and moral aspects of applying certain significant research findings. Political leaders stress commitments to basic human rights. All of us recognize the increasing importance of social service in human communities throughout the world.

The Role of Movement and Sport

Sports and the movement arts frequently play an important role in social service programs. Because play and physical recreation are inherently pleasurable, movement activities are included typically in programs seeking to offer deprived or disadvantaged populations opportunities for meaningful group interaction. For some individuals, sport is a primary channel for developing feelings of self-worth. Well-planned and

Increasing democratization of the arts has brought dance into the daily lives of the masses.

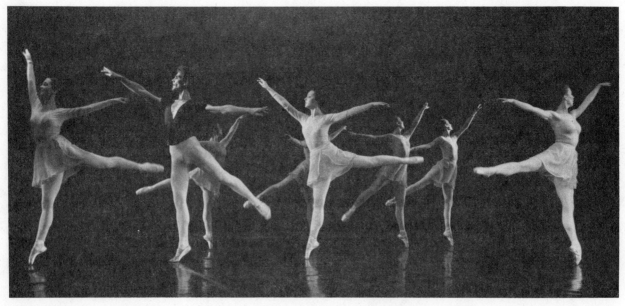

CHAPTER NINE

thoughtfully guided physical recreation programs tend to stimulate total involvement during the play or performance and thus contribute toward emotional and psychological well-being. Social workers and behavioral scientists believe that sport, dance, and exercise are generally wholesome activities when engaged in under the right conditions; consequently, participation is often encouraged with the hope of substituting positive interests for socially undesirable behaviors. As Americans become more and more sports-minded, and as popular interest in dance and other movement arts increases, the social service role of the movement arts and sport sciences is bound to become even more significant.

The movement arts and sport sciences are viewed as a factor in the attempt to solve many social problems, primarily because of the pervasiveness of sport in American society. Because sport has such a powerful impact on the lives of most Americans it is reasonable to try to direct its influence toward societal goals in planning and conducting social service programs.

It is probable that sport in America will continue its popular role in the lives of the masses. Continuing high levels of unemployment extend the non-working time of many and increase the leisure hours of the marginally employed. For the many unable to afford costly hobbies and entertainment, participation in public recreation programs and individual activities requiring nominal costs is feasible. Increasing democratization of the arts and public support for extending opportunities in the broad field of the arts and humanities has brought many forms of dance into the daily lives of lower- and middle-class children, youths, and adults. Overwhelming coverage in newspapers and popular magazines, continuing sport domination of network television, and increasing emphasis on ballet, modern dance, yoga, and fitness exercises, particularly by public broadcasting, keep sport and the movement arts in the public consciousness.

The social service role of the movement arts and sport sciences is heightened by changing philosophies in viewing the body and physical activity. Positive concepts of personal involvement in physical activities and increasing readiness to view the body as self rather than object are more characteristic of Americans than such attitudes were ten years ago. Leonard's[6] popularization of "the ultimate athlete" as "one who joins body, mind, and spirit in the dance of existence" has made a difference. Michener[7] has also stimulated interest in "this enlarging of the human adventure that sports are all about."

Sociologists have provided substantial documentation of changed patterns of family life. Futurists generally predict that current trends will continue — that alternative lifestyles and social arrangements should be anticipated. Many attempting to deal with problems of social transition suggest that the movement arts and sport sciences may be of use in providing local laboratories for positive social interaction.

Ensuring equal opportunity for minorities and women has become an increasingly critical social concern during the past quarter century. Social justice for blacks, ethnic minorities, women, and handicapped persons frequently takes the form of equal access to sport, athletic, and recreational opportunities, and equal employment in occupations relating to sport.

Alert to their potential social service role, school physical education programs attend particularly to the need to develop positive self-images, to assist individuals in establishing satisfying physical recreation interests, to eliminate sex stereotypes relating to participation in physical

Sports are an enlarging of the human adventure.

activities, and to exploit the potential of cooperative group interaction in well-managed competitive sport. Current concepts of social responsibility assign a significant role to public education. Schools in turn must fulfill the important task of developing socially responsible citizens. And all professions, including physical education and dance, must contribute to the solution of major social problems. Social services provided by professionals in the movement arts and sport sciences include day care centers and youth agencies; services for the aging; correctional institu-

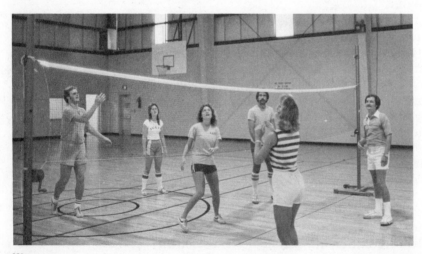

Women must now have equal access to sport, athletic, and recreational opportunities.

CHAPTER NINE

tions and programs for the rehabilitation of delinquents; and legally mandated equal opportunity programs.

American lifestyles have changed dramatically in the past generation. A major change has been the modification of the nuclear family, once the only widely accepted family pattern. Since World War II, single-parent families and families with both parents working outside the home have increased in number.

Preschool Programs. An inflationary economy and the women's rights movement have heightened the need for day care centers, in addition to public nursery schools and traditional preschool programs. As more young children spend more of their waking hours in settings outside their family homes, it becomes especially important to consider whether they are experiencing appropriately developmental environments during these early formative years. Research clearly supports the value of extensive and varied movement experience in the development of the young child. Studies of American child-rearing practices and parental attitudes suggest that, even in "typical" middle-class homes with a male head-of-the-household earning the total family income and the wife devoting full time to the home and family, many children are overprotected, often resulting in limited involvement and no encouragement in stimulating movement activities. Any program designed for the care or education of young children should afford sufficient participation in sound, vigorous physical developmental activities in a safe but stimulating environment. Day care centers should be required to meet this standard for licensing or certification.

Both public and private preschool programs are growing in popularity. In 1971, 4.3 million children were enrolled in nursery schools and kindergartens.[7a] Programs for preschool age children should draw heavily upon the educational potential of movement experiences. Certified early childhood teachers are now expected to possess competencies in movement education essential to the educational guidance of young children.

Social Agency Programs for Youth. Social agencies established to provide services to preadolescent, adolescent, and postadolescent youth have long recognized the value of sport and dance activities. Programs of physical activity are prominent in the overall plans of public, semipublic, and private agencies. Organizations such as the YMCA, YWCA, YMHA, YWHA, JCC, and CYO rely heavily on sport and dance programs to attract and maintain youth membership and participation. Some large individual congregations of organized religious groups employ full-time leaders to direct youth activity programs and coordinate the work of volunteer coaches, sport leaders, dance teachers, and other recreation specialists.

The Scouting movement continues to be strong in this country, with current membership of the Boy Scouts and the Girl Scouts of America totaling over 10 million. These organizations and others, such as the Campfire Girls, play important roles in providing opportunities for young persons to be involved in service-oriented activities and healthful recreation and to develop personal and social skills. Five million young people 9 to 19 years of age are now served by 4-H programs, which offer self-directed education and prevocational experiences as well as recreational and service activities. While sports and the movement arts are not a primary focus in most of these programs, all utilize organized physical activities as an important feature of their group meetings, major conferences or youth rallies, and summer camping programs.

Boys Clubs of America and Girls Clubs of America are organized primarily as a social service in communities recognizing the need for positive peer group identification and responsible adult supervision for disadvantaged youth. Such clubs have been especially effective in large urban communities with significant populations of underprivileged boys and girls. Boys Clubs now enroll a million youngsters in 1000 clubs. Membership in Girls Clubs numbers more than 130,000 in 200 club centers. Sports programs flourish in these club centers and are believed to provide a strong positive influence.

Sociologists, political scientists, economists, psychologists, public health specialists, and educators are all coming to recognize *agism* (or ageism) as a critical social problem. Gunn[8] asserts that agism is "one of the greatest of all social problems in that it will directly affect most of us regardless of race or sex." Every day over 4000 Americans celebrate their sixty-fifth birthday; persons 65 and over now constitute 11 per cent of the nation's population. As a society we desperately need to develop new understandings of the aging process, new perspectives on the problems of the elderly, and new policies for the future.

The conditions of modern life in the United States have created some particular problems for older people. We live in an age that is centered on youth and that places a high value on physical prowess. In assessing the potential influence of the movement arts and sport sciences on the quality of life in the later years, we need to be aware both of services designed to help the aging and of their need to continue to serve others. We must take into account the older person's need for self-respect, the continuing importance of meaningful involvement in the lives of others, and the

NEW PERSPECTIVES ON AGING

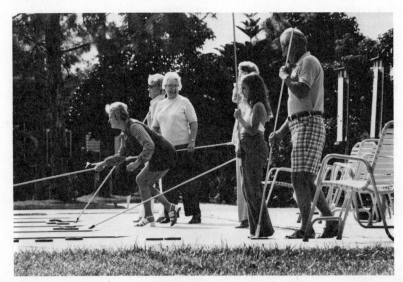

Persons of all ages need to be provided with opportunities to learn new knowledges and new skills

CHAPTER NINE

potential for promoting the full use of existing physical and mental capacities and abilities. Special efforts must be made to overcome false stereotypes that negatively influence both the self-image of the elderly and the reactions of others in our society toward them.

Aging is a fact of life to be accepted; successful adjustment to aging is a realistic goal. Maintaining the ability to be physically independent, to be self-directing, and to do things for oneself as one ages is important to self-esteem. Older people can and do learn. Persons of all ages need to be provided with opportunities to learn new knowledges and new skills. Aging persons need to find substitutes for former activities and to learn to find meaning and satisfaction in these new activities. Older persons can and do change. As unavoidable deterioration in abilities and capacities occurs and living environments are necessarily modified, they need encouragement, concern, and assistance appropriate to their unique needs to continue to lead individually rewarding lives.

Among prevalent sociological theories regarding aging, we concur with the activity theory, which holds that active individuals find life more satisfying than do those who withdraw from the mainstream of society. Recent clinical and research evidence generally supports the thesis that physical and mental deterioration can be slowed by continuing activity. Physical fitness and recreation programs are needed by the elderly. Leslie has provided an excellent summary of the types of programs needed:[9]

> The differences between the types of programs involve the priority given to: (1) a high or low level of physiological stress to which the participants are subjected, (2) an emphasis on the constellation of factors that foster a subjective feeling of well being and self-worth in the participants. Moderate- to high-stress programs that are designed to significantly improve cardiovascular fitness are badly needed but are very expensive and should be under the direction of highly trained personnel. . . . Low-stress programs that emphasize flexibility, muscle toning and balance as fitness variables and emphasize socializing benefits and the development of a favorable self-concept are more feasible to develop. Efforts should be initiated to develop programs with all the above priorities and emphasis but because of the cost and time factors . . . the greatest emphasis should, at this time, be on the low-stress programs.

Although the aging process is characterized by a gradual reduction in dynamic fitness qualities of muscular strength, flexibility, endurance, and neuromuscular coordination, sensible exercise regimens throughout life decelerate these changes. Research supports the positive biological effects of exercise; there is some evidence that training effects can be achieved by persons in their sixties.[10] There is considerable support for the theory that social withdrawal patterns in the elderly can be delayed and even reversed through the physical and mental activities of socializing games and exercise sessions.

Trained leadership is needed to provide programs that educate older persons to the importance of remaining active; training for activity directors to lead programs for the elderly is a critical need. The social service role of the movement arts and sciences has a dual emphasis for the aging, as it has for youth. Problems and difficulties of both the young and the old can sometimes be prevented or ameliorated with physical activity. The unique needs of a youth or an older person can often be met through the opportunity to feel worthwhile to others in a setting in which physical activity is a factor, directly or indirectly.

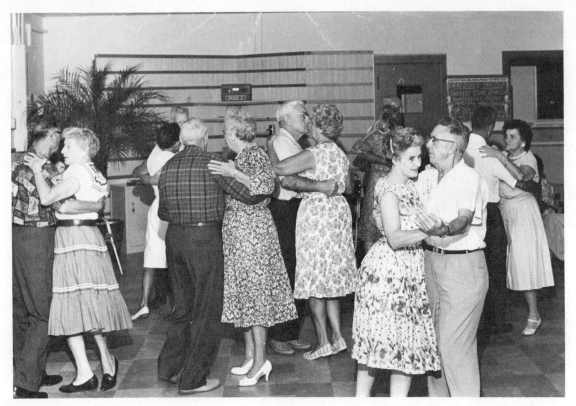

It is believed that social withdrawal patterns in the elderly can be delayed through physical activity and exercise.

Since the era of the New Deal, during the administration of Franklin D. Roosevelt, it has been widely accepted that the federal government is responsible to the American people to provide leadership and substantial financial support in national efforts to resolve major social problems and to improve the welfare of disadvantaged citizens in whatever geographical region they live. Through federal legislation and executive directives, official support is designated for concentrated attention to and federal assistance for particular social problems. In many programs now receiving major federal allocations, sport and recreation play an important role. Even in these days of increasing revolts against taxes, the movement arts and sport sciences will no doubt continue to have an impact on the success of government programs in alleviating crime, delinquency, and recidivism; promoting the civil rights of ethnic minorities, women, and the handicapped; and decreasing underemployment and hard-core unemployment.

Crime and Delinquency, and Offender Rehabilitation. Social agencies at all levels are concerned about high crime rates, and especially about increases in violent crimes. Prisoner rebellions are also of concern. While the causes of crime are complex and controversial, evidence suggests that carefully planned programs of sport and recreation can be a positive factor in fulfilling basic human needs of inmates in correctional institutions. Current policy supports emphasizing rehabilitation and social exposure, for which recreation is viewed as a useful tool. Prison programs of

GOVERNMENT SERVICES TO ALLEVIATE MAJOR SOCIAL PROBLEMS

CHAPTER NINE

supervised physical activity may assist not only in providing needed physical exercise but also in developing a healthy self-respect, better relationships with peers, and recognition that rules and regulations are necessary.

Different types of programs are needed in accordance with the security conditions and the different populations of institutions. More and more, however, officials in prisons and other correctional institutions are recognizing the need for and the potential value of the services of activity therapists. Many institutions now provide a wide variety of activities within the institution. A number also provide for competitive sport programs with other institutional populations and with teams of non-institutionalized individuals. This closer-to-typical adult social interaction is believed to be a positive rehabilitative experience.

Physical Recreation and Rehabilitation. Most programs designed to decrease juvenile delinquency use sport and physical recreation as one method to substitute socially acceptable activities for delinquent or potentially criminal behavior. While scientific evidence of the effectiveness of these programs is still limited, many professionals working with juvenile offenders have found them below average in physical fitness and involvement in physical activity. Low levels of physical fitness may be a contributing factor to the passive approach to life characteristic of drug abusers and to the poor self-concepts that frequently lead youngsters to delinquent behavior.

A Case Study. Collingwood[11] has reported on a Dallas Police Department program for 10- to 16-year-old boys and girls who were arrested. During two of their six months in the Youth Services Program, juvenile offenders received training in physical skills, with attention to emotional and intellectual factors as well. During the four-month follow-up period, each child was put on an exercise application program to be done at home three times a week, and was assisted in becoming involved in a recreation or sport activity.

> Over 1,000 juvenile offenders were referred to the Youth Services Program during its first full year of operation. The 264 youngsters who completed the program's physical training and recreation component averaged a 12% increase in fitness during the first five weeks. About half of those who were put on the home application program followed the physical fitness training routine. There was a 49% increase in involvement in recreation and sports activities.
>
> As fitness and participation increased, recidivism dropped. The usual rate of rearrest is 35%; during the first year of the program, only 2.7% of the youth who completed the program were rearrested.
>
> It seems that a systematic effort to raise the physical fitness levels of delinquents and to involve them in recreation and sports can help to decrease their eventual involvement in crime. While the Youth Services Program also emphasizes emotional and intellectual factors, the importance of physical activity seems obvious.

Ethnic Minority Rights. Sport in America has provided upward mobility and equal opportunity for members of minority groups, but evidence of discrimination against ethnic minorities in this activity continues to exist. Our cultural heritage includes many stories of rugged individualists who achieved fame as athletic heroes. The earliest studies of social class in this country highlight the phenomena of low-status ethnic groups who gravitated toward particular sports, and of individual members of these groups who climbed the social ladder via athletic prowess.

As the civil rights movements of the 1950s and 1960s gained momentum, we began to understand better the importance of competence and skill to the self-image of those struggling for self-worth, identity within an ethnic minority, and belonging to a larger group. Physical skill or athletic excellence became a primary goal for many, especially black youth. Inevitably, many were disillusioned and frustrated, since only the most talented could achieve success and high status as athletes.

Discrimination in Sport.   At the same time, it also became apparent that racial and ethnic discrimination existed in sport itself. Allegations of racism were publicized in the media, with "the revolt of the black athlete" achieving journalistic prominence during the Olympic Games in Mexico City in 1968. In football, for example, there are still charges that blacks and Chicanos are seldom assigned to key leadership positions, such as quarterback; that they must play less desirable positions; that they are "stacked" on the team roster, so that one minority group member is the substitute for another; and that they are treated unequally on trips with respect to lodging facilities and sometimes are discriminated against in other ways. (See illustration below.) Many coaching staffs in all sports still do not have representatives from various ethnic groups in proportion to the number of athletes on the team from the minorities. Few blacks or other ethnic minority group members are head coaches, athletic directors, or game officials. Few are elected to high office in athletic associations, and few are selected for honors bestowed by the coaching fraternity through its professional associations. Aptitude tests required for admission to some colleges are culturally biased against members of minority races yet are crucial to selection for admission. Because blacks and young people of other minority ethnic groups have not had equal access to swimming pools, golf courses, and tennis clubs, very few of them have

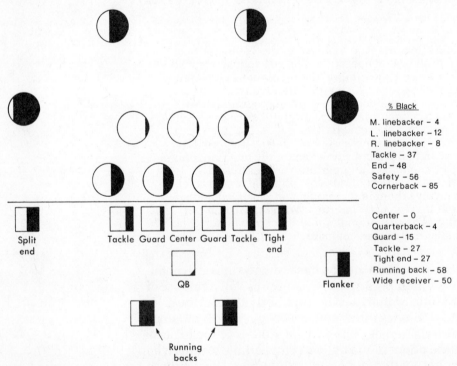

% Black

M. linebacker – 4
L. linebacker – 12
R. linebacker – 8
Tackle – 37
End – 48
Safety – 56
Cornerback – 85

Center – 0
Quarterback – 4
Guard – 15
Tackle – 27
Tight end – 27
Running back – 58
Wide receiver – 50

Split end

Tackle Guard Center Guard Tackle Tight end

QB

Flanker

Running backs

The percentage of black players in each of the starting offensive and defensive positions during the 1974–75 professional football season.

CHAPTER NINE

reached the top levels of either amateur or professional competition in these and a number of other less popular sports.

Signs of racial discrimination are diminishing in our country, however. In this context it is important to recognize the potential sport has for modifying the fabric of American society, and it is encouraging to observe that sport provides a vehicle for social integration and equal opportunity for blacks and other ethnic minorities. A popular, universally understood, and highly visible activity, sport can help the individual develop the confidence needed to participate fully and with satisfaction in today's world.

Women's Rights. The women's rights movement in this country has been compared frequently to the earlier civil rights movement; and many of the difficulties in eliminating discrimination and inequity are indeed similar. But the specific solutions to problems of discrimination on the basis of sex are significantly different in the areas of sport, athletics, and physical education. Our society's traditional attitude that limited participation in vigorous physical activity was in the best interests of women became strongly entrenched because of widespread misconceptions about inherent biological and psychological differences between the sexes in their capacities and in the consequences of sport participation. It has seldom been charged that blacks or other ethnic group members were less suited to take part in rugged athletics than were whites. Yet many have believed this comparison to be true between women and men. American girls and women typically have withdrawn from athletic participation in response to social pressures in support of a "feminine image" that did not include vigorous sports participation.

Sport has long been recognized as a means for developing in the young attitudes and behaviors needed for fully satisfying participation in adult society. Yet the achievement of highly refined motor skills and the development of self-confidence, independence, courage, ambition, and competitiveness considered healthy in men have been considered undesirable for women. In a nation in which sport is such a predominant phenomenon, it is not surprising that the women's rights movement should focus on athletics with the demand that these opportunities no longer be limited to males.

These conditions are changing, as described in a recent *Time* cover story:[12]

> Spurred by the fitness craze, fired up by the feminist movement and buttressed by court rulings and legislative mandates, women have been moving from miniskirted cheerleading on the sidelines for the boys to playing, and playing hard, for themselves.

Athletic programs for women have been dramatically upgraded, both in secondary schools and in colleges and universities. Women are participating in sports in much greater numbers and trying everything from jogging to baseball, ice hockey, and crew. Title IX of the 1972 Education Amendments to the Elementary and Secondary Education Act (ESEA) has supported increased participation of women in sport by providing for the withholding of federal funds from any educational institution practicing sex discrimination, whether such discrimination occurs in the classroom or on the athletic field.

Athletic programs are extremely visible and the changes in women's athletics have caught public attention and imagination. At least equally important are the changes occurring in instructional physical education

Women are participating in sports in much greater numbers.

programs. Changes in attitudes toward women in sport are being reflected in changes in the role of sport and movement activities in the lives of girls and women. School programs are being modified to eliminate sex stereotypes in vigorous physical activities, to extend access to the full range of physical education opportunities to female as well as male students, and to permit most classes to be conducted on a coeducational basis. AAHPERD published a manual to assist local education agencies in implementing the changes.[13]

Services to the Handicapped and Disabled.   Increased knowledge and understanding of the handicapped or exceptional person as an individual with normal needs, interests, and desires has led us to seek better ways of integrating these individuals into society and diverse human activities. In response to an awakened social consciousness, legislation guarantees the rights of handicapped persons to equal educational opportunities, equal employment opportunities, and full access to public services of all kinds. Attitudes are changing and services are expanding to facilitate the movement of exceptional persons into the mainstream of American life.

A major focus of social programs to provide equal opportunity for the handicapped is public education. Public Law 94–142, the Education of the Handicapped Act of 1974, requires that equal educational opportunities be provided to the handicapped in the least restrictive environments possible. Physical education is recognized as an essential educational program for all; regardless of their disability, handicapped individuals need to develop their unique motor abilities. Both functional motor skills and physical recreation skills are important competencies.

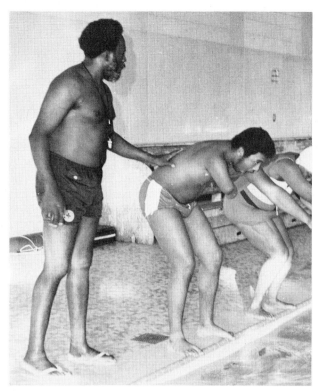

Public Law 94–142 insures equal opportunity for handicapped individuals to develop their unique motor abilities.

Key goals of all programs designed to provide services to the handicapped are the development of basic skills for self-sufficient living and the fostering of feelings of human dignity and individual worth. The movement arts and sport sciences play an important role in working toward each of these goals. Fundamental motor skills allow the young exceptional child to develop personal independence and assist the severely injured and orthopedically disabled in the rehabilitation process. Specialized training in movement activities is a key element in education and treatment in developmental clinics, rehabilitation centers, hospitals, remedial education centers, and schools for special populations. The growth of athletic programs for the handicapped has been phenomenal. The success of such programs as the Special Olympics attests to the value of physical recreational opportunities for the disabled.

Underemployment. During periods of economic depression or recession, when unemployment rates are high and many additional working adults are unemployed, federal government support for the movement arts and sport sciences has usually increased. Such assistance is typically an indirect means of creating additional work opportunities or providing for healthful involvement of discouraged and potentially alienated youth. New Deal programs of the 1930s, such as the Civilian Conservation Corps, the Public Works Administration, and the Works Progress Administration, created public outdoor recreation areas, built gymnasiums, and opened jobs to artists, sport and dance specialists, and recreation leaders. More recently, the Volunteers in Service to America (VISTA) and the Teacher Corps programs have utilized the skills and professional training of physical educators to work with the poor and culturally disadvantaged in many American communities. CETA (Comprehensive Employment and Training Act) programs are currently helping many develop job skills and providing various public services, including supplementary instructional programs in physical education.

Since human beings are social creatures who live and work in groups, communication is a primary human activity. It is vital to our very existence that we learn to communicate effectively with each other. As our world changes, the demands for communication and the nature and forms of communication also change. Technology diminishes distances and crosses geographical boundaries, communications systems become increasingly complex and sophisticated, and human interaction with greater numbers and more diversified groups of persons is required. As changing lifestyles involve us less in primary groups and more in secondary groups, meaningful interpersonal communication becomes a greater challenge. **COMMUNICATIONS**

Western cultures have emphasized verbal modes in knowing and communicating, yet other avenues are available to us. These include music and the graphic arts — and human movement. "Body language" adds a dimension to human communication that is not present in the traditional "language arts" of speaking, reading and writing. Symbolic forms of human movement express ideas and feelings in ways not duplicated by other communicative media. In movement, individuals express messages that do not lend themselves to the spoken or written word. Some persons find communication through dance and sport more satisfying than verbal communication. *The Role of Movement and Sport*

Movement activities play an indirect but important role in communications through bringing people together for participation in sport, dance, or exercise activities or for cultural or sporting events. Such occasions typically provide informal settings for common interests that enhance communication among persons of different ages, backgrounds, occupational specializations, and social classes.

In addition, because of the widespread interest and the popularity of sports, dance, and other movement activities, they have become a major focus for our reading, viewing, conversation, recreation, and social criticism. Thus, the American communications industries unquestionably have a major impact on the nature and quality of the individual's daily human experience through their emphasis on sport.

Historical and comparative studies have documented varying roles of human movement in communication. Dance has provided a means of self-expression and communication in societies throughout history; the various forms of dance have reflected differing needs, lifestyles, and values. Ritual and ceremony have incorporated special dance and sport activities into major life events, both in family and societal patterns.

Research in Movement Arts and Communication. Increasing numbers of sociologists are becoming interested in sport participation as a means of providing identification with a social group or subculture characterized by its own unique forms of expression; as an effective arena for social protest; or as a focus for examining popular values relating to such complex issues as amateurism. Social psychologists, phenomenologists, existentialists, and behavioral and humanistic psychologists are investigating topics significant for understanding and implementing the communications role of the movement arts and sport sciences. Psychological profiles of athletes, analyses of the processes of self-actualization through sport or dance, hypotheses concerning right and left brain functioning, studies of addiction in runners and of the effects of ergogenic aids in competitive sports, and concepts of the inner athlete as "Self 2" in sport achievement have attracted considerable public attention through the mass media. The role of social conditioning in developing sex stereotypes expressed in sport and dance activities is of special interest in this era of growing social awareness.

Physical Education and Communication. School physical education programs have tended to respond to the impact of mass media in undesirable rather than positive ways. Too often the physical education program has been allowed to lose its proper focus on the activity needs of all students in favor of community interest in the success of school athletic teams. Or the curriculum has become a series of repetitive practice sessions of the seasonal sports instead of thoughtfully planned sequences of movement experiences directed toward selected learning outcomes. School programs can and should use special television programs and newspaper and magazine features to enrich learning in physical education, stimulate interest in a wide variety of activities, assist in the analysis of skillful movement, develop appreciation of competent motor performance in sport and dance, and provide real life examples for class activities in value clarification and problem solving.

Physical educators who recognize their responsibilities in the communications area are now giving more attention to dance and other activities that offer greater opportunity for personal integration and self-expression. They are exploring instructional strategies that encourage individual involvement in movement process learning, commitment to continuing participation in exercise, and sport activities as a channel for meaningful personal interaction. They are seeking more accurate and

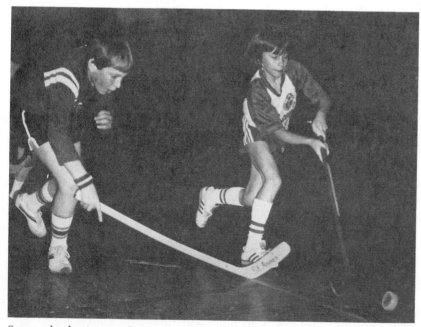

Some school programs have overemphasized seasonal sports instead of carefully planning appropriate movement experiences.

positive communication in and about sport and dance by working to overcome sex stereotypes and by fostering positive concepts about the participation of both sexes. Education about the communications role of the movement arts and sport sciences must be a part of good school physical education programs. Important development of this role may be anticipated in the areas of journalism and broadcasting, dance and sports art, and international understanding.

Because sport is a major interest of the American public, sports communication is a growing specialization within the mass media. Newspaper, magazine, television, and radio coverage of sports events, dance performances, and popular forms of exercise participation continues to rise.

Newspapers. In 1977 there were approximately 1800 daily newspapers in the United States. Almost without exception, the sports section is a major part of the daily newspaper. Many citizens are more interested in the details of yesterday's professional football, basketball, or baseball games than in the international or national news. The standings of local athletic teams often hold greater reader interest than local elections, proposed public building construction, school board actions, or needed reforms in county judicial systems or state constitutions.

Sports writers have created followings of fans who loyally debate the latest team standings in the wire service polls at the beginning of every week and vociferously argue about the predictions for the game outcomes. In recognizing the team of the week, the sportsman of the month, the all-conference athletes, they create popular heroes, assist young athletes to earn college scholarships, control the career choices and modify the private lives of successful athletes; they also build reputations and end careers of many athletes, coaches, officials, managers and athletic administrators.

Newspaper coverage can promote interest in and public support for a city ballet company, a relatively unfamiliar sport like soccer, or a recreational activity such as jogging. Lack of newspaper coverage can also be a determining factor in the failure of such an activity to win sufficient popular interest to become an established part of community life. So important is sports communication that current interpretations of Title IX provisions include equal access to sports information services by women's athletic teams. Through their impact on attendance at local events, newspapers influence spectator sport involvement in every community; such publicity also affects physical activity participation by influencing the allocation of public funds supporting community activities.

Magazines. Eighty-five to one hundred sports magazines are published in the United States today, with magazines such as *Sports Illustrated,* and *Sport,* covering a diversity of sport topics for thousands of readers. *Sports Illustrated* ranked 20th in U.S. magazine circulation in 1977 with a circulation of over 2 million. The top 50 circulation leaders, each reporting circulation over a million, included, in addition to *Sports Illustrated, Sport, Field and Stream,* and *Outdoor Life.* New magazines entering the field in the 1970s included several committed to the promotion of women's sports and the support of women in sport.

Many magazines designed for the advocates of a single sport have also won substantial audiences. Participants and fans subscribe to their

CHAPTER NINE

favorite magazines on bicycling, bowling, fencing, golf, gymnastics, running, skiing, swimming, tennis, yachting, and many other sports. These publications highlight news and information on the major contests, the outstanding athletes, instruction, training tips, equipment, fashions, and sport holidays.

In addition, sports articles are published by at least 500 other weekly and monthly magazines, including most of the circulation leaders. Many have regular sports sections and frequently address a cover story or a major feature to a timely sports topic. In its Bicentennial Year Edition, the 1976 *Almanac and Yearbook, Reader's Digest* devoted 101 pages, or over 10 per cent of the total copy, to sports and games. Clearly, sports have a major impact on the reading public.

Radio and Television. Between 1970 and 1975, the number of radio and television stations in the United States rose from 8127 to 9200. Stations in operation in 1975 included 4488 commercial AM radio stations, 2847 commercial FM radio stations, 850 educational FM radio stations, 759 commercial TV stations, and 256 educational TV stations. Professional and college sport coverage on radio and television easily matches, if not exceeds, that in newspapers and magazines.

Radio coverage consists of daily, and sometimes hourly, reports on sports scores and sporting world highlights. Many stations also broadcast local or major athletic events live, with play-by-play descriptions of the action and extensive commentary. Experienced sportcasters are masters in the art of involving listeners of a sport that may be taking place hundreds of miles away. Such listening has become an important part of the lives of countless Americans, be they commuters tuning in their car radios on the way home from work or fans unable to attend the sport event.

Sports coverage is a very profitable business for the television industry. The preponderance of time allocated for live coverage of the professional and college league sports, especially football, basketball, hockey, and baseball, continues to increase. Addiction to TV viewing of sports is even acknowledged to be a factor contributing to marital difficulties and divorce.

Sports spectaculars are major prime time features on all networks. Many hours of coverage are given to major tennis and golf tournaments, to both summer and winter Olympics and other international sports events, to boxing and wrestling matches, even to state high school athletic tournaments. Every thirty-minute local news broadcast includes a five- to fifteen-minute sports segment.

The impact of television on sport, physical activity, and human movement concepts of the American public is felt in many dimensions. Many films are created to immortalize famous athletes; some offer social criticism on the questionable ethics and morality too often associated with athletics. The athletic prowess of television heroes ranges from Wonder Woman and the Incredible Hulk to the Six Million Dollar Man and the Bionic Woman. Regular programming now includes "athletic" contests among teams of television stars. Commercials, with varying degrees of subtlety, espouse physical fitness and sports participation.

While undoubtedly a major factor in determining the leisure interests and social values of many Americans, the influence of television may or may not be in the best interests of our physical and mental health as individuals and our progress as a civilization. Unfortunately, much of the best programming, from the standpoint of the potential contribution

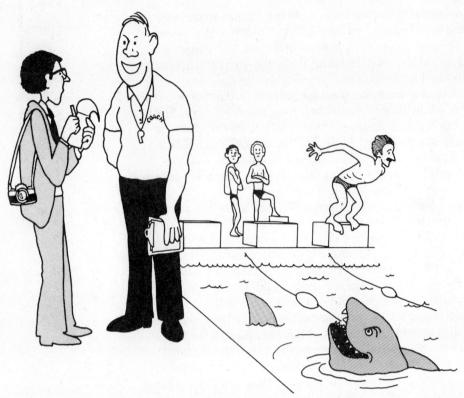

"The TV network people said that the public would never watch professional swimming unless we made it more exciting." From Coakley, Jay, 1978, C. V. Mosby Co.

of the movement arts and sciences, is found in educational television networks. The Public Broadcasting System has created and broadcast many fine programs on dance, yoga, tennis, skiing, conditioning exercise, and other potential lifetime sports.

McLuhan[14] has contributed a particularly intriguing analysis of games as mass media and of the relationships between art and games:

DANCE AND SPORTS ART

> Art and games enable us to stand aside from the material pressures of routine and convention, observing and questioning. Games as popular art forms offer to all an immediate means of participation in the full life of a society, such as no single role or job can offer to any man. . . . Art and games need rules, conventions, and spectators. . . . "Play" . . . implies *interplay*. There must be give and take, or dialogue, as between two or more persons and groups. . . . Sport, as a popular art form, is not just self-expression but is deeply and necessarily a means of interplay within an entire culture.
>
> Art is not just play but an extension of human awareness in contrived and conventional patterns. Sport as popular art is a deep reaction to the typical action of the society. But high art, on the other hand, is not a reaction but a profound reappraisal of a complex cultural state. . . . Perhaps there is . . . a desperate need for games in a highly specialized industrial culture, since they are the only form of art accessible to many minds. . . . Men without art, and men without the popular arts of games, tend toward automatism. . . .
>
> Any game, like any medium of information, is an extension of the individual or the group. Its effect on the group or individual is a reconfiguring of the parts of the group or individual that are *not* so

extended. . . . Art, like games, is a translator of experience. What we have already felt or seen in one situation we are suddenly given in a new kind of material. . . . Games, then are contrived and controlled situations, extensions of group awareness that permit a respite from customary patterns. They are a kind of talking to itself on the part of society as a whole. Any talking to oneself is a recognized form of play that is indispensable to any growth of self-confidence. . . .

That games are extensions, not of our private but of our social selves, and that they are media of communication, should now be plain. If, finally, we ask, "Are games mass media?" the answer has to be "Yes." Games are situations contrived to permit simultaneous participation of many people in some significant pattern of their own corporate lives.

Dance and sports art as communications media take many forms, including dance of all types, literature, photography, and the graphic arts.

Dance. Like games, dance as a folk art is a translator of experience and a means of interplay within the entire culture. Folk dance, including Western square dance, mountain clog, tap, jazz, disco, ballroom, and exotic dance in the United States, as well as the national dances of all countries, brings people together in situations which add additional dimensions to interpersonal communication. Folk dances of all types ritualize or stylize significant events or activities of the culture that created them. Frequently, they lend increased meaning to cross-cultural communications.

Dance as "high art" extends human awareness through direct communication between choreographers and performers, and viewing audiences. Both ballet and modern dance concerts serve as media of aesthetic communication and social criticism, frequently reinforced and extended by dance critics who provide analyses and commentary through the mass media.

Literature. Dance and sport have become increasingly popular as subjects for fiction, non-fiction, and poetry. Biographies of outstanding sports figures and successful dancers have always been popular fare and

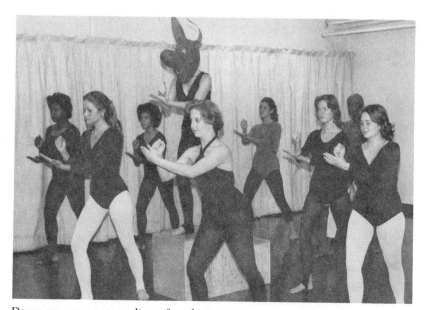

Dance can serve as a medium of aesthetic communication and social criticism.

available in abundance. For sport fiction, one may explore the classic short stories of Damon Runyon or discover for oneself the new wave of sports-fiction writers now holding their own on the best-seller racks, such as Dan Jenkins (*Semi-Tough, Dead Solid Perfect*) or Peter Gent (*North Dallas Forty*). Also widely read and discussed are non-fictional works about sport, such as George Leonard's *The Ultimate Athlete* and James Michener's *Sport in America*. Over 1000 book titles in sports and recreation are now published annually in the United States, not including biographies, fiction, or dance works classified as art titles.

The percentage of sports and recreation books published in the United States has doubled since 1950. Surely these publications are having a growing impact on the American reader, on public attitudes and values regarding sport, and on individual participation in dance, recreational sport activities, and sporting events of all kinds. Those who hope to influence the roles of the movement arts and sport in contemporary or future American society must study the messages concerning dance and sport in current American literature.

Photography. Technology has stimulated a growing interest in "action" photography and increasing recognition of photography as an art. Photographers now create significant volumes of sport art. Much of this sport art is produced for illustration in newspapers and magazines or for television communication; but more and more, sport photography is being recognized as a specialization of photographic fine art.

Sculpture and the Graphic Arts. The human body in motion and persons at play have frequently been central themes for the creative efforts of artists. Since the fifteenth century, painters have been influenced by Leonardo da Vinci's famous illustration of the proportions of the human figure after the first-century B.C. Roman architect Vitruvius.

The organizers of the International Fine Arts Exhibition at Expo 67 in Montreal chose as the exhibition theme, "Man and His World." "Man and Play" was one of ten fundamental themes of the exhibition for better public understanding of the human universality which governs man's artistic expression. An excellent example of the universality of this theme is provided by the comparison of a thirteenth-century Chinese painting, "One Hundred Children at Play," with its western counterpart, "Children's Games," by the sixteenth century Flemish master, Pieter Bruegel.

Dance has been a primary focus for such ranking painters as Edgar Degas and Leo Janssem. The Olympic Games, particularly since the 1968 Olympics in Mexico City, have greatly stimulated collectors and popular appreciation of sport paintings, drawings, lithographs, prints, and posters. R. Tait Mackenzie, and more recently Joe Brown, are especially well-known for their sports sculptures. Popular art now has a tremendous market in sports figures — wood carvings, ceramic figurines, glass and metal sculptures, and mobiles. Not only is the universality of dance and sport in human societies reflected in their artistic expression; their increasing impact is enriching the aesthetic experience of millions of persons throughout the world.

Sports and the movement arts play a very unique role in extending communication among people through language barriers and across the physical and psychological walls created by national boundaries and political ideologies. The dancer makes a personal statement to the recep-

INTERNATIONAL UNDERSTANDING

tive viewer irrespective of language. Through their sports, athletes communicate with each other in ways not open to the average visitor in a foreign country.

International Sport Competition. World class athletes from all continents meet each other in competitions ranging from traditional rivalries in a single sport between two countries and regional competitions in many sports to the highly touted Winter and Summer Olympic Games. In any of these settings, both athletes and spectators have opportunities to become familiar with selected outstanding athletes of other nations; to observe their commitment to sport, their training regimens, their practice routines, their reactions to stress, and their personal interactions, as well as the techniques and quality of their movement performances; and to appreciate national differences in goals, education and lifestyles. More has been said in Chapter 3 about the organization of these competitions and some of the key issues determining their impact on current and future values of Americans. Clearly they will continue to be vehicles of international communication, on both personal and national policy-making levels.

International Education. As physical educators, sport scientists, and performing artists have studied in foreign countries, their mutual interests in the movement arts and sport sciences have provided a basis for increased international communication. American dancers study ballet in Communist countries, primitive dance in "third world" countries, religious dance in the Far East, modern dance in Western Europe, and national dancing all over the world. International students observe and participate in school physical education programs, sports organizations, government sponsored fitness programs, public recreation developments, and professional preparation of teachers and sports leaders. Scholars in physical education, sports medicine, sociology, psychology, history, philosophy, and pedagogy hold frequent international conferences and have organized international professional associations to strengthen communication across national borders. Many of these professional groups distribute scientific journals and other types of publications, establish programs for corresponding fellows, and encourage foreign travel by visiting scholars. All of these efforts reflect the growing role of the movement arts and sport sciences in international communication.

Sport and Dance in Foreign Policy. So significant have sport and dance become in international affairs that governments have made them deliberate instruments of national policy. For more than a quarter-century, cultural exchange programs have been supported by U. S. taxpayers in order to increase international mutual understanding and good will. From their earliest beginnings educational exchanges have involved American physical educators, sports leaders, and dance companies. It is acknowledged on an international scale that dance and sport are significant aspects of all cultures with genuine potential for increasing worldwide understanding.

People-to-People Sports Committee. The People-to-People Sports Committee was established following the recommendation of a 1956 White House Conference. A joint project of the American government and interested private citizens and clubs, its goal is the promotion of international goodwill through sports. Specific projects include sports clinics conducted by American coaches in foreign countries, tours of international sports teams in the U.S.A., provision of sports equipment and training materials to sports organizations in other countries, and sponsoring events featuring talented performers of other nations in this country.

Peace Corps. Established by Congress in 1961 "to promote world peace and friendship," the Peace Corps has been highly successful in volunteer service to people in the developing countries. Peace Corps volunteers are dedicated, adaptable, and imaginative persons willing to live and work in another culture at the same economic level as those served. Physical educators and sports specialists have always been included among Peace Corps volunteers; local recreation and community sports projects have been important vehicles of communication for persons of the host cultures. The Peace Corps continues to be an active program committed to the reduction of dependency within the less developed countries. Today, volunteers are serving in 63 countries around the world, mostly in rural settings, in places as diverse as the remote regions of Guatemala, the bush villages of Senegal, the jungle terrain of Malaysia, the mountains of Nepal and Afghanistan, and the uplands of Kenya.

The Dark Side of Mixing Politics and Sport. Unfortunately, political parties and governments have not always restricted the use of sport as a vehicle to promote national prestige and to legitimate ways of achieving national goals. Recent Olympic Games have been marred by politicizing such as the outrages committed during the 1972 Games in Munich; and participation in or boycotting of international sports competition is becoming an increasingly frequent form of political sanction. Charges and counter-charges of violations of both written and customarily understood rules of international competition plague the world sporting community. Issues relating to excessive nationalism and to professionalism in amateur sports are presently of particular concern. In spite of the many evidences of the misuse of sport as an instrument of national policy, however, these occurrences should not be allowed to overshadow the positive potential of sport and dance toward increasing communication among persons of differing national heritages and toward long-range improvements in international understanding. In the long run, government programs in education and the arts "can create a world-wide common market of ideas, cultural attainments, and human discourse."[15]

LEISURE AND RECREATION

Concepts of leisure have changed dramatically in the past 50 years. An individual's scope of freedom in the modern world has been greatly narrowed and is likely to be more so in the future, as we cope with increasingly complex and interrelated living. Economically, the individual is less and less a free agent: the employer or the self-employed must conform to government controls and accepted methods of competition to succeed in business; the worker is subject to direction and manipulation by the union organization. In politics, especially on a national or statewide basis, the majority of the voters no longer sense a conviction that each citizen's vote is vital. This state of affairs makes it even more important that the individual channel potential influence into those areas of life where freedom of choice remains. Leisure time represents for each of us a great reservoir of freedom; consequently, what we do with this part of life is more important than ever before.

Definition. Leisure has been variously defined. In its simplest terms, it is "discretionary time," unobligated time, time free from work, or time not used for meeting the exigencies of life. In June 1970, a Charter for Leisure[16] was agreed upon at the European Recreation Congress. The document grew out of a symposium convened by the International Recreation Association in Geneva in 1967, in which some sixteen organizations operating internationally in the field of play, recreation, and leisure participated. Three existing documents, the Colmar Charter, the United Nations Declaration of Rights of the Child, and the United Nations Universal Declaration of Human Rights, served as a base. The final document has been translated into five languages; its preface reads as follows:

> Leisure time is that period of time at the complete disposal of an individual, after he has completed his work and fulfilled his other obligations. The uses of this time are of vital importance.
> Leisure and recreation create a basis for compensating for many of the demands placed upon man by today's way of life. More important, they present a possibility for enriching life through participation in physical relaxation and sports, through an enjoyment of art, science, and nature. Leisure is important in all spheres of life, both urban and rural. Leisure pursuits offer man the chance of activating his essential gifts (a free development of the will, intelligence, sense of responsibility and creative faculty). Leisure hours are a period of freedom, when man is able to enhance his value as a human being and as a productive member of his society.
> Recreation and leisure activities play an important part in establishing good relations between peoples and nations of the world.

Leisure Time. Time has become an increasingly important medium of exchange. Yet only recently have time diary studies been undertaken in the United States to examine how Americans organize their everyday lives. In 1965 the United States participated with eleven other nations in a UNESCO study of time usage; a more limited follow-up study was undertaken in 1975.[17] The UNESCO study revealed that both men and women average only about five hours of leisure activity a day. Furthermore, there was a steady decline in the amount of leisure per day of about one hour from adolescence up to retirement. The popular belief of continuous gains in non-work time for the average working person has not been supported by evidence for the period from 1940 to 1965. Surprisingly, however, a preliminary analysis of the 1975 research data shows a gain in non-work time during the decade from 1965 to 1975 of about 10 per cent.

> The leisure activities that gained in popularity during this period were the use of television and other mass media, adult education, and recreation activities, such as sports and walking or driving for pleasure. In contrast, there was a notable drop in visiting and other informal social life.[18]

The prime importance of the use of leisure in enriching individual lives and in influencing the future development of American society cannot be questioned.

A New View of Leisure. New concepts of leisure make it more difficult to predict the future role of movement and sport. After two or three generations in which physically active recreation seemed to be decreasing in contrast to greater emphasis on spectator sports and television viewing, however, a trend toward increasingly active physical recreation appears to be gaining momentum.

The Role of Movement and Sport

Max Kaplan[19] summarizes the new view of leisure as (1) holistic in conception and function, (2) dynamic and developmental in its methods, and (3) futuristic and policy-oriented in its intent. Leisure-time activities and interests are infinite in variety and highly personal. Because a person's interests are limited by experience, it is the responsibility of public education to widen horizons through enriching the recreational environment.

Particular extensions of the scope of leisure are identified by two selected articles from the Charter for Leisure:[20]

> Article 1: Every man has a right to leisure time. This comprises reasonable working hours, regular paid vacations, favorable traveling conditions, and suitable social planning, including reasonable access to leisure facilities, areas and equipment in order to enhance the advantage of leisure time.
>
> Article 4: Every man has a right to participate in and be introduced to all types of recreation during leisure time, such as sports and games, open-air living, travel, theatre, dancing, pictorial art, music, science, and handicrafts irrespective of age, sex, or level of education.

Adapting to More Leisure in the Future. For our future society, an education that prepares an individual for his work will be only half an education. The first function of our schools and colleges is to provide an education that makes a person; vocational or professional education is of secondary importance. In fulfilling its responsibility to educate for leisure, the school should provide the following:

1. Encouragement and instruction leading to the development and maintenance of the organic systems of the body to a sufficient degree that the individual is capable of participation.
2. Introduction and basic instruction in a variety of activities with the potential for development of lifelong leisure interests, including intellectual, social, artistic, physical, and service activities.
3. Opportunities and encouragement to develop skills that will prove satisfying and useful after graduation as well as during the school years.
4. Stimulation of original thought and creative self-expression and guidance of creative energies toward individual self-fulfillment.
5. Encouragement of the development of socially acceptable standards of conduct which make the student a desirable companion, competitor, and humanitarian.
6. Encouragement of desirable attitudes toward play, recreation, leisure, activity, rest, and relaxation.
7. Some appreciation and understanding of the role of leisure and of particular leisure-time activities in one's own and other cultures, including the role of sports and outdoor recreation in the cultures of all peoples everywhere.

The responsibility of the school and its role in the total spectrum of education for leisure is well summarized by the following articles of the Charter for Leisure:[21]

> Article 6: Every man has a right to the opportunity for learning how to enjoy his leisure time in the most sensible fashion. In schools, classes, and courses of instruction, children, adolescents, and adults must be given the opportunity to develop the skills, attitudes, and understandings essential for leisure literacy.

Article 7: The responsibility for education for leisure is still divided among a large number of disciplines and institutions. In the interests of everyone and in order to utilize purposefully all the funds and assistance available in the various administrative levels, this responsibility should be fully coordinated among all public and private bodies concerned with leisure. The goal should be for a community of leisure.

The most obvious role of the movement arts and sport sciences in meeting the recreation and leisure needs of American society is in the education and promotion of physical activities as popular forms of recreation. Sports and dance are high on any list of popular leisure interests. Less evident is the support required of the movement sciences in the pursuit of crafts, hobbies, and amateurism. A growing professional interest is the exciting area of high adventure leisure pursuits and risk recreation. Competitive sport in general continues to increase its dominance on the leisure scene, supplemented by recent growth and publicity of women's competitive sport.

Organized Team Sports. Nearly every public recreation program, semi-public agency sports program, industrial sports organization, and school or college intramural program organizes team competition for boys and men in seasonal sports, with girls' and women's teams becoming more numerous as well. Leagues are common in softball, basketball, and bowling, and less numerous in touch football, volleyball, and soccer. More select clubs offer recreational opportunities in hockey, lacrosse, and rugby. In general, the participants view these activities as voluntary and recreational in nature, even though an obligation for regular participation is assumed and both the activity and its setting are highly structured. When asked to identify the satisfactions of participation, typical responses refer to affiliation, physical benefits, and self-image improvement; catharsis and altruism are less frequent sources of satisfaction. Organized team participation is a more popular form of leisure activity among teenagers and young adults; participants are predominantly male, although this is changing with increased concern for equal opportunity for girls and women.

Individual and Dual Sports. Since World War II, physical educators have been advocating more emphasis on "lifetime sports" in school and college programs. In fact, current educational programs do provide more instruction in tennis, golf, badminton, archery, and other activities viewed as having high potential for adult recreation. These activities have shown tremendous surges in popularity in the leisure community. The "country club sport" concept has given way to free or low-cost public recreation programs. As municipal facilities have expanded and finally passed their saturation points, small business entrepreneurs have opened up racquet clubs, driving ranges, gymnastic clubs, archery ranges, handball courts and skating rinks. Swimming, boating, and other water sports have provided much family recreation; winter sports are thriving, even in areas which seldom enjoy natural snow; and such outdoor activities as hunting and fishing continue to be popular leisure pursuits in all parts of the country.

Dance as Leisure Activity. The arts at the popular level play their most significant role as a "celebration of life." Dance has always held an important place among the popular arts, and many persons who never

LEISURE SPORTS AND DANCE

enroll in organized recreation programs, join sport clubs, or commit themselves to lifelong hobbies engage frequently in recreational dancing. The popular social dance of the era, whether it be the waltz, foxtrot, jitterbug, twist, or disco, has consistently filled many leisure hours for U.S. adolescents and young adults. Folk festivals and ethnic cultural events usually highlight dance activities. Community arts programs have provided leisure satisfactions for many performers who would not classify themselves as accomplished artists but who enjoy participating in ballet, modern dance, jazz, or theatre groups. Clubs are popular in particular areas where specific forms of dance such as square dance or clog have attracted enthusiastic crowds. Continuing education programs have experienced growing demands for classes in jazz, ballet, square, exotic, ethnic, and Middle Eastern dance. Dance, in its many forms, and with its continually changing styles, has always been, and surely will always be, a significant leisure activity.

Crafts such as weaving, pottery-making, carving, and other such popular arts are enjoyed by many as aesthetic experience that goes beyond satisfaction in the end product. In discussing pop art, Arnold[22] supports the value of the art experience in a leisure atmosphere:

CRAFTS, HOBBIES, AND AMATEUR PURSUITS

> The art experience in popular, amateur, or professional form provides one process through which individuals may search for meaning in identity, for solutions to individual or common problems, and for means of recording their experimentations and discoveries. . . . The arts at the popular level do provide enhancement, escape, and intensification of life experiences. . . . Art is a popular experience, and should be a popular expression.

Hobbies are as varied as the persons who pursue them; they include activities as different as gardening, model-building, bird-watching, fine arts, and do-it-yourself home improvement. Hobbyists and amateurs are similar in that they are both practitioners with a serious commitment; they differ in that amateurs maintain ties with professionals in the same pursuits and can relate to a public that finds their contributions of value. Amateurs define as leisure those activities that other people define as professional work. Stebbins[23] identifies the benefits of amateurism as self-actualization, self-expression, self-enrichment, re-creation, feelings of accomplishment, enhancement of self-image, and tangible and lasting products of the activity. He believes that amateurism can fulfill especially valuable roles in the lives of retired persons in that it

> provides worklike activity; offers a possible link with one's former work associates and current friends and relatives; expands one's social circle; promotes transcendence; constitutes a theme in the life review; fosters responsibility; and meets certain needs of other people.

Most crafts and many hobbies and amateur pursuits are dependent upon the movement sciences for their successful conduct. Basic health and fitness underlie all human activity; most of these activities require, in addition, efficient body mechanics and specialized application of particular kinesiological principles. All utilize particular motor skills; many require learning new skills. Thus the role of the movement sciences in providing knowledge for competence in learning and refining new skills throughout life, is extremely important.

One of the most apparent trends in leisure today is the rapidly increasing popularity of leisure activities containing elements of excitement, risk, challenge, adventure, thrill, stress, and danger. Public recreation agencies and leisure service delivery systems have been reluctant to provide for these interests because of understandable preoccupation with problems of legal liability. Yet the attraction of high adventure and risk recreation is undisputed, and the popularity of these pursuits will probably continue to rise in proportion to their availability and publicity.*

The phrase "high risk" in describing particular sports or recreational activities is relatively new in professional literature. Although the concept of professional sponsorship of dangerous or unsafe activities has created conflict and controversy, the positive values of such pursuits are winning increasing acceptance. Because of the negative overtones of the word "risk," this type of leisure activity has been identified by a variety of terms, including high adventure, natural challenge, stress-seeking, thrill sports, rugged recreation, and survival skill, as well as high-risk leisure activity.

The Appeal of High Risk Sports. Many psychologists and sociologists, leisure educators, physical educators, and park and recreation administrators have attempted to analyze the appeal and increasing popularity of high risk sports. It is generally agreed that the human quest for individual self-actualization is a key aspect. A person commits himself or herself to a situation in which a physical and spiritual challenge must be confronted. There is a thrill to the encounter and self-confidence is stimulated through reliance on the powers of self to master the challenge. The moment of greatest stress can produce an intense emotion, a peak

*In 1978, the American Association for Leisure and Recreation devoted one of its two issues of *Leisure Today* entirely to this topic.[24]

A growing number of people are seeking self-actualization through hang-gliding, a relatively new high-adventure activity.

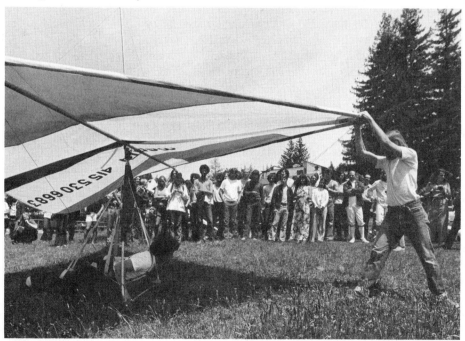

experience in a lifestyle characterized by the typical routines of daily living. Complete involvement demands that the person integrate physical, emotional, social, intellectual, and aesthetic aspects of personality; after the risk has passed and the challenge has been met, a sounder self-concept, increased self-confidence, and great personal satisfaction are the rewards.

The quest for the absolute limits of human ability often leads to choosing an encounter with the natural environment. Natural environments provide challenges in mountain activities such as rock climbing, ice climbing, skiing, and caving; in white-water activities such as canoeing, kayaking, and rafting; and in ocean activities such as surfing and scuba diving. The person who pits self against the elements experiences a freedom of choice, a change of pace and focus in a return to the natural environment, aesthetic satisfaction, and an environmental awareness that may even lead to "cosmic humility."

Some proponents of high adventure recreation also emphasize group cooperation and meaningful interrelating to others, such as that fostered by Outward Bound and Project Adventure. The direct dependence upon other human beings for physical survival, the shared intensity of involvement, and the knowledge that one is personally important to the common goal all make risks worth taking.

The significance of the movement arts and sport sciences to high adventure leisure pursuits and high risk recreation is obvious; an adequate fitness level is of greatest importance in meeting any physical challenge. Specific technical and motor skills must be learned for participation, even at baseline levels. Highly refined skills and high levels of physical fitness are prerequisites for seeking the peak experiences in any activity of genuine high risk.

COMPETITIVE SPORTS

The role of athletic competition in contemporary American society is a subject of intense interest and considerable debate. Controversy exists, both in interpretation of the real impact of current practices and in clarifying the ideal role in achieving desired goals for America. Educators have struggled for years to emphasize the educational aspects of school and college athletics, keeping as their focus education in contrast to entertainment. It is equally confusing to distinguish between leisure or recreation and business in competitive sports: it is clear enough that professional athletes are in business; the extent to which other organized competitive sports are truly recreational is more difficult to determine. Since competitive sports are acknowledged to have a wide leisure appeal, the topic is discussed in this section.

Competition and Cooperation. Competition and cooperation are fundamental elements in the American cultural pattern and are essential to the efficient working of the political and economic systems of American democracy. However, in many governmental as well as private agencies regulation of competition now exists in order that unfair advantage will not be attained by the unscrupulous and dishonest competitor. Also, there are many groups and individuals who believe strongly that cooperation is the basis of successful democratic action. Although the schools use competition as a motive to influence children's behavior, the relative merits of competition and cooperation are argued in educational systems, each having its vocal advocates. Many school practices are strongly influenced by one view or the other.

Perhaps the entire question should be decided not on the basis of a dichotomy of choice — competition versus cooperation — but through an understanding of the essential interrelationship of the two concepts. Sport and athletics, under proper leadership, provide an excellent medium for the development of acceptable attitudes toward both cooperation and competition, attitudes that can have lifelong application. In order to clarify the nature of the cooperation–competition problem, and the role of sport and athletics in attitude and value development in these areas, the following analysis of human nature may be helpful.

Human Traits That Must Be Considered. Six characteristic human behaviors may be described as follows:
1. *Humans are gregarious* — we have a natural need to live in social groups.
2. *Humans are competitive at times and cooperative at other times.*
3. *Play is a spontaneous human activity.* The play of children is a natural response to organic needs; and all sports and athletics have this same natural basis.
4. Through repetition, *humans tend to learn behavior that brings satisfaction*, be it mental, emotional, social, or physical.
5. *Humans must learn ethical or moral standards*—we do not inherit them. We are socialized in early childhood in those cooperative and competitive behaviors that our society values.
6. *Humans are imitative* — we tend to adopt responses suggested by other persons whom we regard as prestigious or influential.

These six categories of behavior provide a partial answer to fundamental questions and problems that accompany the promotion and control of competitive sport and athletics. Conversely, if we fail to take these categories sufficiently into account, we may never arrive at satisfactory solutions.

Characteristics of a Desirable Program

A desirable program of competitive sport has at least three general characteristics:
1. It provides a place for all.
   a. A variety of sports and athletics, appropriate to various interests, degrees of physical power, and stages of development, experience, and skill, should be provided.
   b. There should be adequate equipment and facilities for all.
   c. There should be qualified and interested leadership for the entire program, not for the superior group of performers alone.
   d. The superior performers should not be exploited in such a way as to detract from the ordinary performer.
   e. Competition should be equalized to maintain the interest of players of all degrees of proficiency.
2. It promotes physical well-being.
   a. A medical examination should be required.
   b. Every precaution to prevent accidental physical injury should be exercised and provision should be made to obtain prompt emergency service in the event of a serious injury at practice or in a game at any time of day or night.
   c. No contestant should be permitted or encouraged to sacrifice his or her physical well-being, either in competition or in training.
   d. The rules of healthful living should be taught in connection with activities.

e. Coaches should be models of the exemplary behavior they espouse to their players.

3. It is directed toward the sound social and emotional development of the participants.

    a. The coach, the individual athlete, and the team should make every legitimate effort to win their games. They practice with purpose and train with dedication. They play with intensity and desire according to the rules and ethics of healthy sport competition. They play to win, but not at all cost. When the contest is over, they accept the victory or the defeat with natural emotional reactions, but they do not regard losing as "the end of the world." Neither do they gloat over opponents whom they have defeated. Emotional control should be stressed.

    b. Recreational values should be maintained. Players should enjoy participating in the practices and in the games. Basically, sport should be fun.

    c. Respect for academic and other worthwhile interests should be cultivated. Participation in sport should be scheduled with due consideration to other responsibilities of the participant.

    d. The individual should be helped to find satisfaction in socially desirable behavior and dissatisfaction in poor sportsmanship.

    e. Respect for and friendliness toward the opponent should be encouraged.

    f. Leadership that sets good examples in habits, attitudes, and conduct should be provided.

    g. Material rewards of significant monetary value should not be offered for winning or participating.

    h. The contestant should be helped to see how desirable conduct in athletic contests is similar to that in other phases of life.

Youth Sports

The scope of participation by young boys and girls in a wide variety of athletic competitions is vast throughout the United States, and is presently enlarging at a very rapid rate. One of the reasons for the current expansion is that over the years physical education and community recreation programs had not done the job of fully meeting the needs and interests of elementary age children in sport activities; thus a large gap developed, into which have moved the private groups and sponsors who are motivated to serve youth's insatiable desire for wholesome activity and fun through sport. The Little League Baseball program, with over one million participants throughout the United States and with organizations in several other countries, is one of the most extensive sport programs ever organized under one auspice. Approximately four million youths participate in the various baseball programs sponsored by non-school agencies. The total number of participants in various organized youth sports programs is now conservatively estimated at 20 million.

Seefeldt[25] has described the paradox of this phenomenal growth.

> Parents seem willing, if not eager, to entrust their children to volunteer coaches of agency-sponsored sports who have in general not been educated to conduct specialized movement programs, while simultaneously they reject, at an increasing rate, the bond-issues that are designed to support physical education and competitive athletics in the nation's public schools.

Provoking constant debate among parents, educators, children, and the general public are questions such as the following:

— At what age should intense athletic competition begin for boys and girls?

— What is the best age at which to begin athletic competition in each of the sports?

— How should sport competition be organized for young children — on an informal interschool basis, on an interschool formal league basis, on a play-day and sports-day basis, or in some other organizational structure?

— What are the beneficial and harmful effects of intense participation in sport competition for young children?

— What qualifications should the adult leaders of these programs possess?

— Should schools, community recreation agencies, and outside groups work together to coordinate their programs, facilities, and leadership, and if so, to what extent?

For several years now, these and similar problems have been the subject of many research studies, conferences, workshops, organizational policy statements and platforms, and articles in newspapers and magazines. The Michigan Youth Sports Study, which is now in its third and final phase, has provided some of the most valuable data for seeking solutions to these difficult problems. The study showed that, of the 26 sports included in the survey, baseball, softball, swimming, bowling, and basketball were the most popular sports among Michigan school children. The extent of participation in agency-sponsored competitive sports was somewhat higher for males than females. When the sports were listed in order of popularity, the major difference was in the males' preference for body contact sports as opposed to the females' choice of gymnastics and figure skating.

Key findings on patterns of involvement include the following:[26]

> Competition in some agency-sponsored athletic programs began as early as age 5, but the greatest number of participants across sports begin their involvement at age 8 for both boys and girls. Sports in which competition frequently began at age 5 or 6 were ice hockey, baseball, and swimming for boys, and gymnastics, swimming, and figure skating for girls. Regardless of the age at which competition began, there was usually a steady increase in the numbers who participated at each advancing age until 12 or 13 years. At that point the participation of both boys and girls showed a rapid decline in all of the team sports and many of the individual and dual sports.

Phases II and III of the study will add to the data on the extent and patterns of involvement, and on the opinions of children (both athletes and non-participants), parents, and school officials regarding such issues as qualifications of leaders, conduct of practices, training procedures, and the impact of sports on family life and on the child's values and personality development. The ultimate objective of the Michigan Youth Sports Study and similar research is to enhance the opportunities for children and youth to participate in desirable programs of physical activity.

Intramurals

Many middle schools, most secondary schools, and almost all colleges and universities attempt to provide wholesome athletic and recreational opportunities for a majority of students, regardless of skill, through comprehensive intramural programs. Good intramural programs offer a wide variety of activities in an attempt to suit the needs and interests of all the students. They equalize the competition by ex-

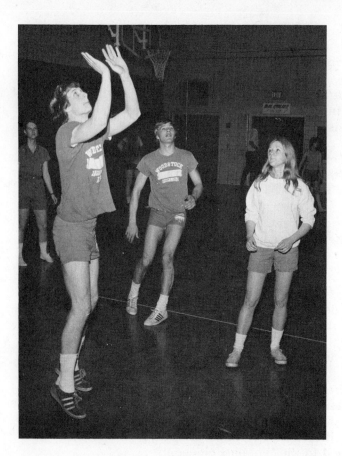

With the advent of Title IX, most intramural programs are coeducational.

cluding the superior groups who are members of school teams. In the main, they promote a sense of responsibility to the team and an interest in wholesome competition marked by fine sportsmanship. Participation in these activities ranges to almost 100 per cent in some schools.

The school administration should provide interested and competent staff leadership to promote, organize, and conduct the intramural program. The intramural director should be assigned sufficient time to perform these duties properly. Many intramural programs fall short of perfection because slight attention is given to the matter of physical conditioning and acquiring greater skill, and not enough thought is devoted to methods of stimulating more general participation. With the advent of Title IX and recognition of the importance of equal educational opportunity, most intramural programs are coeducational. However, leagues of single-sex teams are continued in many of the team sports for maximum participant enjoyment.

"Extramural" Competition.   Another method of extending opportunity for athletic competition to more students has developed in recent years under the name of the "extramural" program. In many cases this is an extension of the intramural program. For example, at the end of the intramural season in a particular sport, intramural teams from one school will travel to a nearby school for contests against intramural teams from that school. In some instances a school will select an all-star team from its own intramural leagues to play the all-star team of another school.

Club Sports.   In recent years there has been a rapid increase in sport clubs nationwide on college and university campuses and, to a lesser extent, in high schools and community colleges. The clubs are organized around sports that are not in the formal institutional sport program, such as sailing, karate, judo, skiing, mountain climbing, cycling, lacrosse, volleyball, bowling, rugby, and fencing. The leadership is provided mainly by interested students and faculty members. Physical education and athletic departments usually cooperate by offering available ground and building space. Sometimes at least partial funding is provided by the school, but most of the expense of operation is borne by the students in the clubs. Many of these clubs use off-campus facilities such as bowling lanes, ice rinks, ski slopes, and so forth. There is every indication that this trend will continue to broaden its scope and influence.

Everyone is familiar with the fact that in past years in secondary schools and colleges there has been a strong emphasis upon competitive athletics for the superior male students who compose the teams that engage in interschool competition. In order to provide more boys with the opportunity to engage in competitive athletics, many colleges and universities have increased the number of athletic teams in recent years in such sports as rugby, crew, and gymnastics. Many community colleges and high schools likewise are expanding athletic programs by having teams in a wide variety of sports, such as cross country, water polo, gymnastics, wrestling, soccer, fencing and softball. Also, more schools are organizing junior varsity, lightweight, and reserve teams in many sports, so that boys of lesser ability will have opportunities to compete against boys of similar skill from other schools. The broadening scope of the program is indicated by the fact that in at least one state more than thirty sports are sanctioned for high school competition. Also, in recent years, girls' and women's interschool sport programs have expanded rapidly in many sections of the country, providing additional opportunities for sport competiton.

Interscholastic and Intercollegiate Athletics

The school program of competitive sport for men had its beginnings and early development between 1852 and 1875. Up to that time, schools and colleges were under the control of administrators who attributed little significance to play, except to consider it more or less a necessary evil. They did not envision it as an educational activity. Play and sport always have been of intrinsic interest to young Americans, even in the early days of the settlers who lived under the influence of the "Puritan work ethic." College boys in the 1800s likewise organized and enjoyed informal sport activities among themselves on and off campus. It was inevitable that sooner or later a group of students from one college would issue a challenge to students in a nearby college.

Beginnings of Men's Collegiate Athletics

In 1852, the first intercollegiate athletic competition took place in the form of a boat race between Harvard and Yale. Regattas were a popular form of athletic competition between colleges on an expanding basis through 1875, and students soon began organizing contests with other schools in additional sports. As enthusiasm and popularity of these sport programs became more intense and widespread, spectators became more numerous, and publicity was developed to "spread the word" even further.

Gradually, athletically inclined alumni began to interest themselves in the athletic fortunes of their alma maters, and as the management of affairs became too complicated for the ever-shifting student control, the graduate manager system developed in American colleges. Soon thereafter professional coaching made its appearance. Although this developing program was not originally under the direct control of the college administration obvious abuses and unpleasant complications that reflected negatively upon the institutions made it necessary for administrations to assume responsibility for athletics.

At the present time, a vast majority of the schools and colleges of this country officially conduct sport programs as a legitimate educational function. They employ well-trained, competent instructors and coaches, many of whom hold traditional academic rank as regular faculty members. With few exceptions, these programs are responsible to the president and the faculty of the institution. In some cases the program still is operated and administered under delegated powers held by associated students' organizations.

Important differences exist in sport competition in American schools and colleges between current programs for girls and women and those for men and boys. The differences between the two programs are in large measure due to sharp contrasts in historical development.

Women's Collegiate Athletics

Background. Oberlin College was the first institution to admit women (in 1833). By 1880, more than half of the liberal arts colleges in the country admitted both men and women. Social customs, then as now, influenced the extent and type of participation by women in physical education and competitive sport.

Intercollegiate competition began at the turn of the century. In 1899, eight years after Dr. James Naismith had invented basketball for men, a committee was appointed to develop basketball rules for women. In 1901, the first basketball rules guide was published by the American Sports Publishing Company, and a standing committee for women's basketball rules became a reality in 1905. As women's sport expanded, student athletic associations were formed to meet the growing interest, the first being created in 1891 at Bryn Mawr to support a tennis program.

Sport days, or informal non-league events, often involving teams from more than two colleges, took place, as well as regularly scheduled games with other colleges. Often women's basketball games were played as preliminaries to men's games. Officiating and coaching frequently were done by men, a development women physical educators generally disapproved of.

In the early 1900s, intercollegiate competition for women suffered from lack of support from women physical education leaders; in fact, from 1920 to 1930 there was a reduction in the number of institutions having such programs and those programs that remained were very limited in scope. Despite this negative picture, a positive development in women's programs occurred when women's competition was inaugurated in the Olympic Games in swimming (1912), fencing (1924), and track and field (1928). When women were made eligible to compete in the Olympic Games, the Amateur Athletic Union (AAU), which had been founded in 1888 to control sport outside colleges and schools, became involved in the coaching and selection of women for the American team. AAU influence on women's sport has been continuous since that time, although there have been conflicts with other groups concerned with girls' and women's sport, chiefly because of differences concerning standards.

CHAPTER NINE

Much of the leadership in the development of sport for American girls and women has come from the National Association for Girls and Women in Sport (NAGWS) of the American Alliance for Health, Physical Education, Recreation, and Dance. NAGWS traces its history to 1917, when the American Physical Education Association established a Committee on Women's Athletics to develop standards and formulate rules for girls' and women's sports. This committee went through a series of name changes over the years and emerged as the National Section on Women's Athletics in 1932. The section achieved division status in 1958 and voted to become an association in the 1974 reorganization of AAHPER.

During World War II, there was a nationwide concern for physical fitness for men and women. Although competition for women was curtailed by wartime conditions, interest in "carry-over sports" increased in schools and colleges, and a national intercollegiate golf tournament for women was initiated in the early 1940s. National competition in tennis followed soon afterward. Telegraphic and postal meets and "extramural" contests (defined as all types of competition except "varsity type" athletics) increased during the 1940s and 1950s.

Girls' Athletic Association (GAA) and Women's Recreation Association (WRA) sport programs continued to expand into the 1950s. But by the end of the decade, these programs were evidencing considerable change in emphasis. The student organizations were giving more attention to the "carry-over sports" and co-recreational activities, and the team sport competitions were being sponsored more often by other groups. This trend was probably accelerated by the development of active student union programs on many college campuses; a number of these programs competed with traditional Women's Athletic Association (WAA) tournaments for student participation. School and college programs in the 1950s reflected the increasing international exchange in expansion of educational gymnastics programs.

In the 1960s, a new concern was expressed from several quarters relative to the restricted opportunities for competition by girls and women with high levels of sports ability. There was impetus to improve America's performances by women athletes in the Olympic Games. It was felt that the sound way to build high competence was to expand opportunities for all girls and women in the secondary schools and colleges. In a joint effort to strengthen girls' and women's sport at the national level, the United States Olympic Development Committee, Women's Division, and the Division of Girls' and Women's Sports (or DGWS, later to become the NAGWS) of the AAHPERD sponsored a series of National Institutes for girls' sports, beginning in 1963. Changes also resulted from the influence of the presidents of some of the major universities who, through their conference commissioners and institutional athletic representatives, stimulated their departments of physical education for women to reevaluate the sport program for women and to upgrade it in terms of high-level competition.

Current Concerns and Challenges. Several factors have influenced, and continue to influence, the development of intercollegiate sport competition for women. Among the more notable influences are changing cultural roles of women in American society, evolving national and international conditions, the women's liberation movement, publicity and mass communications media, professional leadership, medical and

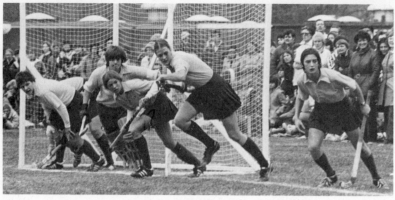

Public acceptance of women's participation in highly competitive sports has changed the traditional concepts of the "feminine image."

biological research, civil rights legislation, and public interest and acceptance of women in sport.

Biological Concerns. Over the years substantial controversy has persisted with regard to whether there are biological limitations that restrict participation in sport by girls and women. Considerable research evidence accumulated in recent years indicates that participation in most events by normal, healthy women is not harmful. Studies concerning menstruation, pregnancy, masculinization, and emotional stress offer the general conclusion that girls need not be barred from competitive sport because of any innate biological or psychological characteristics. The gradual resolution of this issue has supported the trend toward increasing opportunities for competitive sport participation by girls and women.

Sport and the "Feminine Image." Another traditional concern has been the "feminine image" and sport competition. Because of a long history of conflict concerning the female role in America, society has restricted girls' participation in highly competitive sport. This prejudice is finally being overcome, with girls in schools and colleges now enjoying vigorous sport participation. They find that it is not incompatible with female values and interests, and it has become socially acceptable.

Equal Opportunity. Not surprisingly, the recent drive for equal opportunity for women has extended to sport. In the 1970s it was recognized that discrimination against females in athletics exists and that this discrimination should be abolished. Although many professional educators still object to the participation of women on athletic teams established primarily for men, there is increasing support for the principle that qualified athletes should not be excluded from participation in sport because of sex. In practice this has meant participation of girls and women on boys' and men's teams where separate teams were not provided, and where they could demonstrate a level of skill superior to that of male candidates.

The schools and colleges of the United States provide a broad base for sport participation by millions of boys and girls in a long list of sanctioned activities involving many million dollars worth of facilities and conducted by thousands of qualified instructors, coaches, trainers, athletic directors, and physical education administrators. Some high schools report the participation of 60 per cent or more of the total number

CHAPTER NINE

of boys in the student body on one or more of the interscholastic athletic teams. While girls had not had equal opportunities previously, much change has occurred in the past five years.

Title IX of the Education Amendments Act of 1972, forbidding sex discrimination in any educational institution receiving federal funds, has had substantial impact. When the regulations for high schools went into effect in July, 1976, thousands of schools improved their programs voluntarily. During the 1976-77 academic year, 1.6 million high school girls participated in interscholastic sports, a sixfold increase in eight years.

The recent concern for equal opportunity in athletics has also opened up opportunities to the less-gifted boys traditionally squeezed out by win-oriented systems. Through the work of state high school athletic associations and the coordinating efforts of the National Federation of State High School Athletic Associations, the control and administration of high school athletics has been vastly improved in recent years, including a concerted movement to upgrade the quality of junior and senior high school athletic coaching.

At the college and university level, including two-year and community colleges, similar strides have been taken in recent years to broaden the base of intercollegiate athletic competition and to effect better administrative control of these programs. Sports such as soccer, lacrosse, bowling, and skiing have been sponsored by more and more colleges. The inflationary trend of the economy has created serious problems for athletic department operating budgets, however. Deficit budgets result from the expenses of sports that do not generate substantial gate receipts and from new and expanded programs in women's intercollegiate athletics.

Athletic Conferences. The control and administration of college sport is more diverse than in high schools. Although some colleges are "independent" in athletics — that is, they do not belong to any athletic conference — a majority of colleges in the United States do belong to some type of athletic conference. Two national bodies provide overall guidance and control for men's intercollegiate athletics, the National Collegiate Athletic Association (NCAA), and the National Association of Intercollegiate Athletics (NAIA). Most larger schools are under the jurisdiction of the NCAA, while more than 400 smaller schools are affiliated with the NAIA. This division of control is controversial. Many athletic authorities think that all college athletics should be under the control of one organization, in order to provide greater coordination and consistency of policy and practice.

The Association for Intercollegiate Athletics for Women. The controversy over control of amateur athletics has been compounded by the recent dramatic emphasis on national-level sport competition for women. In the 1960s, when women physical educators had achieved some consensus on the need for expanding opportunities for athletic competition for women, the Division of Girls' and Women's Sports formed a Commission on Intercollegiate Athletics for Women. Established in 1966, the Commission sanctioned the First Annual U.S. Intercollegiate Archery Meet and a national swimming meet in 1967, and a gymnastics championship in 1968. One of the notable results of the work of this Commission was the approval of a policy which provided for National Intercollegiate Championships for Women in gymnastics and track and field in 1969, and in swimming, badminton, and volleyball in 1970.

Control of College Athletics

The Commission became functionally independent of DGWS as the Association for Intercollegiate Athletics for Women in 1972. The stated purpose of AIAW is to provide leadership and initiate and maintain standards of excellence in intercollegiate competition for all college women. The Association was established with 278 member schools and now has 825 active members (115 more than the 73-year-old NCAA), conducting 18 national championships annually. The 1979 Delegate Assembly voted for complete autonomy for AIAW, asserting its independence from both NAGWS and AAHPER.

It is estimated that 100,000 women now take part in intercollegiate sports, compared with 170,000 men. Inevitably, renewed concern regarding financial aid for athletes has resulted. Whereas it had been traditional policy to prohibit the awarding of athletic scholarships to women, based on the belief that financial aid for athletes tends to create abuses detrimental to the participants themselves, it is now considered legally untenable to deny financial aid to women athletes when men in the same institution are receiving athletic grants-in-aid. AIAW first allowed athletic scholarships in 1973; in 1977–78, an estimated 10,000 women student-athletes from about 460 schools received scholarships worth approximately $7 million. The largest numbers of grants are being offered in basketball, volleyball, tennis, track and field, and swimming and diving. Estimated expenditures for women's intercollegiate athletic programs are now averaging approximately ten per cent of the reported totals for men's programs; it is assumed that these costs must continue to rise.

A discrimination-free athletic program is exceedingly difficult to define. HEW did not publish a set of regulations to govern application of Title IX of the 1972 legislation, until 1975; these regulations were scheduled to go into effect for colleges and universities July 21, 1978. A review of the regulations directed by HEW Secretary Califano appears to have extended the confusion even longer. Meanwhile, the limited applicable research demonstrates that the virtues of sport, when equally shared, equally benefit both sexes. It is clear that there are not enough qualified women coaches, trainers, and athletic directors. Many of the same problems men have faced over the years are now of crucial concern to women as well.

Spectator Sports as Recreation

It is impossible to estimate the number of Americans who spend a substantial portion of their leisure time as spectators at sports events. High school athletic events provide a focus for community recreation in many cities and towns across the country, drawing regular fans in all kinds of neighborhoods, regardless of the particular sport or the level of participant playing ability or competition. Intercollegiate athletic programs, especially the football and basketball games, attract large crowds of alumni and local team followers, bowl games and national championships accounting for many, many leisure hours. Professional baseball, football, boxing, basketball, and hockey fill huge stadiums and sports arenas every weekend year around. While it is probable that the average American adult spends only a few hours per week in physically active recreation, the total hours spent as a sports spectator, especially when television viewing is included, represent a very major leisure interest.

It is often said that sport is big business in this country. The United States is a leisure economy. Sport, recreation, and vacations are major expenditures for most employed persons, whether wage or salary earners, single or two-income households. We spend plenty of money to enjoy bowling, golf, swimming, and tennis. We finance our power boats, our backyard swimming pools, and our campers. Despite the increased price of admission to major league ball games, attendance figures continue to rise; and enough of us pay exorbitant prices for tickets to championship games to keep the scalpers in business. If necessary, we apply for additional credit cards or higher credit limits; but we seldom give up the big vacation — the two-week ski package, the Southeastern golfing holiday, the Caribbean vacation, the Northern fishing expedition, the Las Vegas casino spree, or the relatively inexpensive family camping trip (which turns out to be very expensive in terms of gasoline consumption). We build our homes with family rooms and construct additions for recreation rooms, hobby-shops, and garage storage for recreational vehicles of all types.

Ours is a consumer economy. The Bureau of Labor Statistics estimates that 30.4 million U.S. families (53 per cent of the total) have at least two earners; their median income is $20,400. Saving is not common. Two-income families, most of whom are in their mid-20s to mid-30s, have been dubbed "America's New Elite"; they are spending more on entertainment, cameras, cars, and travel than single-earner families and more on golf, tennis, and swimming club memberships than older affluent people.

The movement arts and sport sciences contribute to a lively American economy in highly visible ways. The administration of sports and other leisure ventures provides steady cash flows and substantial employment, including some of the highest personal salaries negotiated each year. Tourism has an increasingly important role in the U.S. economy; although physically active recreation is only one of several major categories of attractions promoted, many trips and vacations are planned around sporting spectaculars and special events. Retail sales find big markets in sports equipment and clothing, and the development of facilities for public or private enjoyment of active leisure interests supports the construction industry and many related businesses.

BUSINESS AND ECONOMICS

The Role of Movement and Sport

SPORT ADMINISTRATION

Sport administration, according to Vanderzwaag,[27] "encompasses the administration of those programs involving games of sport and/or sport skills." It includes not only activities, the active participants, and spectators, but also the administration of professional sport, collegiate sport, private sports clubs, commercial recreation, and public recreation.

Professional Sport. Professional sport is a large industry employing many as athletes, coaches, trainers, scouts, officials, agents, medical and paramedical specialists, financial managers, ticket salespersons, sports information specialists, concessions operators and sales personnel, security-guards, and maintenance personnel. They stimulate consumer spending and generate industry income through seasonally scheduled league games; playoffs, bowl games, and other types of championship contests; tournaments and exhibition tours; television contracts; and sales of programs, souvenirs, endorsements, and advertising. The big money-makers are baseball, football, basketball, hockey, boxing, wrestling, golf, tennis, automobile racing, and horse racing.

Collegiate Sport. The economic impact of intercollegiate sports cannot be disputed, despite efforts to maintain amateur standards and educational orientation. Although the athletes are not paid salaries, they are recruited with offers of scholarships or grants-in-aid. Gate receipts and spending by spectators attending athletic contests are a major factor in the economies of many universities and their local communities and universities vie for sponsorship of NCAA championships and for larger shares of the income from television coverage. Financial considerations are also a major factor in the controversies over who shall control amateur sport among NCAA, NAIA, AIAW, AAU, and the sports federations. Those engaged in the administration of intercollegiate sport must carry out most of the same business functions associated with professional sport: budgeting and accounting, scheduling and ticket sales, contest management, sports information, personnel management, facilities management, and government paperwork. The universities with the most successful intercollegiate athletic programs now have annual athletic department operating budgets above $2 million. Setting aside questions concerning whether such programs are educational or entertainment, amateur or semi-professional, they *are* big business.

Private Clubs. The early private sport clubs were exclusive social clubs; admission to the typical country club required a favorable vote of the members, the payment of a large initiation fee which represented an investment in the business, and continuing payment of substantial membership fees. A country club usually provided opportunities for golf, tennis, and swimming, as well as a variety of social activities and other recreational services for its members and their guests. Up until the last quarter century, most American golf and tennis champions developed their talents on the country club courses or courts.

A recent development is the very profitable private sports club. Typically designed to promote a single sport, these facilities have open membership and fees that are usually considerably less expensive than country club memberships. Instruction is generally available for a fee and sports supplies, equipment, and costumes can be purchased at the club. Popular sports organized in the private club sector include swimming and diving, tennis, golf, gymnastics, squash, handball, racquetball, badminton, boating, sailing, scuba, skiing, judo, and karate. Racquetball provides a good illustration of the growing impact of private sports clubs in our economy. In 1970, there were approximately 500,000 participants and about 50 private racquetball clubs; by 1977, this figure had grown to 5,500,000 participants and nearly 300 clubs throughout the United States.

Commercial Recreation. Analyses of consumer spending show that recreation and entertainment represent major expenditures for Americans, with a hefty portion of these going for movement activities. From bowling alleys and skating rinks to organized summer camps and white water rafting, physical recreation has resulted in scores of successful businesses, providing business profits and employment for many. Typically, these businesses are operated on a pay-as-you-go basis, permitting either occasional casual involvement or regular commitments to a "Wednesday-night league" or a series of lessons.

Public Recreation. The administration of public (non-commercial) recreation programs is a significant economic activity. Public recreation programs now provide a broad scope of varied activities such as outing clubs, nature hikes, dance instruction, jogging groups, weight training and yoga, as well as comprehensive programs of competitive sports. Municipal programs are significantly extended by state and national park programs offering camping, backpacking, mountain climbing, skiing, and aquatic activities. Public agency programs are not profit-making; however, they affect the economy substantially in the expenditure of public funds for facilities development, employment of personnel, program operations, park administration, and facilities management.

Tourism is an important element in the world economy. As defined in a recent report published by the United States Travel Data Center:[28]   **TOURISM**

> Tourism is used to denote the collection of productive business organizations and governmental agencies that serve the traveler away from home. At the retail level, they include restaurants, hotels, motels, and resorts, all modes of transportation, rental cars, travel agents, gasoline service stations, national and state parks or recreation areas, and private attractions, among others. The industry also includes those organizations that support the retail activities of the above, including advertising organizations, publications, transportation equipment manufacturers, private and academic research entities, and federal, state, and local travel development agencies.

Tourism spending in the U.S. was approximately $50 billion in 1970, contributing directly $16 billion to U.S. national income, with an additional $12.4 billion contributed by activities that served tourists indirectly. In 1970 tourism accounted for over five per cent of the gross national product. Tourism has been growing at a faster rate than the economy as a whole; it has been projected that tourism expenditures in the U.S. would reach $127 billion by 1980. Tourism, directly or indirectly, is responsible for almost five per cent of total civilian employment in the U.S., one out of every twenty workers.

Spectator Traveling. Major sporting events and leisure sports interests account for a great deal of travel by Americans. Many drive or fly long distances to attend intercollegiate or professional basketball, baseball or football games; to observe the Master's Golf Tournament, the U.S. Open Tennis Championships, the Kentucky Derby, the Indianapolis 500, or the World Series. Airlines offer special charter flights and vacation packages planned around attendance at such events as the Super Bowl or the Olympics. On a lesser scale, many persons take two- to four- or five-day trips to state high school basketball tournaments, NCAA championship events, AAU track competitions, and Olympic try-outs.

Outdoor Tourism. Outdoor camping has become such a popular leisure activity that millions are spent every year in this form of tourism. Expenditures for recreational vehicles, camping equipment, support of road services, and for development and maintenance of camping areas, are still on the upswing. Many persons plan their vacations around specific sports interests: hunting, fishing, skiing, swimming, surfing, scuba-diving, sailing, golfing, mountaineering, or backpacking. They travel long distances (and spend a great deal of money) in order to participate in an activity that is less accessible, satisfying, or enjoyable near home.

Resorts.   Beach resorts, western ranches, golf resorts, and ski resorts are stable elements in the tourism industry. Now some entrepreneurs are promoting special sport "vacations" that emphasize athletic skill development and training as a major goal. Such resorts require the paying guests to maintain severe training regimens, long practice hours, and serious attitudes toward improving performance in such activities as tennis, swimming, or skiing. In some cases, diet and other health practices are also controlled.

The growth in vacation home investment is also stimulating the economy. Ski resorts are proliferating a great many related businesses, extending even to the development of condominium villages.

Equipment.   Sports in America would be big business if for no other reason than because of the production and sale of the great volume of manufactured goods required to support sports participation and to satisfy the demands created by popular interest in these activities. Major equipment purchases are a substantial item in the operating budget of every institution, agency, or business that sponsors a sports program of any type. Most of the equipment is expendable or needs frequent replacement; new models and improved materials often dictate additional purchases. There appears to be no limit to consumer demand for racquets, balls, golfclubs, fishing gear, ski equipment, boats, bicycles, camping equipment and the like. New markets are created every day for the promotion of frisbies, skateboards, snowmobiles, cross country skis, or any other innovation that captivates popular interest.

Clothing.   The manufacture and sale of sports clothing has become a giant industry. Every team has its uniforms, from the professionals down to the average citizen at leisure. Thousands of family budgets include Little League uniforms for the children and bowling shirts for the adults. Swimwear and other items of beach wear are essentials in practically every wardrobe. Tennis, golf, ice skating, ballet, modern dance, and square dance all require substantial purchases of clothing designed specifically for fashionable participation in the chosen activity. The ski industry generates its own fashions each season; different ensembles are now required for different snow conditions; racing outfits are distinct from those of the recreational skier; and cross-country skiing requires new clothing as well as new equipment. Footwear is now designed to increase comfort, improve performance, and ensure safety in an amazing variety of activities, from the obvious requirements of skates, boots, clogs, cleated shoes, and swim fins to subtly differentiated sneakers for jogging, tennis, volleyball, and handball. All-purpose warm-ups no longer satisfy the sophisticated sportsman or sportswoman, who now purchases jogging suits, tennis warm-ups, racquetball suits, and cycling outfits.

Other Sport-Related Businesses.   In addition to the sports equipment

RETAIL SALES

and clothing industries, there are numerous others that contribute to soaring retail sales in sports businesses. The companies specializing in trophies and awards include several that are national in scope. Equipment rental businesses are very profitable in major resort areas. Businesses developed to provide for the care, maintenance and repair of sporting gear are thriving. Popular interest in specific recreational skills has created a large and growing market in training devices, learning aids, instruction manuals, and sports and recreation books.

Another segment of the economy which has benefited from growing public support for sports and recreation is that stimulated by the need for continuing expansion of athletic and recreational facilities. The construction industry and both private and public investment are stimulated by the demand for bigger and better sports arenas and stadiums, more and more swimming pools, new golf courses, and expanding ski areas. Current interests have led to the design and building of running trails, circuit training courses, and commercial recreation and private sport club facilities of the many kinds previously discussed. The development of park facilities, campgrounds, forest preserves, and wilderness areas is an expensive continuing responsibility of both public agencies and private business. The development and maintenance of sport and recreation facilities provides employment for thousands of persons in occupations ranging from unskilled labor to skilled tradespersons, technicians, engineers, designers, and architects.

FACILITIES DEVELOPMENT

SUMMARY

The movement arts and sport sciences have developed in response to human needs and common interests that relate to individual and societal survival and to enhancement of the quality of personal living and enrichment of group life. Sport and the movement arts are pervasive aspects of human societies around the world. The preceding discussions have been focused upon the roles that the movement arts and sport sciences fulfill in contemporary American society. The most important of these roles are played in the broad areas of life in the United States designated as education, health and fitness, social service, communications, leisure and recreation, and business and economics. These roles parallel the ways in which individuals seek personal meaning in movement activities. They provide the basis for the school curriculum in physical education. They also identify societal needs for the preparation of professionals for careers in the movement arts and sport sciences.

FOOTNOTES

[1]"What You'd Better Know Before Joining a Health Club," *Today's Health*, February, 1972, p. 17.
[2]Keith Henschen, "Health Spa Certification," *Careers in Physical Education*, NAPECW and NCPEAM, 1975, pp. 47–55.
[3]Ibid.
[4]Claire Schmais, "Dance Therapy as a Career," *JOPER*, 48:5 (May, 1977), p. 38.
[5]"Medicine," *Time*, August 21, 1978. pp. 40–50.
[6]George Leonard, *The Ultimate Athlete*. New York: Viking Press, 1976, p. 256.
[7]James A. Michener, *Sports in America*. New York: Random House, 1976, p. 451.
[7a]"What Should Higher Education Be Like for the Physical Educator?" *JOHPER*, 43:66–72 (May, 1972).
[8]Scout Lee Gunn, "Labels That Limit Life," *JOPER*, 48:8 (October, 1977), pp. 27–28.

[9]David K. Leslie, "Fitness Programs for the Aging," *Careers in Physical Education.* NAPECW and NCPEAM, 1975, pp. 1–10.

[10]Herbert A. DeVries, "Fitness After Fifty," *JOPER*, 47:4, (April, 1976), pp. 47–49.

[11]T. R. Collingwood, "Physical Fitness, Physical Activity, and Juvenile Delinquency," *JOPER*, 48:6, June, 1977, p. 23.

[12]"Comes the Revolution," *Time*, June 26, 1978, pp. 54–60.

[13]*Complying with Title IX of the Education Amendments of 1972 in Physical Education and High School Sports Programs.* Washington, D.C.: AAHPERD, 1977.

[14]Marshall McLuhan, *Understanding Media.* Chapter 24, "Games: The Extensions of Man," New York: New American Library, 1973, pp. 234–245.

[15]Lucius D. Battle, "Cultural and Educational Affairs in International Relations," *Department of State Bulletin*, XLVII (July 9, 1962).

[16]"Charter for Leisure," *JOHPER*, 43:48–49, 56 (March, 1972).

[17]John Robinson and Geoffrey Godbey, "Work and Leisure in America: How We Spend Our Time," *JOPER*, 49:8. (October, 1978), pp. 38–39.

[18]*Ibid.*, p. 39.

[19]Max Kaplan, "New Concepts of Leisure Today," *JOHPER*, 43:43–46 (March, 1972).

[20]"Charter for Leisure," op.cit.

[21]*Ibid.*

[22]Nellie D. Arnold, "Pop Art: The Human Footprint in Infinity," *JOPER*, 49:8 (October, 1978), pp. 56–57.

[23]Robert A. Stebbins, "Amateurism and the Post-Retirement Years," *JOPER*, 49:8 (October, 1978), pp. 40–41.

[24]"High Adventure Leisure Pursuits and Risk Recreation," *Leisure Today,* (Joel F. Meier, Editor) *JOPER*, 49:4 (April, 1978), pp. 25–32.

[25]Vern Seefeldt, "Competitive Athletics for Children—The Michigan Study," *JOPER*, 49:3 (March, 1978), pp. 39–41.

[26]*Ibid.*, p. 39.

[27]Harold J. Vanderzwaag, "Sport Administration," *Careers in Physical Education.* NAPECW and NCPEAM, 1975, p. 17.

[28]*The Importance of Tourism to the U.S. Economy, 1975.* Washington, D.C.: United States Travel Data Center, 1975.

SELECTED REFERENCES

American Alliance for Health, Physical Education, and Recreation, *Coming to Our Senses: The Significance of Arts for American Education.* Washington, D.C.: AAHPER, 1977.

American Alliance for Health, Physical Education, and Recreation, *Internal Sport in a Social Cultural Setting.* Washington, D.C.: AAHPER, 1975.

American Association for Health, Physical Education and Recreation. *Leisure and the Quality of Life.* Washington, D.C.: AAHPER, 1972.

American Alliance for Health, Physical Education, and Recreation, *UNESCO Conference on Physical Education and Sport: A Report of the United States Delegation.* Washington, D.C.: AAHPER, 1977.

American Alliance for Health, Physical Education, and Recreation. *Leisure Today—Selected Readings.* Washington, D.C.: AAHPER, 1975.

American Alliance for Health, Physical Education, and Recreation. *Adapted Physical Education Guidelines: Theory and Practices for the 70's and 80's.* Washington, D.C.: AAHPER, 1976.

American Alliance for Health, Physical Education and Recreation. *Complying with Title IX of the Education Amendments of 1972 in Physical Education and High School Sports Programs.* Washington, D.C.: AAHPER, 1977.

Bates, Barbara J. (Ed.), "Leisure and Aging: New Perspectives," *JOPER*, 48:8 (October, 1977) pp. 25–56.

Hart, Marie M. (Ed.), *Sport in the Socio-Cultural Process.* Dubuque: William C. Brown, 1972.

HPER Omnibus. Washington, D.C.: AAHPER, 1976.

Jewett, Ann E., "Relationships in Physical Education: A Curriculum Viewpoint," *The Academy Papers.* 1977.

Kando, Thomas M. (Ed.), "Popular Culture and Leisure," *JOPER* 49:8 (October, 1978), pp. 33–64.

Lee, Mabel, *Memories of a Bloomer Girl.* Washington, D.C.: AAHPER, 1977.

Lee, Mabel, *Memories Beyond Bloomers.* Washington, D.C.: AAHPER, 1978.

Leonard, George, *The Ultimate Athlete.* New York: Viking Press, 1976.

Locke, Lawrence F. (Ed.), "Perspective for Sport," *Quest XIX* (January, 1973).

Loy, John W., McPherson, Barry D., and Kenyon, Gerald, *Sport and Social Systems.* Reading, Mass.: Addison-Wesley, 1978.

Meier, Joel F. (Ed.), "High Adventure Leisure Pursuits and Risk Recreation," *JOPER*, 49:4 (April, 1978) pp. 25–56.

Metheny, Eleanor, *Vital Issues*. Washington, D.C.: AAHPER, 1977.

Michener, James A., *Sports in America*. New York: Random House, 1976.

National Association for Physical Education of College Women and National College Physical Education Association for Men. *Careers in Physical Education*. (Briefings 3), 1975.

National Association for Physical Education of College Women and National College Physical Education Association for Men. *Moving Toward Implementation* (Briefings 1). 1975.

National Association for Physical Education of College Women and National College Physical Education Association for Men. *Mainstreaming Physical Education* (Briefings 4). 1976.

Oberteuffer, Delbert, *Concepts and Convictions*. Washington, D.C.: AAHPER, 1977.

Sage, George H. (Ed.), *Sports and American Society: Selected Readings*. Reading, Mass.: Addison-Wesley, 1974.

Siedentop, Daryl (Ed.), "Learning How to Play," *Quest 26* (Summer, 1976).

Siedentop, Daryl (Ed.), "Sport in America," *Quest 27* (Winter, 1977).

Spears, Betty (Ed.), "World of Sport," *Quest XXII (June, 1974)*.

Ulrich, Celeste and Nixon, John E., *Tones of Theory*. Washington, D.C.: AAHPER, 1972.

Ulrich, Celeste, *To Seek and Find*. Washington, D.C.: AAHPER, 1976.

Vanderzwaag, Harold J., *Toward a Philosophy of Sport*. Reading, Mass.: Addison Wesley, 1972.

Vendien, C. Lynn and Nixon, John E., *The World Today in Health, Physical Education and Recreation*, Englewood Cliffs, N.J.: Prentice-Hall, 1968.

Ziegler, Earle F., *Physical Education and Sport Philosophy*. Englewood Cliffs, N.J.: Prentice-Hall, 1977.

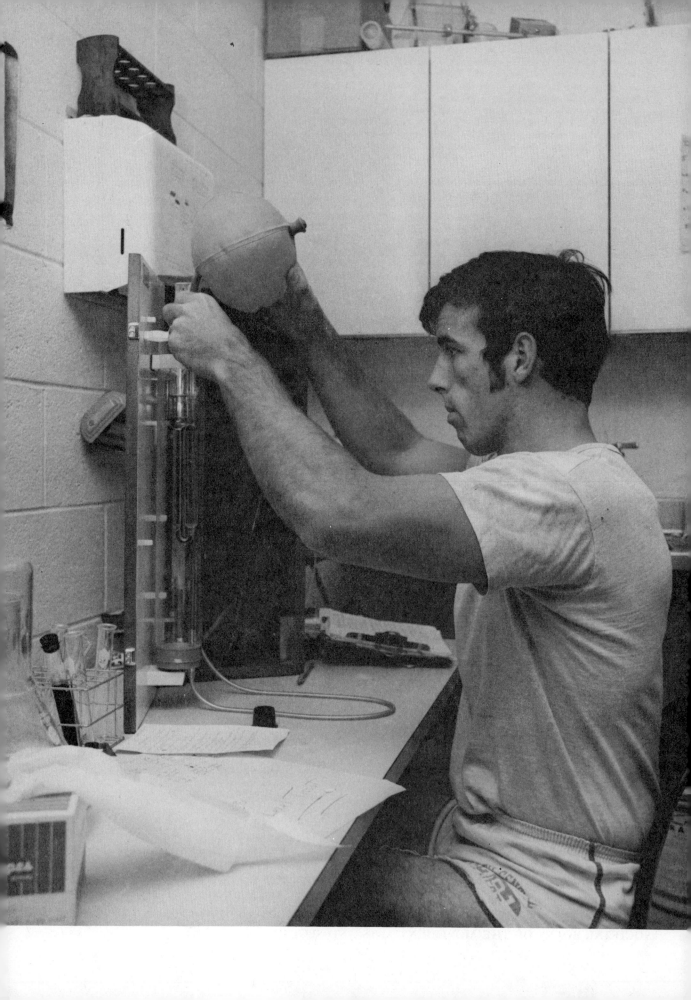

10

PREPARATION FOR ——— ——— PROFESSIONAL LEADERSHIP ———

Traditionally, the study of physical education has been considered appropriate only for those interested in teaching careers. While teaching is still the career choice of most persons with bachelor's degrees in physical education, the field includes an increasingly wide range of occupational specializations. Students interested in numerous and diverse professions focusing on the study of human movement phenomena or the use of movement activities in serving others are now majoring in physical education.

Physical educators in the last decades of the twentieth century will play a part in changing basic aspects of American society. Such changes will involve revitalizing educational programs in terms of national priorities, increasing flexibility in institutional organization and procedure, and restructuring American school and college curricula within the mainstream of modern living.

All responsible persons recognize the potential contributions of physical education in the educational enterprise and are demanding more in professional services from physical educators. Furthermore, greater understanding of the significance of human movement phenomena in contemporary living is opening up new career fields for physical educators. As the need for expertise in dealing with problems involving movement knowledge and skill is increasingly recognized in non-teaching private enterprises and public programs, the demand for qualified specialists grows. We are now looking to professional preparation institutions for competent human movement specialists for non-teaching as well as teaching roles.

The challenge to physical education has become one of quality contribution. In choosing to be a professional physical educator today, the student elects to prepare for any of a number of uniquely diversified, stimulating, demanding, and rewarding careers.

Introduction: The Challenge to Physical Education

Colleges and universities are becoming more and more selective in the admission of students to physical education curricula. The process of selection may assume many forms, beginning with qualifying tests and ending with the elimination of the less competent by the high standards of scholarship and accomplishment demanded by accredited educational institutions. The physical educator has a unique responsibility for contributing in the broadest sense to the wholesome growth and development of others. Thus, sound procedures for the selection, admission, and retention of candidates are essential.

Science Background. One of the first steps in assessment is to determine the extent of high school background and experience. It is desirable that the student's preparation in secondary school include biology, physics, and chemistry, since physical education is a profession for which a scientific background is basic. The lack of such background may not preclude entrance into professional preparation, but it does constitute a deficiency that in many cases may have to be made up at the college level.

Verbal Proficiency. Competence in verbal expression is also a prerequisite for success. The potential physical educator will need skill in reading and writing English sufficiently for intensive study as an undergraduate. If only minimum standards of English composition and reading comprehension were achieved in high school preparation, remedial opportunities may be available in the college setting, but the student will be handicapped in completing the curriculum creditably until the deficiency is overcome.

Physical Activity Background. The student who aims to become a human movement specialist needs a background as a participant in physical activity. It will be particularly helpful if the activity background has been a broad one. In addition to skills in sports in which the individual has particular interest, the prospective student should have had a wide variety of movement experiences and extensive participation in all the common forms of athletic, gymnastic, and rhythmic activities. Competitive sports experience is an asset. Leadership experiences in school clubs and activities, in youth agencies, as camp counselors, playground directors, or lifeguards, are all considered desirable.

Physical education is a professional field encompassing opportunities for individuals of varying backgrounds, personalities, and abilities. It has also become a field offering a wide range of career options. The undergraduate professional curriculum provides a core of common experiences for all those majoring in the field. Sound contemporary curricula also provide for differentiated coursework and related educational experiences designed in accordance with the individual's selected career emphasis.

Programs for professional preparation in physical education are many and varied. All provide for professional specialization in a college or university setting. Such curricula have three major emphases: (1) liberal studies or general education, designed to extend the individual's familiarity with the major fields of organized knowledge, to permit a search for deeper personal meanings in areas of individual interest, and to prepare the student to function effectively as a citizen of society; (2) disciplinary studies, designed to develop knowledge and competence in the field of human movement phenomena; and (3) specialized professional education designed to prepare for responsibilities as a specialist utilizing human movement as the focus and medium. The prospective physical educator will be concerned with all three emphases in preparation at the college level.

Professional Core Requirements. Students majoring in physical education strengthen their general education backgrounds, while establishing the foundations for professional careers, through studies in the biological and physical sciences, the behavioral sciences, and the humanities. To achieve competence in the subject-matter discipline, mastery of a wide variety of concepts relating to human movement phenomena is required. These areas of knowledge include human growth and development, physiology of muscular activity, neural bases of movement, human anatomy, kinesiology, perceptual-motor learning, sport psychology, sociology of sport, rhythmic structure of movement, philosophy of sport, dance philosophy, and history of dance, sport, and related movement activities. Competence in the discipline is acquired through study of the basic concepts, participation experience in many forms of physical activity, skillful performance of selected dance or sport movement forms, and laboratory analysis of human movement phenomena.

Specialized Professional Studies. We recommend that the general education background of physical educators be kept as flexible as is consistent with essential foundation work in basic arts and sciences; most colleges and universities have all but eliminated college-wide requirements for all students. All undergraduate majors in physical education, irrespective of individual career goals, need similar experiences with the subject-matter discipline of human movement. Beyond these minimums, however, the prospective physical educator should pursue a curriculum tailored to the selected career specialization and to personal interests. The department, school or college of physical education should provide systematic orienting, advising, and screening experiences. The student should be assisted in examining the potential of physical education as a professional field, in determining personal suitability for particular professional roles, in becoming acquainted with the designs and resources for the various options, and in developing an appropriate instructional plan.[1]

Students planning careers in the human movement professions need studies in movement analysis, movement performance, and orientation to related professions. Some specializations will require qualification for state certification. Most will require some type of intensive professional, clinical, field, or laboratory experience. Many departments permit major students to assist with large activity classes and to work with officiating and other aspects of the intramural sports program. The professionally oriented student will voluntarily take advantage of every opportunity to become better acquainted with every phase of the department's program.

Opportunities are often available for participation in professional meetings where students and faculty take part, where outside speakers are invited to meet with groups on the campus, and where problems are discussed that have local and national significance. Sometimes student clubs are joined with national professional fraternities whose objective is the advancement of the profession. As a supplement to the more formal professional education program, such group meetings may be very important and advantageous.

Participation in campus recreational activities has many advantages for the prospective physical educator.

Also having many advantages are campus recreational activities. More and more college administrators are recognizing that recreation is an important phase of the services to be offered all students. One aspect of a college recreation program involves participation in physical activities, usually coeducational, including swimming, badminton, tennis, racquetball, and handball, as well as team sports and dancing.

A Personal Professional Library. Early in the professional preparation program the student should start to assemble a professional library, to become acquainted with the literature of the field and reliable sources of information for future guidance. Textbooks could be the foundation for such a library. The quality and quantity of books in the field are growing every year. The American Alliance for Health, Physical Education, Recreation, and Dance has a list of publications, many of which should be in every student's library. A professional library is an indispensable asset and can be gradually acquired and augmented from a modest beginning. The student, with the advice of members of the teaching staff, should be alert to new contributions and add continually to the personal library collection.

Sequencing Requirements. Professional preparation curricula utilize a variety of designs for sequencing liberal arts requirements, professional core requirements, and specialized professional education studies. In most programs, the individual student needs to identify a specialization before entering the third undergraduate year. Decisions should be based upon earlier orientation to the breadth of career possibilities and should lead to increasing depth of preparation in advanced undergraduate studies for the particular career field selected. Most programs also provide

CHAPTER TEN

undergraduates with assistance in the preparation of a professional resumé, writing letters of application, understanding procedures for seeking references, developing job interview skills, analyzing job offers, anticipating payroll deduction procedures, professional association demands, and in-service education expectations.

Much concern has been expressed over the impact of rising educational costs, increasing demands for accountability, and the number of opportunities for professional employment in education. The supply and demand picture for teachers of physical education is not as advantageous today as it was during the 1950s and 1960s. However, the development of new kinds of occupations due to the expansion of physical education as a discipline and service profession, and the upgrading of standards for teacher certification and local employment have maintained openings for qualified individuals seeking teaching positions.

Beginning Professional Experiences. Since economic pressures have affected job opportunities in teaching as in many other occupational fields, the new teachers must be willing to begin their professional experience as necessity dictates. The rate of turnover in the favored suburban systems is often low, and it may be necessary to accept a position in a small town, a rural or semirural community, or a community of lower socio-economic status. Here will be found experience not normally offered in larger systems — the opportunity to organize one's own program, a broader variety of duties and responsibilities, and a chance to become acquainted with the administration of the school as a whole. Under such circumstances the new teacher must be qualified and willing to assume teaching assignments in areas other than physical education, in states where this practice is permitted. The young teacher seeking a first position where the need is greatest may wish to serve in the inner core areas of the large city systems or in other special programs for culturally disadvantaged youth.

As in any field of endeavor, advancement depends to a large extent upon the quality of leadership displayed and the willingness to maintain professional growth through continuing study and self-improvement. Teachers of physical education have exactly the same opportunities for advancement as do teachers in general. Leadership in education for the teacher should not be measured solely in terms of personal advancement from one type of teaching position to another, from the elementary level to the college level, or from instruction to supervision to administration. Leadership in the finest sense may be the day-by-day contribution to the growth of students, to the advancement of the profession, and to the development of the culture of the community as a whole.

Professional Growth. Increased interest in improving instruction in the public schools has led to considerable upgrading in standards for teacher qualification in the current decade. Career teachers are now expected to accept personal responsibility for continuing professional growth. School systems encourage and support the professional growth and development of teachers by sponsoring in-service education programs; by rewarding professional growth through salary advancement, recognition, and status; and by granting leaves of absence for professional reasons. The individual teacher must seek self-improvement through graduate study, workshops, institutes, educational travel, professional conferences, committee projects, research, and professional writing.

Contemporary Challenges. Today's teachers are faced with new challenges. All public institutions are being reexamined and evaluated for their cost effectiveness and public responsibility. American society is demanding not only accountability but also concern for the individuality of each child and the strengthening of interpersonal relationships — all of which require innovation on the part of the teacher. Tomorrow's teachers must be prepared to identify and expand the creative potentials of their students.

The creative physical educator is an innovator who looks for new content to enrich the traditional offerings of the physical education curriculum. Today's physical educator is responsible for creating learning environments that provide varied stimuli, encourage exploration, and motivate students to achieve desired outcomes. Learning opportunities must be designed to facilitate personal variations in movement performance, to stress individual solutions of movement problems, and to encourage inventiveness and extend creative abilities in movement expression. Clearly, the completely structured teaching approach of the physical educator is a thing of the past; the prospective teacher must be prepared to fill a more creative, and thus more difficult, role in today's curricula.

While there is lack of agreement regarding specifics, the general consensus is that education students must be prepared to cope with new and constantly changing social conditions. Racial conflict has made the public school both a target and a tool for civil rights advances. The struggles of ethnic minorities for equal status, affirmative action efforts demanding equal opportunities for women, the prejudices directed against individuals identified with particular religious faiths, and the demands of low-income groups for higher living standards are all reflected in American schools. Schools must face squarely the responsibility to educate for intergroup understanding. Teachers must learn to facilitate the development of social responsibility and understanding, and skills for finding constructive solutions to social problems. The school has a vital role in working toward greater integration of our pluralistic society, and the prospective teacher faces a crucial challenge in preparing to pursue this goal effectively.

Opportunities are increasing for students to be challenged and stimulated through experiences with new organizational patterns and instructional media and devices. Educators of the future will need more intensive study of techniques for modifying learning behaviors, more practice in those teaching strategies most adaptable to one's style of teaching, and more experimentation with procedures for eliciting creative responses in learners and for influencing attitudes in desirable directions.

The trend in undergraduate teacher education and certification is toward competency-based programs and requirements. The AAHPER Professional Preparation Conference held in New Orleans in January, 1973, used this approach to develop possible competencies relating to basic human movement understandings; physical education movement patterns; and professional competencies in methodological, administrative, curricular, and co-curricular analysis, and in evaluation.[2]

Physical education teachers need experiences and competencies required by all teachers in areas such as human development, learning, school and society, communications, and media and technology. They

Preparation for Teaching

share with other physical education specialists interests and undergraduate preparation in movement analysis, movement performance, and study of the human movement professions. As physical education teachers they require extensive professional laboratory experiences in working with individuals and groups in both movement and non-activity settings and specialized competencies in the guidance of movement learning.

Professional preparation programs need to help prospective educators to redefine roles in relationships with parents, elected community officials, and individuals in the other public service professions. Physical education teachers need to give particular attention to the roles they play in supporting the professional efforts of their colleagues in the fields of health education, safety education, dance education, leisure education, and guidance. They need to learn to work with the paraprofessionals who serve as teacher aides, audio-visual technicians, equipment specialists, and computer programmers.

The recommendations of knowledgeable and concerned student professionals for strengthening undergraduate teacher education curricula are of particular interest and importance. At the 1973 AAHPER Professional Preparation Conference, the Student Action Council presented seven resolutions.[3] These included recommendations for more practical exposure to teaching situations; inclusion of coaching and officiating preparation for prospective women teachers; more sport psychology and sociology; more encouragement for students to become involved in professional organizations; increased emphasis in health education, motor learning, adaptive methods and skills, and mathematics for research potential; and immediate and thorough reviewing and restructuring of

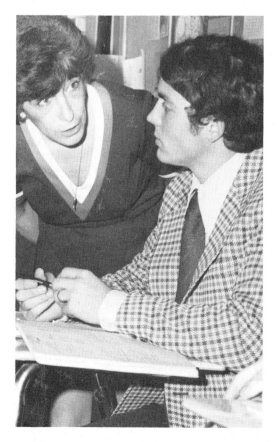

Physical educators play a large part in supporting the professional efforts of their colleagues.

current undergraduate programs. Teacher educators should give prompt and careful attention to these recommendations.

Specialization. This is an age of specialization. Although greater emphasis is being given to a more comprehensive general education for all teachers, regardless of their special field of study, tomorrow's physical educator also will be expected to qualify as a specialist within the profession. In addition to an understanding of human growth and development within the total life span, and of the learning process as it applies to the whole range of learning behavior from the preschool child to the adult, teachers will be expected to develop particular understandings and skills for working effectively with the population of the community in which they choose to teach.

Knowledge and understanding concerning the nature of human movement and considerable insight into principles and key concepts of movement are basic. Specific abilities are also needed to apply these general principles and utilize movement skill and understanding in teaching and coaching others. Further individualization in the undergraduate program depends on the student's professional plans; the following list provides an indication of the numerous capacities in which one could serve:

— preschool teacher
— elementary or middle school teacher
— high school teacher-coach
— college or university instructor or professor
— dance teacher
— aquatics expert
— gymnastics specialist
— teacher of the elderly, the disabled, the handicapped, the retarded, the bilingual
— urban teacher, or teacher of the rurally isolated

Again, this list is meant to be only an indication of the possibilities in the teaching of physical education; it is by no means exhaustive.

Elementary School

It is well recognized that to be most successful physical education must lay its foundations in the elementary school. Basic skills and attitudes are learned in this period, and hence it is important that those in charge of the physical education program provide for the development of these essential attitudes and skills.

Opportunities. Educators generally agree about the necessity of fundamental training in physical education at the elementary school level, but school administrators do not always insist upon expert knowledge in their teachers. Thus, elementary school physical educators usually are employed either as members of a single school faculty teaching children on a full-time basis, or as central office consultants, guiding classroom teachers in the improvement of physical education instruction. As educators have become convinced that movement education in the elementary school years is basic to sound developmental experiences for all children, and not just useful in learning athletic skills early in life, facilitating the release of emotional tension, or even establishing sound habits of play, more school systems are allotting adequate funds for elementary school facilities and competent instruction.

Professional Preparation. The elementary physical education specialist studies motor development and child psychology in depth. This curriculum option includes considerable emphasis on the philosophy, content, and instructional strategies of movement education. Specific materials and teaching techniques in creative dance and thorough knowledge of educational gymnastics are needed. The elementary educator must learn to analyze and modify games and to guide children in designing and playing new games. It is assumed that he or she will be knowledgeable and skillful in teaching the exceptional children who are "mainstreamed" into the physical education class. Clearly the physical educator must be prepared to work with other educational specialists as a member of the elementary education team.

Middle School

Plans for school organization vary in different systems; but the majority of plans include a middle or junior high school unit of two to four years. Educators and child development specialists have come to recognize that preadolescents have unique needs that cannot be met in either elementary or high school settings.

Opportunities. The middle school offers particular job satisfactions for teachers. In the large cities, physical education specialists are engaged to teach only physical education. In smaller communities they are often required to teach other subjects and must qualify for an appropriate certificate. Many middle school physical educators also have coaching and intramural assignments.

Professional Preparation. Middle school physical educators need professional preparation similar to that required of the elementary school specialist, with additional emphasis on the sensorimotor, intellectual, and socio-emotional development of the preadolescent. Special attention must be given to the developmental rationale and educational philosophy underlying the middle school concept. Skills and knowledges relating to the popular team games, dances, gymnastic activities, and individual sports activities appropriate for boys and girls of this age group are also important. Competence in organizing and coaching intramural and competitive sports activities is also expected.

Secondary School

Opportunities. The secondary school physical educator needs to be a generalist in order to give leadership through a complete program of movement activities. Most junior and senior high schools employ only one to four physical educators. The physical education staff is expected to provide instruction in team sports, individual and dual sports, gymnastics, aquatics, and dance. Whether male or female, the secondary school physical educator should be prepared to coach as well as teach.

Professional Preparation. Professional preparation should emphasize adolescent development and learning, sociology, psychology of sport, and leisure counseling. While preparing to meet state certification in physical education, the undergraduate student should achieve, in addition to broad preparation in the field, a specialization that will permit supplementing the particular strengths of other physical education staff members effectively. This specialization may be expertise in a selected activity area for teaching and coaching; a special competence, such as the organization and administration of intramurals; or qualification as an adapted physical education specialist to provide educational services to exceptional children.

All secondary school physical educators should develop basic competencies in health education, safety education, and guidance. All will need minimum coaching skills and competence in a variety of different teaching and evaluation skills. During the early 1980s, particular attention must be given to the physical education of the handicapped and to the development and administration of coeducational programs that assure equal educational opportunities for all secondary school boys and girls.

Opportunities. Positions in colleges and universities are usually of five types: (1) activity class work; (2) teacher education courses in those institutions offering a major in physical education; (3) administration of intramural programs; (4) the coaching of athletic teams; and (5) teaching and guiding research in graduate programs directed toward higher degrees. Frequently, the college or university physical educator is responsible for some combination of these assignments. *College and University*

Professional Preparation. In junior colleges or community colleges, the emphasis is usually placed upon teaching activity classes or continuing education classes, conducting intramurals, and coaching. A master's degree and a fifth-year-level teaching credential are usually required. A doctor's degree is preferred for teachers of the undergraduate professional theory courses and is generally a standard requirement for the assignment of graduate program responsibilities. The undergraduate student looking toward a position in a college or university should anticipate qualifying for admission to graduate school and earning a graduate degree. Since teaching experience may also be a prerequisite for the desired college position, it is wise if the undergraduate professional preparation curriculum also meets all certification requirements.

No longer may a teacher achieve advancement and success on the strength of athletic performance as an undergraduate. Rather, successful teaching requires dedication, with knowledge, vision, and professional skills. The college or university physical educator is a scholar, an adviser, a coach, an artist, a researcher, an administrator, an evaluator, an author — yet always a *teacher*, "because that is his essence, that is his commitment, that is his love."[4]

Teacher education curricula, as we have known them, need significant changes. Individuals will be required to develop diverse talents and widely varying skills for living and working in a world of change. As our world becomes more technologically advanced, ecology-aware, ethnically conscious, and globally interdependent, we will need professionals oriented toward education as a problem-preventing enterprise, a complex of useful services attuned to unlimited possibilites. *Future-Oriented Teachers*

Professional preparation curricula for physical education teachers will have to go beyond the development of competencies of presentation, group organization, coaching, and testing. Teacher educators will strive to help people appreciate the different meanings of movement, to present physical activity as an essential aspect of a complete life, to contribute to answering the important questions relating to the movement sciences, and to seek creative fulfillment in the movement arts. Future teachers will be prepared to provide educational services beyond school settings and oriented toward continuing their own education.

Undergraduate students who prepare for careers as health educators, fitness specialists, therapists, or athletic trainers need to include in their programs additional study in the biological sciences (anatomy, physiology, kinesiology, physiological chemistry, exercise physiology, physiologi- **HEALTH AND FITNESS EMPHASES** cal psychology); psychology (social psychology, personality, counseling, human relations and group development, motor learning); and health and safety education (personal health problems, prevention of injuries, mental health, adult fitness). In addition, they will enroll in professional courses specific to the specialization desired. Each will serve an appropriate type of internship.

Health Education. It is generally acknowledged that anyone teaching health education should have a major in that field. The undergraduate curriculum leading to certification in health education requires a solid science background with professional specialization in the following:

— personal health and fitness
— alcohol, narcotics, and drug education
— mental health, human sexuality, and death education
— community health organization, interpretation of public health statistics, and health care delivery systems
— curriculum development, health instruction, and school health services
— first aid, CPR training, driver and traffic safety, industrial and fire safety, and safety in sports

The importance of employing fully qualified health educators in secondary schools has become generally accepted. At the present time, however, too many physical education teachers are still teaching most of the health education in junior and senior high schools. Of course, a number of responsibilities pertaining to health do form a legitimate part of the physical educator's assignment; these include:

— promotion of a vigorous activity program that will contribute to individual health and fitness;
— incidental instruction regarding fatigue, rest, conditioning, warm-up training, diet, sleep, injuries, and other such matters;
— attention to emotional health;
— cleanliness of the physical education plant, safety in the use of facilities and in the operation of the program, and adequate provisions for first aid and emergency care;
— complete cooperation with school medical personnel in the conduct of health examinations and the application of their findings;
— the wise use of information regarding health matters that should receive the attention of medical personnel, and referral of serious health problems to proper community health agencies.

The undergraduate program of physical educators should prepare prospective physical educators to fulfill these responsibilities.

The health instruction program should be assigned to a fully certified health educator. Assignment of this responsibility to any teacher whose preparation does not include adequate education in this subject is apt to result in a poor quality of teaching and an adverse reaction on the part of students. The assumption of administrators that a teacher can adequately teach physical education and at the same time plan and direct curricular experiences in health for the school population demonstrates that inadequate importance is attached to both areas.

Fitness Centers. Whether employed in an agency fitness program, a corporate health center, or a commercial health spa, the fitness specialist will require the scientific background described previously. It is hoped that licensing or certification will become a standard to protect the public by ensuring adequate qualification of personnel operating fitness centers. Preparation need not include teacher certification, although an undergraduate physical education major is appropriate. The program should include, in addition to the common core experiences and a strong background in the biological sciences, extensive knowledge of posture, body mechanics, conditioning, weight training, fitness exercise, care and prevention of injuries, aquatics, motor learning, and physiology of the aging. A minor in business administration would be helpful, including studies in management, marketing, accounting, risk and insurance, and advertising. Desirable electives might be selected from departments of leisure studies, sociology, psychology, and journalism.

Therapy. Professional preparation of therapists occurs primarily at the graduate or post-baccalaureate level. However, this does not preclude initiating some specialized preparation at the undergraduate level. Most accredited physical therapy and corrective therapy programs identify physical education as a recommended baccalaureate program for admissions purposes. The potential recreation therapist should earn the bachelor's degree in recreation and leisure studies. The occupational therapist might choose any of several undergraduate majors, including both physical education and recreation. The dance therapist should select dance as the undergraduate specialization, if available; physical education in a program with a strong dance component would be a second choice.

Prospective therapists at the undergraduate level may be encouraged to develop skills and competencies related to the assessment and analysis of motor function and movement patterns, a general orientation to disease and disability, and an overview of characteristics of special populations. Professionals in these fields will need many movement skills, familiarity with all types of physical activity recreation, and ability to use a wide variety of teaching methods, especially those appropriate for independent learning and small group settings. In-depth study of disabling conditions, evaluation techniques, and therapeutic procedures and extensive field or clinical experience will normally be left for graduate level preparation.

Sports Medicine. Individuals involved in sports medicine represent a variety of professions, including physicians, physiologists, therapists,

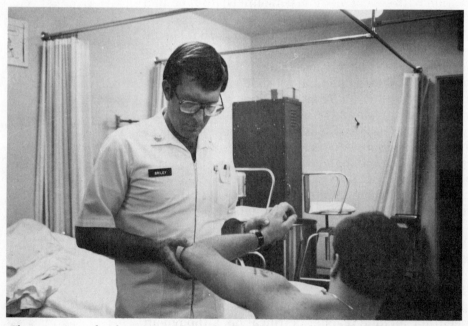

Therapists must develop competencies related to assessment and analysis of motor function.

psychologists, physical educators, coaches, and athletic trainers. Undergraduate professional preparation for physical education teaching and coaching and for therapy have been discussed previously. The other fields are graduate specializations, with the exception of athletic training.

The significant role of the athletic trainer is abundantly recognized by national associations concerned with health, physical education and athletics, sports medicine organizations, and medical societies and associations. It is well understood that the athletic trainer is crucial in preventing injuries, in recognizing and evaluating injuries, and in providing appropriate paramedical services when injuries occur. The demand for qualified athletic trainers is evident in that every major league professional sports team and every major university athletic program employs at least one full-time athletic trainer on its staff. Although their potential value to high-school athletic programs is recognized, financial considerations have limited the ability of many school districts to provide athletic trainers. Trainers also work in sports medicine clinics, in student health centers, and with athletic training supply companies.

Professional Preparation for the Athletic Trainer. The recognized certification of an athletic trainer is based on meeting the qualifications established by the National Athletic Trainers Association, including passing a professional examination. Those who desire NATA certification may prepare through completion of a NATA-approved athletic training program, completing a physical therapy curriculum, or serving an apprenticeship in the profession. Since athletic training is not a teacher certification field, most candidates are certified in health and physical education, although other teaching fields are acceptable.

Courses specifically required in an approved athletic training program include

— anatomy, physiology, physiology of exercise, applied anatomy and kinesiology, and psychology;
— first aid and safety, nutrition, personal, community, and school health;
— remedial exercise, therapeutic exercise, adapted exercises, or corrective exercise;
— techniques of athletic training, including a minimum of 600 clock hours of laboratory practice.

Also recommended are laboratory physical science, pharmacology, histology, pathology, physical education administration, psychology of coaching, and coaching techniques. The NATA publication, *Athletic Training Careers,*[5] is recommended for further information.

SOCIAL SERVICE OPTIONS

Teaching is usually viewed as a social service profession. Those interested in studying the movement arts and sciences as a basis for social service careers generally major in physical education or recreation, whether they plan to teach or to complete non-certification programs. It is wise to select substantial supporting study in sociology, psychology, political science, economics, social work, and public administration to strengthen this orientation. In most instances, undergraduate physical education curricula have enough flexibility so that the student's advisor can assist in planning an individual specialization option by thoughtful selection of courses to meet university liberal arts requirements and judicious choices of electives within the professional program and among free electives.

Children and Youth. Undergraduates looking forward to working in agency programs for children and youth will include advanced study in motor development, child and adolescent psychology, perceptual-motor learning, and special education, in addition to the recommended offerings in the social sciences. Many professional preparation programs now offer undergraduate options in adapted physical education for those interested in directing their energies into service with special populations.

The Aged. Geriatrics is a growing medical specialty. The recognition that many medical problems associated with aging can be prevented, minimized, or at least delayed has led to the recent development of interdisciplinary studies of gerontology and the expansion of programs and career opportunities in working with the aged. Of special interest to physical educators is the need for qualified individuals to direct low-stress exercise-activity programs for the elderly. Leslie[6] discusses the rationale for such programs and suggests the following for academic content as a specialization option within an undergraduate physical education program: biology of aging, sociology of aging, health and aging, fitness and therapeutic programs for the elderly, and recreation programs for the elderly. He further recommends field experience in such settings as nursing homes, retirement centers, Golden Ager-type organizations, recreation departments, YMCAs and YWCAs, university extension programs, and programs sponsored by such groups as the American Association for Retired Persons and area agencies on aging.

HEW Programs. Health, education, and welfare programs supported by public funds will vary with each political administration. Physical educators interested in providing services to delinquents, minorities, the handicapped and disabled, the poor, or any other group needing special assistance may tailor the elective portions of the undergraduate curriculum to their unique special interests. Offerings that might receive consideration could be found in almost any department. Some of the most relevant courses are those in social work, community planning, public administration, law and social problems, crime and delinquency, special education, ethnic studies, and women's studies.

Professional preparation oriented toward communications specializations may be directed toward either sports communication or communication through dance. Either curriculum should be strong in analysis, understanding, and interpretation of movement, speech and language arts, literature and the fine arts, and the social and behavioral sciences.

COMMUNICATIONS SPECIALIZATIONS

Sports Communication. Interdisciplinary curricula made up of physical education, journalism, and communications are growing in popularity. A number of institutions have developed programs that permit the student to declare a major in one department and to include in the undergraduate program a substantial number of courses in the cooperating department. To these interdisciplinary programs, physical education contributes such traditional offerings as history and philosophy of sport, sport psychology, sociology of sport, and coaching courses. Typical journalism courses are reporting, broadcasting, mass communications, public relations, and advertising. Curriculum patterns also show titles such as photojournalism, film for television, persuasive communication, and factual television. Courses jointly developed, specifically for new programs in sports communication, include sports information, sports literature, and sportscasting. Practicum experiences are essential; students experience a variety of assignments with the local mass media —

campus publications, and radio and television stations. Cooperative arrangements between media personnel and university personnel in both communications and physical education have facilitated the upgrading of media coverage of sports, especially girls' and women's sports.

Dance. Dance as communication assumes levels of knowledge and performance ability that require in-depth academic concentration. The undergraduate student looking toward such a career would ordinarily require a major in dance as a performing art. Teacher certification is not inappropriate, but a complete physical education program usually would not permit sufficient depth of study in dance. The undergraduate dance major requires thorough study in the scientific analysis of human movement, in addition to history and philosophy of dance, cultural anthropology, drama, theatre, music, dance literature and criticism, choreography, and a high level of ability in many types of dance performance.

RECREATION LEADERSHIP

The insistent demand for recreation in modern American life has brought about the realization of the community's responsibility to provide not only space and facilities, but also trained leadership. During recent years, many curricula in colleges and universities have been developed for the professional preparation of recreation workers, and steps have been taken to standardize educational qualifications for such positions. These curricula emphasize a broad liberal arts background pertinent to an understanding of the needs and aspirations of individuals and groups in a democratic society, an understanding of the significance of leisure in our culture, and skill in and an appreciation of a wide variety of leisure-time activities.

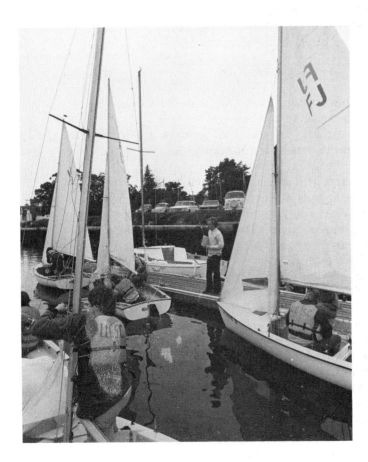

Recreation leaders must understand the needs of individuals and groups in today's society.

In the past, many positions in recreation were taken by professional physical educators or by people who had no formal training in physical education but rather learned through practical experience on the playground. Now more and more of such recreational positions are being filled by professionally prepared recreation personnel. Many part-time positions in community recreation are available after school hours and in the summer months, and these positions offer the physical education major good experience. Such positions include playground leader, special activity leader, camp counselor, assistant camp director, waterfront director, and lifeguard.

The undergraduate student wishing to enter recreation as a profession is strongly urged to enroll in a professional curriculum in recreation and leisure studies. The best programs in this field are now accredited by state or national agencies and offer certification to the qualified graduate with a baccalaureate degree in recreation. Specializations within the field include park management, public recreation administration, camping, outdoor recreation, and therapeutic recreation.

As the demands for both professional sports entertainment and recreational sports participation have grown, career opportunities in these fields have increased. At the same time, teacher educators, observing trends toward tax economies and possible tightening of the educational job market, are proposing additional options in undergraduate professional preparation for those interested in business or careers requiring knowledge and performance abilities in the movement arts and sports sciences. Professional preparation for the management of exercise and fitness programs, operation of health spas, and sports communication have already been discussed. Other vocations toward which undergraduate programs can be directed include coaching, athletic administration, and sports management.

SPORTS MANAGEMENT AND BUSINESS ADMINISTRATION

Concern for adequate professional preparation of those responsible for the coaching of school and college athletic teams is increasing among physical educators, especially those most directly involved in teacher education. Since the 1920s, the accepted preparation for coaching has been an undergraduate major in physical education. Since the number of sports and teams increased to a point where the demand for coaches exceeded the supply of physical education teachers, efforts of the professional associations have been directed toward specialized preparation for coaching aspirants and state certification of high school coaches. This trend has made it possible for physical educators to include or to minimize coaching preparation in bachelor's and master's degree curricula and has encouraged teachers in other academic fields to become qualified and certified coaches if they so desire.

Professional Preparation. Recommendations for strengthening the coaching profession through certification standards were provided in 1970 by the AAHPER Task Force on Certification of High School Coaches and endorsed by the National Council of Secondary School Athletic Directors.[7] The 1973 AAHPER Professional Preparation Conference[8] identified the following special competencies needed by coaches: background in the medicolegal, sociological, and psychological aspects of coaching; theory and techniques of coaching; and kinesiological and physiological foundations of coaching. In spite of continuing concerns of

Coaching

professional educators, the adoption of specialized certification requirements for coaches has been slow. Noble and Corbin[9] have recently reported findings of a 1976 survey of all 50 states, Puerto Rico, and Washington, D.C. Although most states required that a coach be a certified teacher, and two (Indiana and Wisconsin) made coaching certification available, only five (Minnesota, Nebraska, Iowa, Wyoming, and South Dakota) had minimum certification requirements in addition to teacher certification.

The movement toward equal opportunity for girls and women in sport has concurrently opened up opportunities for women in the coaching field. Coaching now represents a realistic career option for men and women at secondary, community college, college and university levels. Full-time positions in coaching are increasingly available in colleges and universities, and in public and private enterprise.

Athletic administration is combined with educational administration in many secondary school and some college and university positions. However, the trend is toward separating the administration of athletics from the supervision and administration of physical education. Athletic directors require practical experience in coaching; but a successful coaching record is not in itself sufficient recommendation for appointment to a position as an administrator of athletics.

Athletic Administration

In addition to coaching, officiating, athletic training, and directing athletic programs, career opportunities in sports administration include such positions as financial manager or business manager, publicity director, ticket manager, general manager, intramural sports director, sports club manager, director of sports marketing, and supervisor of sports facilities and equipment. Vanderzwaag[10] has proposed that the undergraduate program for professional preparation of sports administrators include basic sports studies and seminars in history, philosophy, psychology, and sociology of sport; business administration courses in accounting, finance, marketing, management, and economics; an integrating sports administration seminar; and an internship in a sports organization such as a collegiate athletic department, collegiate intramural sports program, high school athletic program, professional sports team, or a league office or commissioner's office in professional sports.

Professional Preparation. Since athletic administrators are usually expected to gain prior experience as full time coaches or teacher-coaches, specific professional preparation for this field is usually graduate-level preparation. An approved program of professional preparation at the graduate level for those who plan to go into athletic administration at the secondary school or college level has been developed by a Joint Committee on Physical Education and Athletics of the AAHPER, the NCAA, and the National College Physical Education Association for Men.[11] A study reported in 1978[12] based on questionnaires sent to 261 institutions offering a master's or a doctoral program in physical education and related fields found 20 institutions offering graduate courses of study in athletic administration and sports management; with the exception of one Ed.D. (Doctor of Education) program, the degree offered was a master's degree. The emphasis varied with two-thirds of the programs emphasizing athletic administration and most of the others emphasizing sports administration.

Young persons interested in the management of a private sports club, the operation of a sporting goods business, the development of a commercial recreation facility, or the promotion of tourism, are apt to find the best undergraduate preparation in a school or college of business or in a program sponsored jointly by business administration and health, physical education and recreation. An example of the type of innovative undergraduate program now becoming available is a program in professional golf management developed at Ferris State College in Big Rapids, Michigan, in cooperation with the Professional Golfers' Association of America. This is a 4½-year program leading to a Bachelor of Science degree in Marketing. It requires 34 months in college and 20 months of on-the-job internship, providing preparation in golf course maintenance, design and construction of golf courses, operation of a golf shop, public relations, teaching skills, and organization and conduct of golf events. George Washington University[13] offers programs in tourism including courses in business, economics, environmental education, and leisure education, with such topical offerings as travel marketing and advertising, tour package development and wholesaling, resort management, management of conventions and trade shows, travel data collection, and consumer education. The expansion of such programs with a wide variety of specializations can be expected.

GRADUATE STUDIES

Choosing a Graduate School and Program

For the student who is ambitious of greater responsibility or who may be especially interested in pursuing research, the graduate curricula now available in physical education offer ample opportunity, challenge, and reward.

The curriculum designed for each individual should depend to a large extent upon individual needs; that is, a specified pattern for all graduate students should not be attempted. Included in the graduate program will be education in methods and techniques of research, as

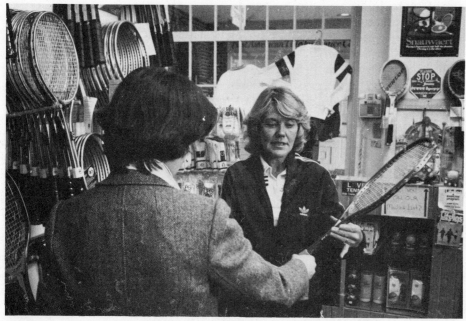

Management of a sporting goods business provides an alternative career for the physical education specialist.

well as seminars offering advanced work in areas such as curriculum, supervision, administration, history, philosophy, sport psychology, sociology of sport, motor development, perceptual-motor learning, kinesiology, biomechanics, physiology of exercise, and measurement and evaluation.

Graduate specializations in physical education may be developed in any of the above subdisciplinary fields. To choose the appropriate institution for graduate study, the student should first review the programs of those graduate schools most respected for graduate work in physical education, then select the college or university that offers the best program with faculty members who can provide expert guidance in the student's desired specialization. Programs should be tailored to individual student career goals.

Careers selected by physical educators may require graduate study in departments other than physical education, interdisciplinary programs developed cooperatively by several university departments, or particular specializations centered in physical education. For example, careers in health education, tourism, and the sporting goods industry suggest degree programs in health, leisure studies, and business, respectively; similarly, physical therapy curricula are provided in allied health science departments, often in cooperation with a medical school. The best preparation for careers in sports communications, sports management, and work with the aging is probably through interdisciplinary curricula. Specializations in athletic training, adapted physical education, and fitness leadership are usually offered by physical education departments. The vast majority of today's graduate students in physical education are choosing careers in higher education, administration, or research.

HIGHER EDUCATION

All universities and many colleges define their missions as threefold: teaching, research, and service. Those who aspire to careers in higher education must prepare themselves to make contributions in all three areas. Although most two-year and many four-year colleges have positions in physical education for which the master's degree is the basic qualification, advancement to the top ranks within a university normally requires progress toward a doctoral degree.

The student interested in becoming a college or university professor will select a specialization within the broad field of physical education that will permit development of an area of scholarly expertise in which the individual can teach courses for undergraduate students, conduct research, and ultimately teach graduate students and guide their research. In addition, the program should include studies in curriculum development, since most faculties are charged with decision-making relative to courses and curricula. Teaching effectiveness, instructional strategies, and educational evaluation should be studied to strengthen individual teaching competence.

Professional Preparation. Each graduate student should become sufficiently familiar with the organization and administration of higher education to function effectively as a member of the college or university community of scholars. Prior to completing the degree program, advanced students should ensure that they have

— conducted research;
— developed skills for independent research in a well defined area of scholarly specialization;

— published in one or two refereed journals;

— acquired a fundamental knowledge of curriculum development;

— had some successful experience in classroom presentations;

— gained an awareness of tools and procedures for evaluating teacher effectiveness;

— had opportunity for involvement in university and professional association service.

Graduate study in physical education may be directed toward academic administration or athletic administration or some combination of both. Careers in administration and management may focus on public school opportunities, college and university administration, or upon business settings.

School district organization and arrangements for staff leadership and supervision vary greatly from district to district and state to state. Departments of physical education with three or more faculty members generally appoint a member of the staff as a *department chairperson;* this position may be part-time, requiring only a few hours free from teaching responsibilities, or it may be a full-time position, depending upon the size of the program and the number of faculty members to be supervised. Larger districts usually arrange for supervision of instruction and curriculum development in physical education through the appointment of one or more individuals to the central office staff; these positions carry such titles as *curriculum associate, curriculum consultant, supervisor,* or *director of physical education.* In some states county supervisors or state directors are appointed.

School administration also offers advancement opportunities for qualified physical educators. In fact, a disproportionately large number of school principals are educators whose initial preparation was in physical education. At the college and university level, administrative positions include department and division chairs, deanships, and so on, up to and including college presidencies. All positions in educational supervision and administration require considerable teaching and staff experience, in addition to advanced graduate study in the appropriate areas. Still more extensive administrative training will be expected of those students looking ahead to college or university administration.

While athletic administration is combined with educational administration in many schools and colleges, the trend is toward separation of these responsibilities. Today it is generally agreed that athletic administration and sports management are sufficiently unique to require specialized training at the graduate level. A recent survey[14] found 20 United States universities that offer a graduate course of study in athletic administration and sports management. In addition to interscholastic and intercollegiate athletic administration, these programs offer specialized preparation for professional sports administration, private and public recreation sports administration, arena/auditorium management, and the sporting goods industry.

Physical education professionals are evidencing increasing interest in physical education as an area of study and research. It is probable that future developments will include increased opportunities for investigating, organizing, and developing knowledge in the field and extensive opportunities for applying such knowledge in educational, recreational, and therapeutic settings. Many graduate degree programs in colleges and universities currently emphasize research preparation; and a few undergraduate curricula are already offering options that permit the student to build a strong background for a career in research. It is anticipated that greater opportunities will become available for primary contributions in physical education research in university, private foundation, commercial industry, and government contexts.

Most higher education institutions now encourage graduate professors to devote a significant part of their time and creative effort to personal research interests. The average assistant professor is expected to demonstrate some degree of research productivity to achieve career advancement in academia. These and other factors have increased interest among physical education graduate students in developing research specializations. It is important to note, however, that almost all university research positions require the individual to gain experience and seniority while in positions in which research is not the full-time responsibility. Consequently, those seeking careers in university research should qualify for the less specialized roles in higher education described above. The more highly specialized research competencies are normally acquired on the job.

Professional preparation in the future will be more in-service education than pre-service education. Our entire society is placing increasing value on continuing adult education. A baccalaureate degree will be obsolete within a very short time if it is not continuously supplemented with newly discovered knowledge and the stimulation of innovative

CONTINUING EDUCATION

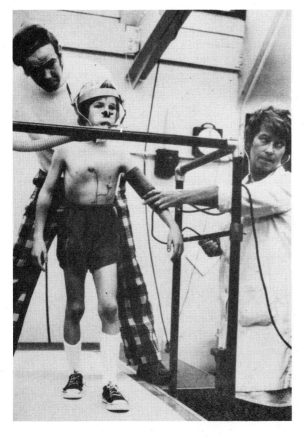

It is probable that future developments will open up increased opportunities for research positions for the qualified physical educator.

ideas. Futurists project that eventually adults in this country will move in and out of organized educational experiences throughout their lifetimes; in other words, individuals will be continuously updating their knowledge and strengthening their professional skills, resulting in widely diversified career patterns. For educators, this will mean that a terminal degree will not signify the end of a graduate study program but will instead be a potential beginning to a new career.

Career physical educators must accept individual responsibility for continuing professional growth. Growing interest in increased teacher effectiveness has led to upgrading standards. Schools and colleges support the professional growth and development of teachers by sponsoring in-service education programs, by granting professional leaves of absence, and by rewarding professional growth through promotion and merit pay increases. In the last analysis, however, it is the individual physical educator who must take the initiative to enroll in graduate programs, to become actively involved in the work of professional associations, to read and contribute to professional publications, and to participate in workshops, seminars, and professional conferences.

Progress in any field is closely tied to the quality of professional leadership available. Progress does not come about by chance or accident, but through the concerted efforts of interested and committed individuals. Each physical educator has the personal responsibility of striving constantly to improve local conditions and to increase individual professional effectiveness. Cooperation in professional organizations makes it possible to achieve much more through group efforts. Soon after entering the professional preparation curriculum, the student should become acquainted with the various professional organizations and with the contributions of the individual leaders in these organizations. Active membership in organizations concerned with the promotion of the profession, with the establishment of higher standards for programs and certification, and with the improvement of employment conditions should begin with undergraduate student membership and continue throughout a professional career.

It would be impossible and inappropriate to attempt to list here all the national organizations directly or indirectly concerned with promoting the various phases of health, physical education, and recreation. A few of the more prominent in developing professional leadership will be cited.

ORGANIZATIONS PROMOTING PROFESSIONAL LEADERSHIP

History. The original organization, called the American Association for the Advancement of Physical Education, was founded in November, 1885, by a group of 35 men. They were called together by Dr. William G. Anderson, then of Adelphi Academy, Brooklyn, who in 1902 became medical examiner and director of physical education at Yale University, where he remained until his retirement. Through most of its recent history, the organization was entitled the American Association for Health, Physical Education, and Recreation (AAHPER). In 1974, as a result of reorganization, this became the American Alliance for Health, Physical Education, and Recreation. The current name, the American Alliance for Health, Physical Education, Recreation, and Dance (AAHPERD), was adopted in March, 1979. Today the Alliance is the largest professional association in its field and occupies a top-ranking position among professional education groups.

American Alliance for Health, Physical Education, Recreation and Dance

Organization. The Alliance now serves 50,000 members. Its headquarters are currently located in the NEA Building in Washington, D.C., but will be relocated in Reston, Virginia; the ground-breaking ceremony for the new Alliance Center was held in June, 1978. To improve regional services, six district associations have been formed on a geographical basis. The Alliance has official organizational structures in each of the 50 states, as well as in Guam, Puerto Rico, and the District of Columbia; each is represented in the Representative Assembly of the national organization. The Alliance is structured to administer professional programs and projects through seven associations: *National Association for Sport and Physical Education; National Dance Association; Association for Research, Administration, Professional Councils, and Societies; American School and Community Safety Association; Association for the Advancement of Health Education; National Association for Girls and Women in Sport;* and *American Association for Leisure and Recreation.*

There are 21 national organizations affiliated with the Alliance, many of which sponsor programs at the national convention. These are

American Academy of Physical Education
American Association of College Baseball Coaches
American College of Sports Medicine
American Corrective Therapy Association, Incorporated
American School Health Association
American Youth Hostels, Incorporated
Boys Clubs of America
Canadian Association for Health, Physical Education, and Recreation
Delta Psi Kappa
Health and Physical Education Directors Associations of YM-YWHA's and Jewish Community Centers
National Association for Intercollegiate Athletics
National Association for Physical Education in Higher Education
National Athletic Trainers Association
National Intramural Association
National Soccer Coaches Association of America
Phi Epsilon Kappa
Physical Education Society of the YMCA's of North America
Sigma Delta Psi
Society of State Directors of Health, Physical Education, and Recreation
United States Volleyball Association
Young Women's Christian Association of the U.S.A.

Publications. The first official publication of the Alliance appeared in 1896; it continues under the title of *Journal of Physical Education and Recreation* (JOPER). The *Research Quarterly* began publication in 1930. During the past decade, the publication activities of the Alliance have been considerably expanded, to include *Health Education,* published six times a year, and *Update,* a newspaper published monthly from October through June. The current list of over four hundred publications ranges from leaflets to rule guides, filmstrips, loop films, research abstracts, monographs, and books. The first volume of the five-volume *Encyclopedia of Physical Education, Fitness, and Sports* is now in print. This series, sponsored by AAHPERD Research Council, is being published by Addison-Wesley Publishing Co.

Conferences. The Alliance sponsors many professional meetings, in addition to its annual conventions. Recent events of national significance include student seminars; national institutes on coaching and athletics; symposia on federal support programs; regional and national conferences on elementary school, secondary school, and college physical education, dance, aquatics, and school health; and national and international seminars and meetings on undergraduate professional preparation, graduate education, perceptual-motor development, and many topics of timely interest.

International Involvement. The broad scope of Alliance services includes participation in international professional efforts, as the following examples will indicate:

1. Formation of the International Council on Health, Physical Education and Recreation in August, 1959, marked a significant development in the international orientation of the profession. The ICHPER is an integral part of the structure of the World Conference of Organizations of the Teaching Profession.

2. The International Relations Council of the Association has sponsored a project for the collection of books for foreign libraries. During the years since its inception, books have been sent to Yugoslavia, Iraq, India, Pakistan, Taiwan, the Philippines, Burma, Liberia, Thailand, and Colombia. The Council planned the 1967 National Conference on International Relations Through Health, Physical Education, and Recreation, which approved a series of recommendations directed toward increasing the depth and breadth of international interest and work throughout the whole structure of AAHPERD.

3. The Youth Fitness Test has been translated and officially adopted for use in Japan, Burma, Pakistan, Saudi Arabia, Portugal, Mexico, Cuba, Ecuador, Colombia, and Peru.

4. The Alliance is represented by officers and staff in international planning sessions for the Department of State's American Specialist Program, the Agency of International Development (AID), International Union for Health Education of the Public, and many other organizations. As a result of this cooperation, highly qualified personnel are being sent all over the world. Many have written their experiences in the pages of the journal.

5. The Alliance was co-host to the Fourth International Congress of Physical Education and Sports for Girls and Women held in Washington, D.C., August, 1961.

Students are referred to the April, 1960, anniversary issue of the *Journal of Health, Physical Education and Recreation* (JOHPER), the former title of JOPER, for historical information on the Alliance and biographies of early leaders, and to current issues of *Update* and JOPER for most recent information. The Alliance also publishes an Annual Directory of Supplies and Equipment and current publications reviews and listings in JOPER and in *Health Education*.

As stated in its constitution, the American Academy of Physical Education "shall be concerned with the art and science of human movement.... The academy shall promote its purposes by: Extending knowledge in this field; transmitting knowledge about human movement; fostering philosophic considerations regarding issues, values, and pur-

American Academy of Physical Education

poses; electing to membership Fellows of outstanding achievement; bestowing honors for outstanding contributions to this field; conducting and sponsoring scholarly and social meetings."

The Academy was originally conceived in 1926 by five leaders in physical education but was not officially founded until 1930, when a constitution was adopted by 29 charter members. Each year since 1950, the Academy has sponsored a special speaker at the AAHPERD Convention in honor of its founder, R. Tait McKenzie. He was one of the great pioneers of our profession, serving as president of the AAHPER during several of its formative years and as first president of the Academy. From its inception, the Academy has directed its efforts toward the expansion of scholarship in the fields of health, physical education, and recreation. Membership is limited and by invitation only, on the basis of contributions through research, writing, and exceptional service. The R. Tait McKenzie Lecture[15] is one of the Academy's many contributions to the profession. Publications which have resulted from national meetings, originally titled *Professional Contributions,* and more recently, *The Academy Papers,* are an invaluable addition to any professional library.

On July 1, 1978, NAPEHE came into being as the result of the decision of the National Association for Physical Education of College Women and the National College Physical Education Association for Men to join forces as a single professional association for all college and university physical educators. Each of the two associations had a unique and distinguished heritage, including a common heritage of several significant joint undertakings during the past quarter of a century. *National Association for Physical Education in Higher Education*

History. The National College Physical Education Association for Men traces its history to 1897, when it was organized as the Society of College Gymnasium Directors for the purpose of advancing the work of physical education in institutions of higher learning. Membership in the early years of its existence "was restricted to directors of gymnasiums, and they were concerned primarily with growth, development, physical examinations, anthropometric tests, and systems of gymnastics." In 1908, the name of the organization was changed to the Society of Directors of Physical Education in College, and teachers in college departments for men were admitted to membership. Later, in 1933, the name of the organization was changed to the College Physical Education Association, and in 1962 the organization became known as the National College Physical Education Association for Men (NCPEAM).

Although meetings of women college directors were held as early as 1910, no definite society was formed until 1915. This organization was known as the Association of Directors of Physical Education for College Women, and its membership was designed to include "Directors or Heads of Departments of Physical Education for College Women in colleges and institutions of similar standing in the eastern section of the United States." Two years later, and no doubt inspired by the professional spirit engendered in the eastern association meetings, the midwestern society was organized and, for a similar reason, was followed by the formation of the western society in 1921. At a joint meeting in 1924, these three societies were merged into one, to be known as the National Association of Directors of Physical Education for College Women. The activities of this new association were broadened to include review of administration and organization policies; study of the problems and promotion of the interests of departments of physical education for women; presentation of research papers; and cooperative effort "in advancing the standards of education and the ideals of the profession." During World War II, membership was opened to all teachers in college and university women's physical education departments, the scope of the organization was extended, the word "directors" was removed from the association's name, and it became the National Association for Physical Education of College Women (NAPECW).

Publications. As independent Associations, each was responsible for numerous publications. NAPECW published its *Biennial Record* regularly; NCPEAM published an annual *Proceedings*; and both Associations published newsletters. A joint semiannual publication, titled *Quest*, first appeared in December, 1963. *Quest* was initiated in order to provide a creative, literary contribution to the profession and, in the words of the first editor, Donna Mae Miller, is "committed to publishing scholarly papers of philosophical and scientific interest." *Briefings* was initiated as a joint venture in 1975 as a series of monographs designed to provide preliminary information on topics of emerging concern for college physical educators. NAPEHE will continue the publication of *Quest, Proceedings* of the annual conferences, and a quarterly *Newsletter*.

Over the years both Associations have held many successful conferences and workshops. In 1967, NAPECW sponsored the First Annual Amy Morris Homans Lecture, to pay homage to one of the early pioneers in the profession. Miss Homans established the Boston Normal School of Gymnastics in 1909 and later moved it into Wellesley College. She originated NAPECW and had a tremendous impact on an entire generation of professional leaders. Each year, an outstanding speaker is selected to deliver this address at the annual luncheon during the AAHPERD Convention.

Though necessarily quite small in membership, this organization occupies an important place in professional leadership throughout the country. "Because of the strategical position of the state officers, the society from its beginning took cognizance of national problems and endorsed and sponsored worthy procedures by unanimously passing resolutions on vital tactics and policies."[16] Since its founding in 1926, the society has maintained close contacts with the National Education Association, the American Alliance for Health, Physical Education, Recreation and Dance, and other key professional associations, and has been particularly helpful in influencing national thinking in the field of health, physical education, and recreation. Informal programs, maintained on a committee basis, cover a wide range of topics, including state certification, school curricular requirements, safety education and athletic policies and programs.

Society of State Directors of Health, Physical Education, and Recreation

The purposes of the society are

> (1) to promote sound programs of health, safety, physical education, and recreation throughout the United States; (2) to study problems in these areas and seek solutions to them; (3) to provide a basis for exchange of ideas and programs among members of this organization; and (4) to cooperate with other professional organizations in furthering the development of programs in health, safety, physical education, and recreation.

A recent statement of "Basic Beliefs" is an important contribution which offers guidelines for school health, physical education, and recreation programs.[17]

CHAPTER TEN

A group of representative physicians, physical educators, and physiologists founded the American College of Sports Medicine in 1954 for the following purposes: (1) to promote and advance scientific studies dealing with the effect of sports and other motor activities on the health of human beings at various stages of life; (2) to cooperate with other organizations concerned with various aspects of human fitness; (3) to sponsor meetings of physicians, educators, and other scientists whose work is relevant to sports medicine; (4) to make available postgraduate education in fields related to the objectives of the College; (5) to initiate, encourage, and correlate research; and (6) to publish a journal dealing with scientific aspects of activity and their relationship to human fitness.

American College of Sports Medicine

The College is affiliated with AAHPERD and the Fédération Internationale de Médecine Sportive. It holds an annual national convention, and the College's regional chapters conduct scientific meetings on a regional basis. It publishes a regular newsletter; a quarterly journal, *Science and Medicine in Sports*, began publication in 1969.

The Encyclopedia of Sport Sciences and Medicine, a volume of approximately 1500 pages, including 1200 articles by 550 authors, was published in 1972 and is a major contribution to the profession. Subjects are drawn from many facets of sport sciences, ranging from growth and development, physiology, psychology, and sociology, to safety of participation, rehabilitation, orthopedics, pharmacology, and measurement and evaluation. The work has an international flavor, since the authors are citizens of 35 different countries, and the 6000 bibliographic references include many international publications.

Membership in certain international organizations is on an association as well as an individual basis. The individual physical educator may gain a great deal through participating in programs sponsored by international groups and through reading publications of these organizations and reports of their conferences. Even if individual participation in international activities must be limited, the significance of physical education in international relations and the impact of international factors on the future development of the profession make the work of these associations important.

International Organizations

The *International Council on Health, Physical Education and Recreation (ICHPER)* was founded in 1958. World Congresses are now organized every two years. AAHPERD is a national member of ICHPER, and its immediate past-president serves as the official delegate to the ICHPER Assembly. The Council publishes annually: four issues of the ICHPER Bulletin; a newsletter reporting significant professional developments and activities; four issues of *Gymnasion,* a journal treating professional issues of international concern; proceedings of each international congress; and other research reports as developed and made available. In its 20 years of existence, ICHPER has strengthened the profession at the international level immeasurably, providing channels for communication among physical educators of different nations, and a framework for operation with other educational bodies through its relationships with the World Confederation of Organizations of the Teaching Professions.

The *International Association of Physical Education and Sports for Girls and Women (IAPESGW)* is an organization with members from more than 50 countries.

Its purpose is to bring into active cooperation and participation women of many countries working in the fields of Physical Education and Sports; to cooperate with other organizations in encouraging the particular services which women contribute to society; to strengthen international contacts; to afford opportunities for the discussion of mutual problems; to promote the exchange of persons and ideas among member countries, and research into problems affecting Physical Education and Sports for women.

The IAPESGW was founded in 1949 and held its first Congress in Copenhagen. Congresses have been held at four-year intervals since that date in Paris, London, Washington, Cologne, Tokyo, Teheran, and Capetown.

The *International Olympic Academy (IOA)* is located in a permanent setting near Olympia, and houses the Museum of the History of the Modern Olympic Games as well as living facilities, library, and sports facilities for the participants. Although it was founded in 1949, the first session convened in 1961; annual sessions have been held each succeeding summer. The general activities of the IOA embrace lectures, seminars, question and answer sessions, general discussions, tours, films, and recreation. Subject matter is selected and programs are conducted in accordance with the general purpose of continuation of the high ideals and true spirit of the Olympic movement. English and French are the two official languages of the Academy.

U.S. Department of Education

In the fields of school health and physical education, the work of the Department of Education is largely consultative, advisory, and promotional. The staff engages in compiling and disseminating information concerning all phases of health education, physical education, and recreation, and in sponsoring and conducting conferences on numerous problems relating to these three areas of education. A bibliography of the publications of this office is available; many of the pamphlets are provided without charge, and for the others a nominal charge is made. The official publication of the office is *American Education*.

Federal support to education expanded tremendously during the 1960s, particularly through public funds appropriated under the Elementary and Secondary Education Act of 1965 and the Higher Education Act of 1965. Funds allotted to these programs were administered initially through the U.S. Office of Education. The National Institute of Education (NIE) came into being in August, 1972, as a separate agency within the Department of Health, Education, and Welfare. Title III of the Education Amendments of 1972 established the NIE to provide leadership in the conduct and support of scientific inquiry into the educational process.[18]

Professional Fraternities

Delta Psi Kappa, Phi Delta Pi, and Phi Epsilon Kappa are national professional fraternities. Each is interested primarily in developing among its members, and the profession in general, high ideals and a desire for service, and each sponsors a professional magazine. The official publication of Delta Psi Kappa is *The Foil* (semiannual); of Phi Delta Pi, *The Progressive Physical Educator* (semiannual); and of Phi Epsilon Kappa, *The Physical Educator* (quarterly). These organizations have done much to stimulate professional leadership.

PROFESSIONAL PUBLICATIONS

The professional physical educator will begin building a professional library during the undergraduate years. This is also the time to form the habit of regularly reading professional journals. Recommended reading

394

CHAPTER TEN

for all physical educators are the *Journal of Physical Education and Recreation, Update,* and *Quest.* In addition, each person will want to subscribe to more specialized journals in areas of interest and responsibility and to the state association journal. Many education journals and a number of coaching magazines provide good reading. Periodical literature is the best source for keeping up with current issues and concerns.

Every person who wants to continue his or her education throughout a full career will read reviews of new professional books and select those most likely to be of interest and help. Publishing companies are glad to place educators on mailing lists to receive announcements of new books and instructional materials. Professional associations provide their members with frequent mailings concerning available materials. Professional conventions usually provide for book exhibits that permit the prospective purchaser to examine new books conveniently.

Professionals also have the responsibility to contribute to the literature of their profession. Physical education students, both undergraduate and graduate, are encouraged to submit ideas and articles to *JOPER* and to state association publications. Each member of the profession should, from time to time, share innovative ideas, opinions, and research findings through contributions to the professional literature.

Those interested in continuing their education usually seek opportunities for advanced study in graduate school or in less formal settings. In addition, they participate in professional associations. They read and contribute to professional literature. They also take advantage of selected opportunities to attend conferences and other types of professional meetings.

WORKSHOPS, SEMINARS, AND CONFERENCES

Professional seminars and workshops are sponsored by colleges and universities, professional associations, school districts, commercial firms, and government agencies. The wide variety of topics covered provide current and timely assistance for strengthening professional abilities. Clinics provide the latest performance, instructional, and coaching techniques in a wide range of activities.

Most professional associations sponsor annual conventions, presenting lectures, panel discussions, small group discussions, demonstrations, and exhibits of many kinds. In addition, numerous professional conferences on topics of current interest are offered by associations, universities, and public and private agencies. Much can be learned at such meetings. All of these can make highly valuable contributions to continuing professional preparation.

Physical education is now an appropriate undergraduate major for college or undergraduate students interested in any of a broad spectrum of professions focusing on the study of human movement phenomena or the use of movement activities in serving others. The undergraduate professional curriculum provides a core of common experiences for all those majoring in the field. Sound contemporary curricula also provide for differentiated coursework and related educational experiences designed in accordance with the individual's selected career emphasis.

SUMMARY

Teaching continues to be the career choice of most persons studying for baccalaureate degrees in physical education. Teacher education students must be prepared to cope with new and constantly changing social conditions. The school has a vital role in working toward greater integration of our pluralistic society, and the prospective teacher faces a crucial challenge in preparing to pursue this goal effectively.

The trend in undergraduate teacher education and certification is toward competency-based programs and requirements. Although greater emphasis is being given to a broad and comprehensive general education for all teachers, regardless of their special field of study, tomorrow's physical educator will also be expected to qualify as a specialist within the profession.

Professional preparation curricula for future physical education teachers will have to go beyond the development of competencies of presentation, group organization, coaching, and testing. Teacher educators will strive to develop abilities needed to help people appreciate different meanings of movement, to give leadership in accepting physical activity as an essential aspect of a complete life, to identify and research important questions relating to the movement sciences, and to seek creative fulfillment in the movement arts. Future teachers will be prepared to provide educational services beyond school settings and oriented toward continuing their own education throughout the years of full-time employment. Undergraduate students preparing for non-teaching careers will need to include in their programs additional courses specific to their particular area of study; they will need in-depth specialization in addition to their physical education backgrounds.

Recent efforts of the professional associations have been directed toward specialized preparation for coaching aspirants and state certification of high school coaches. It is no longer assumed that all physical education majors will complete coaching emphases. Coaching now represents a realistic career option for men and women at all educational levels, in public agencies and in private enterprise.

Graduate specializations in physical education may be developed in a number of subdisciplinary fields. Most graduate programs in physical education are oriented toward advancing careers in higher education, administration, or research.

Career physical educators must accept individual responsibility for continuing professional growth. Growing interest in increased teacher effectiveness has led to upgrading in standards. Schools and colleges support the professional growth and development of teachers by sponsoring in-service education programs, by granting professional leaves of absence, and by rewarding professional growth through promotion and merit pay increases. In the last analysis, however, it is the individual physical educator who must take the initiative to enroll in graduate programs, to become actively involved in the work of professional associations, to read and contribute to professional publications, and to participate in workshops, seminars and professional conferences.

FOOTNOTES

[1] Ann E. Jewett and Marie R. Mullan, "A Conceptual Model for Teacher Education," *Quest*, XXIII:76–87 (June, 1972).

[2] American Association for Health, Physical Education and Recreation. *Professional Preparation in Dance, Physical Education, Recreation Education, Safety Education, and School Health Education*. Report of New Orleans Conference (January, 1973).

[3] "Student Action Council Resolutions" *JOHPER*, 44:55 (April, 1973).

[4] Celeste Ulrich, "The Physical Educator as Teacher." *Quest*, VII:58–61 (December, 1966).

[5] National Athletic Trainers Association, *Athletic Training Careers*. Lafayette, Indiana: NATA, 1974.

[6] David K. Leslie, "Fitness Programs for the Aging," *Careers in Physical Education*. NAPECW and NCPEAM, 1975, pp. 1–10.

[7] American Association for Health, Physical Education and Recreation. *Certification of High School Coaches*. Washington, D.C.: AAHPER, 1970.

[8] American Association for Health, Physical Education and Recreation, *Professional Preparation in Physical Education and Coaching*. Washington, D.C.: 1974.

[9] Larry Noble and Charles B. Corbin, "Certification of Coaches," *JOPER*, 49:2 (February, 1978), pp. 69–70.

[10] Harold J. Vanderzwaag, "Sport Administration," *Careers in Physical Education*. NAPECW and NCPEAM, 1975, pp. 17–27.

[11] Joint Committee on Physical Education and Athletics, AAHPER, NCAA, and NCPEAM, Robert Weber, Chairman. "Professional Preparation of the Administrator of Athletics." *JOHPER*, 41:20–23 (September, 1970).

[12] Bonnie L. Parkhouse, "Professional Preparation in Athletic Administration and Sport Management," *JOPER*, 49:5 (May, 1978), pp. 22–27.

[13] Donald E. Hawkins, "Tourism," *Careers in Physical Education*. NAPECW and NCPEAM: 1975, pp. 56–61.

[14] Bonnie L. Parkhouse, op. cit.

[15] "R. Tait McKenzie Lecture," *JOHPER*, 32:73 (October, 1961).

[16] Schrader, Carl L., "The History of the State Directors' Society." *J. Health and Phys. Educ.*, IV:3 (December, 1933).

[17] *School Programs in Health, Physical Education, and Recreation: A Statement of Basic Beliefs*. Kensington, Md.: Society of State Directors of Health, Physical Education, and Recreation, 1972.

[18] U.S. Department of Health, Education, and Welfare. *The National Institute of Education: A Brief Outline of Its History, Status, and Tentative Plans*. Washington, D.C.: Department of Health, Education and Welfare (NIE 73–25000), February 23, 1973.

SELECTED REFERENCES

American Association for Health, Physical Education and Recreation, *Preparing the Elementary Specialist*. Washington, D.C.: AAHPER, 1973.

American Association for Health, Physical Education and Recreation, *State Requirements in Physical Education for Teachers and Students*. Washington, D.C.: AAHPER, 1973.

American Alliance for Health, Physical Education and Recreation, *Professional Preparation in Dance, Physical Education, Recreation Education, Safety Education, and School Health Education*. Washington, D.C.: AAHPER, 1974.

American Alliance for Health, Physical Education and Recreation, *Careers in Activity and Therapy Fields*. Washington, D.C.: AAHPER, 1976.

American Alliance for Health, Physical Education and Recreation, *Professional Preparation in Adapted Physical Education, Therapeutic Recreation and Corrective Therapy*. Washington, D.C.: AAHPER, 1976.

American Alliance for Health, Physical Education and Recreation, *Recreation and Leisure Time Careers*. Washington, D.C.: AAHPER, 1976.

American Alliance for Health, Physical Education and Recreation, *Professional Preparation of the Intramural-Recreational Sports Specialist*. Washington, D.C.: AAHPER, 1977.

Gage, N. L., *Teacher Effectiveness and Teacher Education: The Search for a Scientific Basis*. Palo Alto, Calif.: Pacific Books, 1972.

Jewett, Ann E., "Future Projections for Professional Preparation." Southern District American Alliance for Health, Physical Education and Recreation Conference Proceedings, February, 1978, pp. 169–178.

Jewett, Ann E. and Mullan, Marie R., "A Conceptual Model for Teacher Education," *Quest XXIII:* 76–87 (June, 1972).

Joyce, Bruce R., Weil, Marsha, and Wald, Rhoada, "The Training of Educators: A Structure for Pluralism." *Teachers College Record*, 73:371–391 (February, 1972).

Locke, Lawrence F. (Ed.), "Teaching Teachers." *Quest XVIII* (June, 1972).

McCarty, Donald J. (Ed.), *New Perspectives on Teacher Education*. San Francisco: Jossey-Bass, 1973.

National Association for Physical Education of College Women and National College Physical Education Association for Men, *Careers in Physical Education*. (Briefings 3). 1975.

National Association for Physical Education of College Women and National College Physical Education Association for Men, *Continuing In-Service Education: Professional Direction or Dilemma*. (Briefings 5). 1977.

National Athletic Trainers Association. *Athletic Training Careers*. Lafayette, Indiana: NATA, 1974.

Nixon, John E. and Locke, Lawrence F., "Research on Teaching Physical Education," *Second Handbook of Research on Teaching*, Travers, Robert M. W. (Ed.). Chicago: Rand McNally, 1973, pp. 1210–1242.

Reid, Marsha A. (Ed.), "Careers in Recreation: A Look at the Potential," *JOPER*, 50:4 (April, 1979), pp. 33–64.

Siedentop, Daryl (Ed.), "Graduate Study in Physical Education." *Quest 25* (Winter, 1976).

Smith, B. Othanel, *Research in Teacher Education: A Symposium*. Englewood Cliffs, N.J.: Prentice-Hall, 1971.

Woods, John B., Mauries, Thomas J., and Dick, Bruce V., *Student Teaching: The Entrance to Professional Physical Education*. New York: Academic Press, 1973.

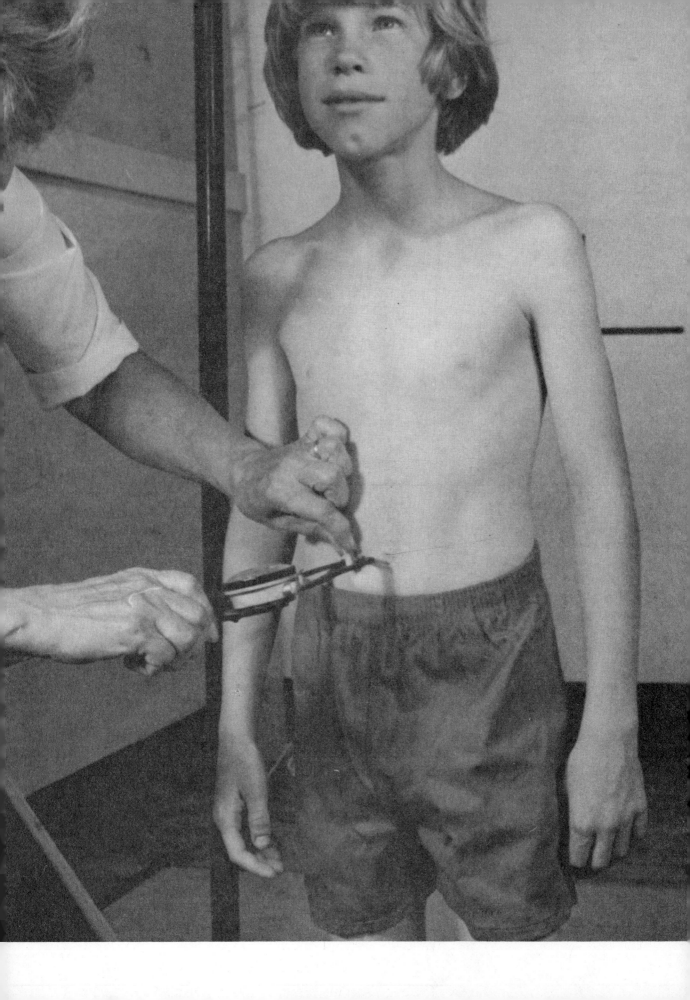

EVALUATION AND ────── RESEARCH

11

Evaluation is one of the central components of the educational enterprise. Although many definitions have been ascribed to this word over the years, there is general agreement that it means the totality of the processes deliberately employed to assess the extent to which objectives have been attained in the areas of pupil behavioral changes, curriculum efficiency, and teacher effectiveness. Informally, evaluation probably is occurring most of the time, particularly in the teacher's mind. Formal stages of overtly planned evaluation programs take place at scheduled intervals, such as administering a physical fitness test, taking the height and weight measurements of each pupil, and making out the final course grade for each student. Teachers informally observe their classes in action every day and gain impressions about each pupil's behavior, physical skills, and attitudes toward the program, toward other pupils, and toward the teacher. Of course, students also make a large number of similar covert evaluations throughout the time spent in the physical education class.

EVALUATION IN PHYSICAL EDUCATION

Measurement refers to that phase of evaluation that is concrete, identifiable, quantifiable, and capable of accurate assessment through the use of valid, reliable measuring instruments, with the results being recorded in our numerical system. Thus, physical education teachers can measure the time a student takes to swim 50 yards with the crawl stroke, the distance an 8 pound shot is thrown, and the score attained in a Columbia round of archery competition.

Role of Measurement in Evaluation

There are other areas of pupil progress toward objectives that are not yet measurable by such objective tests. In such cases, the teacher must render a subjective judgment, which should be based on many observations of pupil behavior in the area of concern. Subjective judgment is required to assess leadership, cooperation, and similar behaviors. Tests are available to assess student interests, attitudes, personality, sociometric relationships, values, and similar components of human behavior. These tests to date have achieved varying degrees of validity and reliabili-

399

ty. In general, they cannot be regarded as having high validity and objectivity, so they must be used and interpreted with caution. However, they may provide valuable insights and "leads" for the perceptive teacher to attain a greater understanding of students.

Modern measurement and evaluation books in physical education describe tests and cite the degree of validity, reliability, and objectivity of each. The teacher who desires to do a thorough task of test selection, administration, and interpretation should study this evaluation literature as a valuable guide to one of teaching's most fundamental functions. Most physical education major programs now require a course in measurement and evaluation in physical education. In order to make intelligent selection and use of tests, teachers must have a basic knowledge of statistics. The typical measurement and evaluation course in physical education starts with an introductory section on the most useful statistics. The teacher who has not had such a course should enroll in one as soon as possible, for it is impossible to be an effective teacher without knowing how to select, administer, interpret, and evaluate tests and test results, and to develop a valid grading plan.

The Teacher as Evaluator

Another reason for a thorough knowledge of measurement and evaluation is that the physical educator must have the competence to construct tests. This admonition applies particularly to the preparation of knowledge tests. It is virtually impossible to use a state or national standard knowledge test at the end of a teaching unit, because each teacher has taught the course in a unique way and has planned the content and instructional methodology without reference to how the test maker would have performed these tasks. Obviously, these tests should accurately cover the knowledge taught in the unit, so teachers now tend to build and administer their own objective knowledge tests at the end of instructional units. It is possible to construct a departmental test of knowledge if two or more teachers work together on its preparation, and if they come to close agreement in planning and teaching the unit to several classes of pupils.

It is also recommended that the physical educator take at least one course in basic computer science. There are many ways in which the capabilities of the computer can be employed to expedite the work of the teacher in test scoring, analysis of data, reporting, and performance research. School districts are using computers in a variety of helpful ways.

In recent years Benjamin S. Bloom[1] and others have popularized a distinction between two types of evaluation, namely, formative and summative. *Summative evaluation* has existed in education for many years. It is based on the theory of the curve of normal distribution of test scores involving a large number of pupils taking the test. Typically, the well-known letter grades A, B, C, D, and F, are assigned to students based on their relative placement on the test in relation to the normal distribution of test scores of similar students who have taken the same test in the past. Thus, this type of evaluation is *norm-referenced*. Through their scores students compete with others taking the test, or with those who have previously taken the test. In each case the individual's score is compared with the table of norms composed of all of the scores of the students included in the norming group. Typically, this type of evaluation is made at the end of an instructional unit or at the termination of a course. Occasionally it is used at mid-term or with periodic quizzes over material covered in a class at certain time intervals.

FORMATIVE AND SUMMATIVE EVALUATION

Summative Evaluation

Uses. It is apparent that such information about pupil performance and progress frequently becomes available too late to be useful in helping the pupil to adjust study habits or specific learning problems. Summative evaluation generally is used:

— to determine final course grades and pupil numerical ranking in a class or school;

— to establish pre-requisites for admission into a higher level course;

— to assess specific types of skills and abilities needed for satisfactory performance in a specific occupational role;

— to provide students with information concerning their comparative levels of performance so that they may plan for further development and success;

— to compare the progress of two or more groups of students who have been exposed to different pedagogical or curricular approaches.

Formative evaluation is a more recent concept that emphasizes the guidance function of test scores and other evaluative techniques concerning student performance and learning. This type of evaluation is *criterion-referenced*. Specific behavioral descriptions of desirable student behaviors are spelled out. These behavioral, or performance, objectives become the criteria that the pupils strive to master.   *Formative Evaluation*

Assessment of pupil progress can be made at any time during the instructional sequence — from the first day, when "entering behavior" may be determined, and throughout the course as many times as the teacher deems useful. Each pupil's test result is compared with the criterion measure that was previously stated. Achievement of the criterion at the specified level reflects mastery of that objective and readiness to move to the next higher level of behavioral objectives. Hence, formative evaluation is criterion-referenced. Again, each student's performance at any given time is compared *only with his or her past achievement*, so that the degree of progress since the previous test administration becomes evident. The student is not compared competitively with the other students in his class or in the norm group as in the case of summative evaluation. The pupil is given prompt feedback about performance with respect to specific learning objectives. Based on this information the pupil's study program can be adjusted and revised each time any formative evaluation is made so that progress can be maximized. This concept promotes the individualization of both learning and instruction. It also removes the threat and fear of being graded competitively and comparatively in relation to the other students, which is inherent in the summative evaluation model, and thus provides an important psychological benefit for the students who typically score at the lower end of summative test norms. Each pupil receives the advantages of diagnosis and of specific aid in optimizing possibilities for achieving mastery of the behavioral objectives that have been set. Of course, the objectives themselves can be modified in light of the evidence provided by the formative evaluation. Where summative evaluation emphasizes the apparent final product of learning, formative evaluation emphasizes guidance of the learning process itself.

Uses. Bloom says that the main purpose of formative evaluation is to indicate the extent to which mastery learning has occurred and to enable the teacher and the pupil to know precisely where the pupil is not mastering the task. Also, formative evaluation data facilitate revisions in teaching procedures and strategies, in terms of both the group and the individual, and reveal deficiencies. The teacher can compare the results of formative evaluations from previous years with present results to determine areas wherein instructional competence can be improved. Clues also are provided concerning ways to improve the amount of learning and the rapidity with which the pupils achieve the performance objectives. Bloom calls this the "quality control" of instruction. Frequent formative evaluation throughout the course provides an opportunity to assess many more of the major units in the instructional sequence than does periodic summative evaluation, which at best samples only a small proportion of those units offered throughout the course.

Finally, there is some evidence to indicate that formative evaluation data may be correlated positively with summative test scores. If so, final summative test results can be predicted with some accuracy from on-going formative evaluation data. If the prediction at a given time in mid-course is that the end of course test results will be inferior, the teacher is forewarned and can attempt to take appropriate remedial steps to improve the instruction in the desired directions.

Because formative evaluation is a relatively recent concept, physical education evaluation literature is limited in this respect. The leading reference in this area is Margaret J. Safrit's[2] *Evaluation in Physical Education*. This book discusses the concepts of summative and formative evaluation in the context of physical education instructional programs and provides concrete illustrations of how to teach and evaluate through the proper applications of these concepts and principles. All teachers and coaches interested in improving their evaluation techniques are referred to this excellent source.

In summary, the total combination of all of the possible types of measurements, the observational data and inferences drawn from them, and the resulting educational implications and conclusions represents the highly complex art of evaluation. As evaluative data are generated, teachers direct their thoughts to the program objectives. These objectives are revised, reformulated, and readjusted to the realities and needs revealed by the evaluation. So, it is a continuous process, circular in nature, in which teachers, department staffs, and school faculties *formulate objectives, conduct programs* designed to assist pupils to accomplish those objectives, *evaluate pupil achievement* with respect to the stated objectives, and in turn, review, restate, and revise the original objectives. The cycle is never-ending.

Summary.

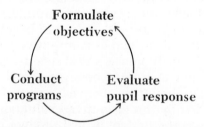

The program can be assured of steady improvement if this philosophy of evaluation is accepted wholeheartedly by the teachers in concept and in action.

Baumgartner and Jackson[3] have summarized very effectively the meaning of educational measurement and evaluation:

> *Measurement* is the collection of information upon which a decision is then based; *evaluation* is the use of measurements for making decisions. . . . In the context of contemporary education, then, evalua-

tion is a dynamic decision-making process focusing on changes in pupil behavior, i.e., learning. This process involves (1) collecting suitable data (measurement), (2) judging the value of these data according to some standard, and (3) making decisions based on these data and the alternative courses of action available. The ultimate function of evaluation is to facilitate rational decisions in an effort to improve student learning.

Evaluation serves six major purposes: diagnosis and guidance, motivation, classification of pupils, appraisal of knowledge, efficiency of instruction, and evaluation of student achievement. In addition, tests in themselves can provide one form of practice in the skills being taught. Finally, data generated from tests can be employed in research designs that are developed to provide new knowledge or to seek new solutions to current physical education problems.

PURPOSES OF EVALUATION

The starting point in physical education evaluation is to determine the specific needs of each pupil. What can we do in our program to minister to these needs?

Diagnosis and Guidance

One of the greatest challenges facing the physical education teacher today is how to individualize the program so as to assist each pupil in making optimal progress toward the important objectives of this field. Typically, physical education teachers instruct five periods per day and have pupil contacts numbering between 200 and 250 students per day. By its very nature, physical education has the most complex logistical problem of any subject in the curriculum. Large numbers of students must be instructed every period of the day, in many kinds of facilities, employing diverse types of equipment and supplies. It is little wonder, under these conditions, that the need to individualize the program for each pupil stands out as a current major problem and challenge.

The starting point in individualizing physical education is an accurate assessment of the present status, "entry behavior," and the individual needs of each pupil. Once this accurate individual assessment has been made, the physical education staff then is in position to provide maximal guidance to each pupil in the physical education experience.

While many of the tests mentioned in other categories can be used for the purposes of motivation, physical education literature describes several that are designed primarily to inform students of their individual standing in relation to a group. Such tests offer scoring scales by which students can keep accurate account of their improvement and make performance comparisons in various activities. Students are not always conscious of their weaknesses in particular phases of an activity, and objective scales offer a means of encouraging effort and practice. Motivation may thus go on indefinitely.

Motivation

One of the most promising trends in recent years in some schools is the intensive use of a cumulative Pupil Physical Education Profile Record. With this concept, the pupils have a major role in testing themselves and their peers in the basic elements of the activities that will comprise the semester's or year's program in physical education. They are then responsible for noting their status at the time of testing on the Profile Record form. Each test is scored in percentiles based on test scores of hundreds of similar pupils in the school or district. State or national percentile norms also can be included on the form for the information of each pupil. The plan avoids the embarrassment that was present under the old system of posting the test results of all members of a class for everyone to see.

Responsibility for maintaining the file rests with the individual student. Teachers counsel students individually about their status and their progress and offer suggestions as to how the pupil can work to improve. Schools that have adopted similar plans uniformly report an increased interest in physical education and a high degree of enthusiasm and morale among the students. Discipline problems decline and the learning process seems to accelerate.

Classification

Classification, as a function of evaluation, is the arrangement of pupils into groups according to relevant criteria. There is little agreement within the profession as to the best grouping procedures. The following classification plans seem to be most prominent:

— school grade
— age-height-weight scale
— physical fitness or physical performance test
— specific sport skills tests
— teacher subjective judgment of sport skills
— student interest

There are variations of these plans, and there are other systems not in general use. Also, there are embellishments involving elaborate point systems for a variety of positive and negative behaviors that can be observed or measured during class, usually with respect to physical fitness.

Schools that have adopted programs based on the principles of individualized instruction have broken tradition with the long standing concept of moving groups or "squads" of students through an instructional unit of physical education. Despite our knowledge that individuals enter such squads with varying achievement records, and that each pupil learns at his own distinctive rate, we have too long permitted the squad tradition to hamper efficient learning opportunities. Individualized physical education programs are based on the premise that each student should learn at a personal rate and in a variety of uniquely appropriate ways. Formative evaluation is preeminent in this system; thus, the progress of each pupil is frequently evaluated in relation to self-established goals. The pupils are no longer "grouped" in the old sense of the term.

It behooves each physical educator to give careful thought to the implicit as well as the explicit assumptions underlying the selected grouping practices. We recommend that, when necessary for one reason or another, grouping is best accomplished with the pupils' interests and abilities in mind. We believe there should be several curricula, for various groupings of boys and girls; and that it is the responsibility of each teacher to capitalize on the unique interests, abilities, and personality of the pupil in helping each to make maximal progress toward physical education goals.

Knowledge Appraisal

This phase of evaluation has expanded rapidly in physical education programs at all educational levels throughout the country. Among the standardized physical education knowledge and understanding tests now available is a series based upon the AAHPERD instructional manual entitled *Knowledge and Understanding in Physical Education.*[4] Three examinations are available for upper elementary grades, junior high school, and senior high school, with two forms available for each test. The Educational Testing Service of Princeton, New Jersey, is the source and publisher.

Teachers must master the techniques and the statistical assumptions of knowledge test construction, because a majority of the tests they use will be constructed by themselves or by local committees. Knowledge tests may cover an individual activity containing questions about terminology, history, leaders, equipment, scoring, rules, strategy, etiquette, field or court dimensions, skill analysis, and similar relevant factors. Knowledge tests may also concern basic knowledge related to physiological principles governing learning, motivation, and personality development. Likewise, kinesiological principles of movement are suitable topics for knowledge tests. There is a considerable trend throughout the country to test for these kinds of knowledge in consonance with the new philosophy of emphasizing the teaching of the "why" of physical education as well as the "how." With the development of the concept curriculum approach in physical education, as explained in an earlier chapter, we may safely forecast increased importance for knowledge-type testing in physical education in the future.

Teaching Efficiency

In the school system of a large city, it is often desirable for the administration to make a careful check on the efficiency of the instruction in the various schools of the district. Evaluation is a valuable aid in such a survey, but it must be used with caution. If tests are used as a basis for determining pupil progress, thus reflecting the efficiency of instruction, good judgment must be exercised in equalizing all outside factors that may have a bearing on the situation. These factors may include the experience of the teachers concerned, the experience and ability of the pupils, the type of community and heritage of the pupils, working conditions in the physical education facility, and the content of the course of study.

Test results provide the teacher with valuable information about personal strengths and weaknesses. They also indicate areas in the instructional unit where more emphasis should have been placed and spots where less attention is required. Likewise, the teacher can determine the range of performance by the pupils in each class, and with this knowledge can better prepare instructional strategies to meet the individual needs. It is believed that most experienced teachers will admit that they learn as much about themselves as they do about their pupils as they review the results of tests they administer.

Grading

Evaluation in physical education is quite closely identified with the entire problem of credits, marks, and promotion. The legitimacy and value of assigning grades in any school subject may be a debatable point, but at present it is a function of the school and, as such, must be properly accomplished.

In most schools and colleges, credit toward graduation is given for the successful completion of courses in physical education. Since student progress in nearly every school activity is evaluated, it appears not only administratively desirable but necessary for teachers of physical education to give careful consideration to the manner in which their evaluation is made. Too often grading has become a system of rewards and punishments rather than a positive aspect of student achievement evaluation.

Grading, like grouping, is a highly controversial subject among physical educators. There is little uniformity or agreement in practice. The system used ultimately depends upon the way in which each student in the class is perceived in terms of the teacher's personal philosophy of education and value system. Some schools or colleges will put pressure on individual teachers to persuade them to join in a common grading system, even though a teacher might not agree with certain underlying assumptions. Other institutions will give the teacher great freedom to derive an individual grading system. Generally, some over-all faculty consensus is desirable for the purposes of grading in a school and the spread of grades to be awarded, without restricting the teacher to a formula that must be followed.

We strongly believe that teachers must have complete faith in the integrity and individuality of each and every pupil, whatever his strengths and weaknesses. We must work with each child where he or she is today, and build on that base to make optimal educational growth through physical education experiences toward worthwhile objectives and pupil goals. Grades should be viewed as positive educational tools to facilitate growth, development, and desirable educational behavioral changes. In too many cases grades in physical education are used to control pupil conduct and even to punish pupils for errant behavior. Threatening a student with a low grade for failure to comply with certain expectations may not be very effective, and in some cases it may even be detrimental. It is a negative reinforcer of dubious value.

The Disadvantages of Letter Grading. It is probable that highly competitive, publicly announced letter grading is more harmful to many children than has been realized in the past. Many physical education teachers have been guilty of subjecting low-scoring pupils to public ridicule and embarrassment by posting these grades on a bulletin board or by making them the overt basis for grouping or forming teams. Regrettably, severe damage has been caused to the self-concept and self-confidence of many pupils by such public exposure.

We wonder if perhaps the traditional letter grading system has outlived its usefulness in physical education. If in fact our primary concern is to help each student become a self-directing, self-responsible person, experienced and knowledgeable in a variety of movement activities, skillful in a self-selected few, and highly motivated toward lifelong active participation, then the ultimate meaning of letter grades is subject to question. This statement may apply particularly to pupils who, by most grading systems, are doomed to receiving C, D, and even F grades, owing to the way the grading system is set up. If we sincerely want to help each pupil be as "physically educated" as possible and have a voluntary attitude toward physical activity participation for a lifetime, then we will eliminate the negative influences that impede such development. Perhaps a pass–no credit system, consisting of an individual profile of fitness achievement, sports achievement, knowledge achievement, and teacher judgment of social behavior, constitutes the most desirable form of course reporting in physical education. As such, it would combine record keeping with pupil counseling and motivation.

Fair Grading. If grades are to be assigned, however, it is the responsibility of the physical educator to determine them knowledgeably and

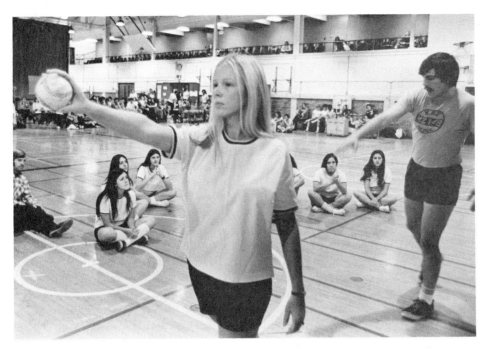

Cognitive factors in grading include knowledge of physiological and kinesiological principles.

fairly. Grading is a two-step process. The first step is the selection of measurements that will be used as a basis for the grade; the second is the calculation of the grade. Since the instructional objectives must be the basis for evaluation of student achievement, the measurements must be directed toward these objectives. Grades become both unfair and meaningless if the measurements do not relate to important educational objectives. Baumgartner and Jackson[5] recommend asking three questions when selecting testing instruments for grading:

> (1) What are the instructional objectives? (2) Were the students taught in accordance with these objectives? and (3) Does the test reliably and validly measure the achievement of these objectives?

Appropriate Grading Factors. There is considerable controversy concerning the factors used in physical education grading. The factors basic to the accomplishment of the objectives established for the lesson, the unit, and the course of physical education assessable by measurement and by teacher judgment can be grouped in three major categories:

1. *Motor (and physical) factors.* Skills in activities, fitness status, motor ability, postures, and game performance.
2. *Cognitive (mental) factors.* Knowledge and understanding of rules, strategy, performance, techniques, history, physiological and kinesiological principles, learning principles, health, safety, and equipment.
3. *Affective (social) factors.* Social behaviors in the physical education environment, attitude, appreciation, sportsmanship, cooperation, citizenship, leadership, and social relationships.

The teacher must decide which of the factors to include in determining the student's grade. The primary consideration should be the selection of attributes which are truly major objectives of the physical education program. Additional questions to consider are whether all students have equal opportunity to demonstrate their ability relative to the factor and whether it can be satisfactorily evaluated. The teacher must also determine the relative "weighting" to be given to each of the factors selected, based on their priority of importance and the proportional time that has been devoted to their development in the instructional program.

Inappropriate Factors. At times teachers also have included in the grading system such factors as attendance, uniform cleanliness, absences, tardiness, profanity, failure to take showers, and similar behaviors. We believe these factors are inappropriate in a grading system. We regard them as matters of departmental policy, not as grading criteria. We do not downgrade the importance of hygienic practices and guidelines for controlling student conduct, nor the role the physical educator can and should take in promoting desirable behaviors in these regards. However, we believe they are in the province of school administrative policies, and that violations should be handled through established school guidance and disciplinary channels. If grades are affected by these factors, they become confusing to students, parents, and administrators alike. It is not intended that the physical education grade serve as a reward for good behavior. Good teachers can manage these disciplinary and control problems without having to resort to the threat of lowering the grade.

Calculation of Grades. The second step in the grading process is the calculation of the grade. The measurements attained to assess the factors selected by the teacher as most relevant to the major educational objectives can be used to assign grades in a number of different ways. Grading methods to be considered include natural breaks, teacher's standard, rank order, normal curve, and norms. Each method has unique advantages and disadvantages; consequently, no single method is best for all situations.

Advance planning of the grading system is essential. The students are entitled to know at the start of the course how the grades are to be determined. Furthermore, grading is a much less time-consuming process for the teacher if the system has been carefully planned in advance.

PROGRAM EVALUATION

Educators generally agree that curriculum or program evaluation is a comprehensive activity that goes beyond evaluation of individual student achievement. Barrow and McGee[6] distinguish between product evaluation and process evaluation. In their view, program evaluation is process evaluation that focuses on the processes or procedures of physical education. The process may be measured directly, or it may be measured indirectly through product evaluation, which emphasizes tests of student achievement. Baumgartner and Jackson[7] take the position that the key question in program evaluation is whether students are meeting the important instructional objectives. They recommend the use of formative and summative evaluation procedures in a sound plan for program evaluation. Safrit[8] takes a broad view of program evaluation, emphasizing formative evaluation and a wide variety of measures to assess achievement of highly diverse curriculum goals.

Student Achievement Data. Everyone agrees that data on student achievement are needed to assess the effectiveness of a physical educa-

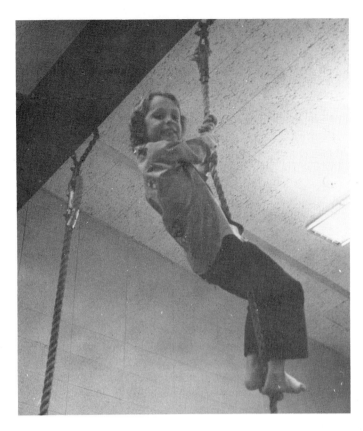

Skills tests are used to collect data for evaluation.

tion program. Tools most frequently used for collecting these data include knowledge tests, sports skills tests, and performance rating scales. Motor performance tests available to the physical educator include tests of muscular strength, muscular power, endurance, perceptual motor development, basic motor patterns, speed, flexibility, and balance. Additional tools used in fitness testing include tests of aerobic work capacity and body composition. Sociopsychological measures include attitude scales, sociometrics, behavior rating scales, semantic differentials, and self-concept measures. Comprehensive program evaluation also includes assessment of teacher-pupil interaction, learning climate, class management procedures, curriculum requirements, aspects of the "hidden" curriculum, and such physical characteristics as facilities, equipment, and supplies.

Formative program evaluation uses all types of available data to determine the extent to which the program goals are being met. Program standards can be set in a number of ways: based on minimum levels of anticipated achievement; based on selected measures for particular groups of students or for a given percentage of students; or in terms of mean performance of all students. Ongoing evaluation activities will suggest to the teacher the need for program modifications, or for review of criterion standards or the instructional objectives themselves.

Summative program evaluation should include evaluation related to all important program goals. Program success relative to student achievement can best be evaluated according to norms of some sort. Often local norms, especially in a medium to large district, or in situations in which comparable data on earlier similar groups of students are available, are most satisfactory for program evaluation. Several states have developed state norms for particular tests. National norms are available for the AAHPERD Youth Fitness Test[9] and for the AAHPERD sports skills tests in archery, basketball, football, softball, and volleyball.

As a result of widespread dissatisfaction with the performance of public school systems in this country in recent years, several state legislatures have passed laws requiring that schools become strictly accountable for their educational endeavors. This notion of accountability has been adapted from industry by business and professional men and women who compose local school boards and state legislatures. Teacher effectiveness is the focus of concern by the critics of public education. It is no longer sufficient that teachers be certified; they must also demonstrate their professional competence.

Product Evaluation

Pretest, Posttest.   Most of the initial state laws enacted on this subject require that the effectiveness of each teacher be evaluated by assessing the gains in student learning over the course of a semester or a school year. Usually, a *pretest, posttest evaluation* is expected. The teacher is responsible for preparing behavioral objectives that can serve as criteria of pupil learning. At the beginning of the school year the teacher and principal confer and negotiate until agreement has been reached upon the suitability of the proposed performance objectives for each of the teacher's classes. The pupils are then given a pretest. At some designated point in time prior to the end of the semester or year the pupils are administered a posttest. The differences in pupil scores indicate the degree of effectiveness the teacher demonstrated in the intervening time period.

Competency-Based Education.   This particular approach to teacher accountability has had many harsh critics. As a result, there has been a trend toward the identification of more broadly conceived performance-based objectives and the use of criterion-referenced standards in a generic model popularly designated as *competency-based education* or CBE. A competency-based curriculum is directed toward the achievement of specified competencies; the curriculum guide becomes very much like a job analysis as the technique was developed in industry. Particular tasks are to be performed and a specified level of performance is expected. Students are evaluated in terms of their achievement of the competencies. And teachers are evaluated according to the success of their pupils relative to the standards established.

Competency-based education quickly led to *competency-based teacher education*. A CBTE program identifies specific competencies or skills to be demonstrated, provides instructional alternatives to facilitate the student's progress, and holds the student accountable for the achievement of the specified goals. CBTE has excellent potential for personalization of learning experiences and increased motivation of students. It offers all involved persons opportunities to participate in program design and provides specific criteria by which to measure success or failure. Although difficulties with this program do exist, the most crucial of these can be overcome through careful consideration of local guidelines for stating competencies and selecting criteria.

Process Evaluation

Teacher competency is subject to process evaluation as well as to evaluation of the product outcomes as measured by specific student achievements. There is much current interest in various approaches to analyzing teacher behaviors. Some observers focus on analysis of the time spent engaging in instructional activities versus management activities. There are numerous systems that record aspects of teacher-pupil interaction, such as comparing the relative amounts of time the teacher spends in individual instruction, small-group instruction, and total class instruction. Teacher evaluation can be based on teacher and student behavior within the learning environment, which can be assessed as positive, neutral, or negative. Observation systems are used to contrast teacher initiatory and reflexive behaviors; this type of analysis is helpful to the teacher who wishes to minimize directive behavior and encourage pupil self-direction by trying to respond more frequently to the needs, requests, inquiries, and suggestions of the students. Excellent growth has occurred for many teachers through studies of teacher feedback to students.

It is often helpful to seek supplementary information about teacher effectiveness through student evaluations. But most important to instructional improvement is the teacher's self-evaluation. Today's teachers clearly need to educate themselves to a high degree of sophistication about the latest techniques, statistical analyses, principles of test construction, and other aspects of evaluation that apply to their subject matter field and to the teaching and learning responsibilities they carry.

RESEARCH IN PHYSICAL EDUCATION

EARLY RESEARCH ACTIVITIES

Physical education is a relatively young field in the family of scholarly disciplines. By nature and tradition it has been an activity-oriented field. Young people enter this profession primarily because of their desire to work with boys and girls through sports, dance, and fitness activities. Most want to be teachers and coaches of youth. In the early days of the profession, very few physical educators dedicated their efforts to a research role. Some of these early research leaders were medical doctors who had been placed in positions of administration in college and university physical education programs. Establishing the first physical education research laboratories, they developed anthropometric measurements, strength tests, and posture tests. They published their results and altered their physical education programs in the directions indicated by research findings.

Gradually, the number of physical educators interested in research increased. Persons with basic graduate preparation in related fields such as psychology, child growth and development, physiology, and kinesiology became faculty members in physical education departments and fostered research relevant to their specialized interests.

Although the number of young men and women entering the field expanded rapidly in this country, the percentage who selected a career in research remained very small. It became obvious that the way to increase the number of qualified research experts in physical education was to develop an interest in research among young, active teachers, coaches, and administrators. In effect, they had to be recruited and retrained with a research emphasis at the advanced graduate level. In some respects, this system for attracting qualified researchers into physical education differs from that of most other fields of knowledge, especially those which have held a place in the university curriculum for a long period of time. In many other fields, undergraduates decide that they want to become researchers, and they pursue an undergraduate and a graduate program that prepares them for this type of career, often under the tutelage of senior research professors. They continue in graduate education immediately upon receiving the bachelor's degree and remain in master's and doctoral programs until they receive their advanced degrees.

The physical educator typically entered the field of teaching and coaching either at the end of the bachelor's degree work or after one graduate year of preparation leading to a master's degree or a teaching credential. Prior to World War II, a small number of these teachers and coaches did return to graduate school in order to complete doctoral degrees in physical education. Some of these persons prepared themselves for positions in research, while others turned to teacher preparation and departmental administration roles.

Since World War II, there has been a boom in enrollment in physical education preparation at all levels in hundreds of colleges and universities. More and more institutions are establishing physical education research laboratories. Research facilities are now considered essential for top quality professional preparation. Interdepartmental research programs are being developed. Young people are learning about research opportunities in their undergraduate programs, and more physical educators are electing a career in research at an early age. Physical educators are obtaining funds to sponsor their research from governmental agencies and private foundations.

The scope and variety of studies in physical education broaden each

PHYSICAL EDUCATION RESEARCH TODAY

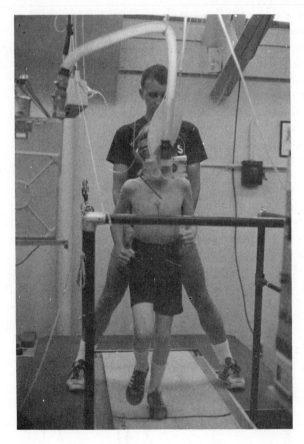

More institutions are establishing physical education research laboratories.

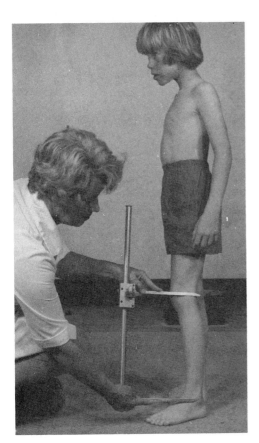

Growth and development is a major concern of physical education research today.

year. Perusal of the table of contents of recent issues of the *Research Quarterly*, and the topical index provided in the yearly report, *Completed Research in Health, Physical Education, and Recreation*, published by the AAHPERD, indicates the great diversity of subjects covered in the research literature of physical education. Research reports by physical educators also appear in the scholarly journals of many other fields.

In a recent book, Clarke and Clarke[10] have clearly described the current status of research endeavors by physical educators. A review of this book emphasizes the breadth of the investigations reported and the variety of research methodologies employed. It is clear that today physical education can be regarded as a multi-disciplinary field of broad scope, relying on the foundational fields of knowledge for much of its theoretical formulations and scientific and philosophical underpinnings. Physical educators are now receiving advanced research preparation in doctoral and postdoctoral programs across the country, not only in physical education itself but also frequently in Ph.D. major and minor programs in several other disciplines. Likewise, interested scholars and researchers from related fields study various phenomena central to the body of knowledge of physical education and make significant contributions to it.

A brief review indicates that physical education research today delves into many diverse topics:

— philosophical inquiry
— history and historiography
— child growth and development (maturation, body types, growth patterns)

EVALUATION AND RESEARCH

- psychological foundations (motor learning, behavior modification, motivation, concept formation, attitudes, non-verbal communication, personality, self-concept, and body image)
- exercise physiology (physiological control systems that adapt the organism to exercise stress under various environmental influences)
- biomechanics of human movement (gravity, resistance, air pressure, leverage, flexibility, stability, acceleration)
- neurological foundations (motor learning, reaction and movement time, kinesthesis, memory, retention, transfer, mental practice, specificity of motor skills)
- sociology (socialization, norms, social stratification and mobility, sport in institution, religion, economy, mass communications, leisure, work, women in sport, social problems)
- nutrition (diets for athletes)
- anthropology (competition, cooperation, acculturation)
- political science (sport as an instrument of national policy, international good will, propaganda, health, rehabilitation, ritual and ceremony)
- economics (spectator sport, leisure time expenditures, newspapers and magazines, motion pictures and television)

Other disciplines could be added to this list; the preceding examples are only intended to point out the diversity of research topics.

BASIC PROBLEMS IN PHYSICAL EDUCATION RESEARCH

The Need for a Theoretical Framework

Certain persistent problems have faced physical education researchers over the years. One of these is that the knowledge and central concerns making up the physical education discipline have never been clearly identified, described and organized. Professional organizations, individuals, and university faculties have studied this problem in recent years, and progress is being made toward identifying and describing a theoretical framework of physical education for scholarly study and research. A theoretical framework is essential to any field of study because it provides an orientation for the researchers in that field, giving their work relevance and priority. Arriving at a common acceptance of the nature and scope of the body of knowledge that is unique to physical education will enhance significant research and extend our knowledge in this field. Practical solutions to educational problems, developed through applied and field research, will improve the quality of countless everyday educational decisions.

The Need for Alternatives to the Laboratory Experimental Model

Another problem in the development of physical education research has been the overemphasis upon the experimental model. Indeed, progress in physical education in the post World War II period depended almost solely upon experimental research. At the time, science was generally being emphasized throughout education; the public was impressed with programs based on the scientific method, and physical educators in the colleges and universities were enamored of laboratory studies in which the selected research variables could be well controlled. Given this context, the exercise physiologists and the biomechanics researchers made genuine progress in strengthening selected foundations of physical education.

While the excellent work being done in human performance laboratories today is essential to our continuing forward movement as a profession, physical educators in the past decade or two have recognized the importance of alternative models for research as well. As we gradually developed the theoretical framework of our field, it has become clear that certain aspects of the field needing research do not lend themselves to the laboratory experimental model, but require the use of research models more like those used in anthropology, sociology, social psychology, history, and philosophy. Some outstanding research in areas such as motivation of athletes, socialization of women in sport, analysis of the hidden curriculum in physical education, teacher effectiveness, ethnic differences in perceptions of movement activities, constructs of creativity in movement behavior, and children's play behavior, has resulted. Our continuing progress as a total profession will require that researchers seek new knowledge in many diverse areas, utilizing the wealth of research models appropriate to the many important problems, and developing new research models when called upon to do so.

The Need to Apply Modern Measurement Advances

As a group of professionals, physical educators have adjusted to the need for research specialization. We are making progress in defining and elaborating a theoretical framework of physical education. More and more scholars have come to accept the significance of research studies utilizing the many models and procedures providing viable alternatives to the laboratory experimental model. However, one of the key difficulties today is the need for increased sophistication in measurement, computer programming, and statistical analysis. Research instrumentation is far more advanced than anyone could have predicted when the first physical education research laboratories were established. Measurement theory is highly sophisticated; developments in computer science have made statistical analysis highly advanced and relatively inexpensive. We must capitalize upon all of these advances in the best interests of physical education research. Researchers need to understand the potentials of the various resources available to them. They need to utilize supporting research services in areas in which their own expertise is insufficient. They need to communicate to professionals who are not research specialists that these tools are not to be feared, but to be put to work to further knowledge and strengthen the base for effective practice.

The Communications Gap

Physical education research is making excellent progress. But the physical education profession continues to be concerned about the problem of acquainting teachers, coaches, and administrators with recent research findings of significance for school practices. Practitioners in physical education should know the major research publications. They should be able to interpret research results and apply them to their teaching practices. Most graduate programs attempt to solve this problem by offering some type of course in research review, critique, and analysis. But this is insufficient. The profession needs to extend its best effort and thought to the question of how to bridge the gap between research findings and school practices. Practitioners need to be convinced of the value of devoting some of their time to keeping up with recent research and applying the most relevant and valid findings to on-going programs. Researchers must find meaningful ways to communicate their results to practitioners.

Professor Lawrence F. Locke[11] and others believe that very little progress will be made in bridging the gap between the researcher and the practitioner until a third type of specialist becomes available, namely, an interpreter of research. Since few such experts exist at the moment, it may be more feasible to encourage the researchers and the writers in the profession to accept more responsibility for publications that will communicate more effectively with the practitioner. Two excellent examples of such publications are the *Physical Fitness Newsletter*, published by H. Harrison Clarke, and the *Learning and Physical Education Newsletter*, by John N. Drowatsky. Also of interest is the series published by AAHPERD, *What Research Tells the Coach About (Baseball, Distance Running, Football, Sprinting, Swimming, Tennis, and Wrestling)*.

Not only do physical educators have an obligation to keep informed of selected research findings from the literature within the profession; but also they must keep up with recent information from closely related fields. Our traditional teacher education programs have advocated this for some time, particularly at the undergraduate level, through courses in "foundations" or "principles." Physical education principles generally are evolved from validated generalizations produced by scholars and researchers in physical education and related fields. Attempting to keep up-to-date with these principles and generalizations can be a difficult challenge, as can be seen upon perusal of even one principles book. A recent approach to this dilemma is the *Foundations of Physical Education* series,[12] which consists of books written by physical education scholars who also are noted authorities in one related field of knowledge. These authors have selected recent "relevant generalizations" from their respective fields of knowledge and have described them for the physical educator. The physical educator in turn can formulate principles and desirable practices, based on the validated generalizations. This series is another attempt to bridge the gap between research and practice.

Research is a challenging and fascinating career in physical education. Young people entering the profession should be aware of its potentialities as a possible career goal. Many teacher education programs now are providing research experience to undergraduate students, so there is more opportunity to become acquainted with this type of professional activity. In terms of conceptualization of significant problems, research design, methodology, instrumentation, data analysis, and formulation of conclusions and recommendations, research in physical education today is more highly sophisticated than ever before.

The diversity of phenomena that physical education researchers investigate has brought about an era of research specialization. Doctoral students interested in a career in research now choose a concentration in areas such as exercise physiology, neurological bases of human movement, biomechanics, motor learning, history of physical education, sociology of sport, philosophy of physical education, curriculum development, teacher behavior and other relevant specializations. Some outstanding doctoral programs are highly interdisciplinary in content. A student may take as much as one-third to one-half of the total program in one or more departments outside of physical education, such as physiology, psychology, neurology, sociology, history, philosophy, or anthropology.

Commendable progress indeed is being made throughout the United States and many other countries of the world in physical education research. There still remain many unanswered questions and unsolved problems to occupy the time, energies, intelligence, and talents of in-

THE PRESENT AND FUTURE OF PHYSICAL EDUCATION RESEARCH

terested and qualified students. An idea of the unlimited possibilities in physical education research can be obtained by reviewing such publications as (1) *Research Quarterly* of the American Alliance for Health, Physical Education, Recreation and Dance; (2) *Completed Research in Health, Physical Education, and Recreation* (yearly), published by the American Alliance for Health, Physical Education, Recreation, and Dance; (3) *Journal of Sports Medicine and Physical Fitness;* (4) *Microfilm Bulletin,* School of Physical Education, University of Oregon; (5) *Education Index;* and (6) *Bridging the Gap,* Department of Physical Education, City University of New York.

A field of knowledge is dependent upon research for its development and extension. Only through the research of its own professionals can physical education knowledge increase and strengthen its impact upon our world. Only with continual extension of its research base can a profession grow and affect desirably the lives of those whom the profession serves. Research in physical education must have the continuing strong support of all educators who believe in the future of the discipline and its profession.

SUMMARY

Evaluation refers to the totality of the processes deliberately employed to assess the extent to which objectives have been attained in the areas of pupil behavioral changes, curriculum efficiency, and teacher effectiveness. Measurement refers to that phase of evaluation which is concrete, identifiable, and capable of accurate assessment through the use of valid, reliable measuring instruments. Both summative and formative evaluation are used in physical education. Summative evaluation, the traditional type, is norm-referenced; typically, it is used at the end of an instructional unit or at the termination of a course. Formative evaluation is criterion-referenced; it is a more recent concept which emphasizes the guidance function of test scores and other evaluative techniques concerning student performance and learning.

Evaluation serves six major purposes: diagnosis and guidance, motivation, classification of pupils, appraisal of knowledge, efficiency of instruction, and evaluation of student achievement. Educators generally agree upon the importance of curriculum evaluation or program evaluation as a broader, more inclusive activity which goes beyond evaluation of individual student achievement. Formative program evaluation uses all types of available data to determine the extent to which program goals are being met. Summative program evaluation includes evaluation related to all important program goals using local, state, or national norms.

The trend in evaluation of teacher competency is toward the use of criterion-referenced standards. Specific competencies or skills to be demonstrated by the teacher are identified and the evaluation program provides specific criteria by which to measure success or failure. Teacher competency is subject to process evaluation as well as to evaluation of the product outcomes as measured by specific student achievements. Most important is the teacher's self-evaluation. Today's teachers clearly need to educate themselves to a high degree of sophistication about the latest techniques, statistical analyses, principles of test construction, and other aspects of evaluation which apply to their subject matter field and to the teaching and learning responsibilities they carry.

Physical education research today delves into many diverse topics. One of the most persistent problems which has faced researchers over the years is that physical education has never been clearly identified and described as a scholarly discipline with its own body of knowledge and central concerns. Substantial progress is now being made, however, in the development of a theoretical framework of physical education as an area of scholarly study and research. Another problem has been overemphasis upon the experimental model. Continuing progress as a total profession will require that researchers seek new knowledge in many different areas, using the wealth of research models appropriate to the many important problems, and developing new research models when called upon to do so. Another key problem is the need for increased sophistication in measurement, computer programming, and statistical analysis.

Research in physical education today is much more sophisticated than ever before. But the profession needs to extend its best effort and thought to the question of how to bridge the gap between research findings and school practices. Practitioners need to be convinced of the value of devoting some of their time to keeping up with selected recent research and of applying the most relevant and best validated findings to the improvement of ongoing programs. Researchers must find meaningful ways to communicate their results to practitioners. A field of knowledge is dependent upon research for its development and extension. Only through the research of its own professionals can physical education knowledge increase and strengthen its impact upon our world.

FOOTNOTES

[1]Benjamin S. Bloom, J. Thomas Hastings, and George F. Madaus, *Handbook on Formative and Summative Evaluation of Student Learning*. New York: McGraw-Hill Book Company, 1971.

[2]Margaret J. Safrit, *Evaluation in Physical Education*. Englewood Cliffs, New Jersey: Prentice-Hall, Inc., 1979.

[3]Ted A. Baumgartner and Andrew S. Jackson, *Measurement for Evaluation in Physical Education*. Boston: Houghton-Mifflin, 1975. pp. 1–3.

[4]AAHPER, *Knowledge and Understanding in Physical Education*. Washington, D.C.: 1973.

[5]Ted A. Baumgartner and Andrew S. Jackson, op. cit., p. 320.

[6]Harold M. Barrow and Rosemary McGee, *A Practical Approach to Measurement in Physical Education*. Philadelphia: Lea and Febiger, 1979.

[7]Ted. A. Baumgartner and Andrew S. Jackson, op. cit.

[8]Margaret J. Safrit, op. cit.

[9]*AAHPER Youth Fitness Test Manual*. Washington, D.C.: 1976.

[10]David H. Clarke and H. Harrison Clarke, *Research Processes in Physical Education, Recreation, and Health*. Englewood Cliffs, N.J.: Prentice-Hall, 1970.

[11]Lawrence F. Locke, *Research in Physical Education: A Critical View*. New York: Teachers College, Columbia University, 1969.

[12]*Foundations of Physical Education* series, John E. Nixon, (Ed.). Englewood Cliffs, N.J.: Prentice-Hall, 1968.

SELECTED REFERENCES

American Alliance for Health, Physical Education and Recreation, *Assessment Guide for Secondary School Physical Education Programs*. Washington, D.C.: AAHPER, 1977.

American Alliance for Health, Physical Education and Recreation, *Proficiency Testing in Physical Education*. Washington, D.C.: AAHPER, 1974.

American Alliance for Health, Physical Education and Recreation, *Sports Skills Test Manuals* (Archery, Basketball, Football, Softball, Volleyball). Washington, D.C.: AAHPER.

American Alliance for Health, Physical Education and Recreation, *Evaluating the High School Athletic Program*. Washington, D.C.: AAHPER, 1973.

American Alliance for Health, Physical Education and Recreation, *What Research Tells the Coach About (Baseball, Distance Running, Football, Sprinting, Swimming, Tennis)*. Washington, D.C.: AAHPER.

American Alliance for Health, Physical Education and Recreation, *Testing for Impaired, Disabled, and Handicapped Individuals.* Washington, D.C.: AAHPER, 1975.

American Alliance for Health, Physical Education and Recreation, *Knowledge and Understanding in Physical Education.* Washington, D.C.: AAHPER, 1973.

Barrow, Harold M., and McGee, Rosemary, *A Practical Approach to Measurement in Physical Education.* (3rd ed.) Philadelphia: Lea and Febiger, 1979.

Baumgartner, Ted A., and Jackson, Andrew S., *Measurement for Evaluation in Physical Education.* Boston: Houghton-Mifflin, 1975.

Bloom, Benjamin S., Hastings, J. Thomas, and Madaus, George F., *Handbook on Formative and Summative Evaluation of Student Learning.* New York: McGraw-Hill Book Company, Inc., 1971.

Clarke, David H., and Clarke, H. Harrison, *Research Processes in Physical Education, Recreation, and Health.* Englewood Cliffs, N.J.: Prentice-Hall, Inc., 1970.

Clarke, H. Harrison, *Application of Measurement to Health and Physical Education,* (4th ed.) Englewood Cliffs, N.J.: Prentice-Hall, Inc., 1966.

Completed Research in Health, Physical Education and Recreation, Volumes IX through XX, Washington, D.C.: American Association for Health, Physical Education and Recreation, 1967–1979.

Franks, B. Don, and Deutsch, Helga, *Evaluating Performance in Physical Education.* New York: Academic Press, 1973.

Glass, Gene V., "The Many Faces of 'Educational Accountability'." *Phi Delta Kappan,* 636–639, June, 1972.

Haskins, Mary Jane, *Evaluation in Physical Education,* Dubuque, Iowa: William C. Brown and Company, 1971.

Johnson, Barry L., and Nelson, Jack K., *Practical Measurements for Evaluation in Physical Education.* Minneapolis: Burgess Publishing Company, 1969.

Locke, Lawrence F., *Research in Physical Education: A Critical View.* New York City: Teachers College, Columbia University, 1969.

Mathews, Donald K., *Measurement in Physical Education.* (4th ed.), Philadelphia: W. B. Saunders Company, 1973.

Neilson, N. P., and Jensen, Clayne R., *Measurements and Statistics in Physical Education.* Belmont, Calif.: Wadsworth Publishing Company, 1972.

Nixon, John E., and Locke, Lawrence F., "Research on Teaching Physical Education." *Second Handbook of Research on Teaching,* Travers, Robert M. W. (Ed.), Chicago: Rand-McNally, 1973. pp. 1210–1242.

Research and Practice in Physical Education. Champaign, Illinois: Human Kinetics Publishers, 1976.

Safrit, Margaret J., *Evaluation in Physical Education: Assessing Motor Behavior.* Englewood Cliffs, N.J.: Prentice-Hall, Inc., 1979.

Sheehan, Thomas J., *An Introduction to the Evaluation of Measurement Data in Physical Education.* Reading, Mass.: Addison-Wesley Publishing Company, Inc., 1971.

Weber, Jerome C., and Lamb, David R., *Statistics and Research in Physical Education.* St. Louis: The C. V. Mosby Company, 1970.

Zeigler, Earle F., Howell, Maxwell, and Trekell, Marianna, *Research in the History, Philosophy, and Comparative Aspects of Physical Education and Sport: Bibliographies and Techniques.* Champaign IL: Stipes Publishing Company, 1971.

INDEX ─────

Physiology, definition of, 160
exercise, 160–176. See also *Exercise physiology.*
Piaget, Jean, 154–155, 201–202
Ping Pong diplomacy, 107
Play, 87
infant and, 154
learning, 151
and evolution, 119–120
Playback television, 256–257
Playgrounds, 89
Political ideology, sport and, 132–133, 341–342
Pop Warner football, 91
Portland time study, 295
Positive self-concept, 157
Positive transfer, 213
PPCF, 52, 245–248, 263–264
Practice, 207–208
massed versus distributed, 208
opportunity to, 210
whole-part, 214–215
Presage criteria, 289
Preschool child, development in, 155
Preschool Programs, 264, 325
Presidential Physical Fitness Award Program, 180
President's Citizens Advisory Committee on Fitness of American Youth, 179
President's Council on Physical Fitness, 181
President's Council on Physical Fitness and Sport, 54, 61, 179–181
development education, 98
President's Council on Youth Fitness, 179
Preventive medicine, 320–322
Primitive times, 77–78
Private clubs, 360
Problem-solving, 304
Process knowledge, 11
Product knowledge, 11
Professional certification, 90
Professional leadership, preparation for, 367–397
Professional sport, 359
Program(s), evaluation, 408–410
HEW, 380
selective and elective, 253
social service, 325–326
Program Evaluation and Review Technique (PERT), 231
Program Planning and Budgeting System (PPBS), 231
Progressions, 249
Proprioception, 197
Psychological foundations, 191–225
Psychological needs, 38
Psychology, definition of, 191
sport, 215, 217–223
Psychrometer, Sling, 165
Public Law 94–142, 60, 239, 253, 332
Public recreation, 361
Public school expenditure for physical education, 138
Public Works Administration (PWA), 89
Publications, 394–395
of American Alliance for Health, Physical Education, Recreation and Dance, 389
Pupil. See also *Student(s).*
Pupil Physical Education Profile Record, 403

Purpose concepts, 52
Purpose Process Curriculum Framework (PPCF), 52, 245–248, 263–264
Pye and Alexander framework, 263

Race, upward social mobility, 131–132
Racism, 133
Radio, 337
Radio telemetry, 166
Reception skills, 265
Recreation, 342–348
commercial, 360
leadership, 381–382
public, 361
therapy, 320
Regional championships, 106
Rehabilitation, offender, 328–329
Reinforcement, 289
Reinforcer, 19
Religion, sport and, 134–135
Renaissance, physical education during, 84
Research, 386–387, 411–417
anthropological approach, 120–122
cross-cultural, forms of, 94–99
in biomechanics, 168–176
in comparative physical education, 99–101
in exercise physiology, 165–167
in sociology of sport, 140–142
increased emphasis of, 92–93
interpretation of, 415–416
sociological, 125
Research Quarterly, 171, 389, 413
Resorts, 362
Resource(s), centers, 258
learning, 256–259
Resource Center on Media in Physical Education, 257
Response, conditioned, 19
Responsibility, student, 260
Results, knowledge of, 208
Retarded, mentally, National Physical Fitness Award Program for, 183
Retention, 212
Review of Sport and Leisure, 142
Rhythms, body, 120
Role(s), 129
of coach, 218–219
of sport, 125–126
sex, 130–131
Roman empire, physical education in, 81–82
Royal Central Institute of Gymnastics in Stockholm, 86
Running, cinematographical study of, 172
in secondary school, 271
Ryder Cup, 107

Safety in extramural sports, 92
Scales, 166
Scheduling, modular, 258
staffing and, 253–256
Scholarships, athletic, 137
Scholasticism, 83
Scholastics, effect of sport on, 127–128
School, non-graded elementary, 252